A
Passion
for Birth

A Passion for Birth

My life: anthropology, family and feminism

Sheila Kitzinger

pinter & martin

A Passion for Birth: My life: anthropology, family and feminism

First published by Pinter & Martin Ltd 2015

© 2015 Sheila Kitzinger

Sheila Kitzinger has asserted her moral right to be identified as the author of this work in accordance with the Copyright, Designs and Patents Act of 1988.

ISBN 978-1-78066-170-4

British Library Cataloguing-in-Publication Data
A catalogue record for this book is available from the British Library.

The publishers would like to acknowledge that this book is not in any way connected with Passion for Birth™ childbirth educator workshops. Passion for Birth™ is a registered trademark held by Teri Shilling in the US and used with permission.

Index Helen Bilton

The publishers are grateful to The Estate of the late Louise Bennett-Coverley for permission to reproduce her poem 'Census' on page 103 and Deborah Ross for permission to use her untitled poem on pages 85–86.

Photographs courtesy of the Kitzinger family unless otherwise stated. Photograph of Birthrights Ralley courtesy of Anthea Sieveking; Launch of *Freedom and Choice in Childbirth* courtesy of Chris Lord. All efforts have been made to contact the copyright holders, and the publishers will gladly correct any omissions in future editons.

Set in Minion

Printed and bound in the UK by TJ International Ltd, Padstow, Cornwall.

This book has been printed on paper that is sourced and harvested from sustainable forests and is FSC accredited.

Pinter & Martin Ltd
6 Effra Parade
London SW2 1PS

pinterandmartin.com

sheilakitzinger.com

CONTENTS

INTRODUCTION

This is the story of my half century of activism and research with women in more than 30 countries, and producing 24 books that are translated into 23 languages. It is written at a brisk pace that flows from its subject matter – birth and women's and babies' rights. It is not an autobiography so much as lightning flashes that shine on the most significant experiences in my life – as I struggle alongside women around the world and in every culture for women's empowerment.

Writing about memories is not easy. People from the past invade my dreams and wake me, and I live jostled by a crowd of ghosts who at times seem more real than human beings around me now. There is a persistent clamour of voices demanding that I remember them and shifting pictures that reshape my recollection of individuals and events to form new patterns, a vivid kaleidoscope of colours, one flash photograph overtaking and eclipsing another. It is more vivid than anything on TV, or anything that I have reconstructed, usually without realising it, because it made a coherent story. But as for the effect that these incidents had on my development, feelings and thinking – how can I evaluate them honestly? What part do they play in my personality, commitment and enthusiasm? How did they rush together to create the energy that suffuses me, and drives me on the adventures in which I find myself – about babies, birth, women, social justice and challenging powerful institutions?

Birth, cookery and flower arranging used to be next to each other on the shelf in libraries and bookshops. They were domestic subjects, to do with woman and home. Like knitting and embroidery, they were reserved for women busy indoors, while men ran the world. In the last 40 years the subject of birth has burst these confines and become a political issue, and one that affects us all. This came about because of the energetic action of women, and some exceptional men, in the UK and internationally who committed themselves to positive change in childbirth. I am one of those women. A theme of this book is my work to humanise birth and acknowledge it as a major life transition.

The right to knowledge about our bodies and minds in childbirth and to decide what hospitals and professional caregivers do to us and our babies is a fundamental human freedom.

In these pages I describe personal experiences that have shaped me, from childhood, and tell how from the 50s on enormous changes have taken place, how they came about and why. I have juggled motherhood, lecturing, campaigning and anthropological research, painting, cooking, writing, listening to women overwhelmed with problems, counselling – and being there for my family.

My life has never been split between work on the one hand and personal experiences and relationships on the other. I don't go off to an office – and have rarely done so in the past. I need not comply with a pattern dictated by an institution. Nor obey its rules. This means that I never know what any day will bring and my life must look very untidy. My autobiography can't fit into neat boxes.

With 600,000 births a year in the UK, women are eager for knowledge not only about what is done to them but as a real life *experience*.

Language is never neutral. It reflects a view of the world. From the time that my first book *The Experience of Childbirth* was was published I have worked to create a language for women's intense experiences. Birth isn't just pain, which is a side-effect of the work of the uterus and the opening of the cervix, bony pelvis and soft tissues. Yet pain has eclipsed other aspects of birth to such an extent that women don't realise that if they are not free to move around, can't get themselves into upright positions, are not surrounded by loving people who treat them as women – not just skeletons and muscles – and if they are in an alien environment, they suffer more pain, feel they have no control over it, and believe that nothing they can do will change it. When that happens pain turns to *suffering*. Until I started writing women really had no language for the sensations of giving birth. Now we have moved on from medical language to one that is women's own.

I describe people who had most impact on me, some of them international celebrities, others less well known, how I have combined research and activism with motherhood, and explore links between my mother's radical beliefs, her pacifism and feminism and those of my daughters, three of whom are lesbians. And I show when and how I became fascinated by birth, how this has influenced my personal life, and the impact of anthropological research.

I describe the powerful influence of my mother, pioneer feminist, pacifist and worker for racial equality.

A chunk of the book is about my first field research in Jamaica and the effects of being immersed in another culture, seeing into the lives of women in a peasant society, and exploring birth, midwifery, sex, families and religion in the hills and in the shanty town down by Kingston harbour.

Everybody's memory is selective, and depending on what is happening in the present, our emotions at the time, and the people to whom we talk, it throws up different stories. I am often astonished when reminded of individuals I have encountered and incidents that have occurred. *'I'd forgotten that!'* I can't pretend to create a complete account of my life and give the whole unvarnished 'truth'. But this is how it looks for me here and now.

The American way of birth, dominated by obstetricians who expect women to behave like obedient children, started to colonise the rest of the world in the 60s. Pregnancy became treated as a pathological condition terminated by delivery in an environment of intensive care. As a result today childbirth is a medical crisis. Obstetricians actively manage labour with the sophisticated technology of ultrasound, continuous electronic monitoring and an oxytocin drip – perhaps with an elective Caesarean section so that the product of pregnancy, like any product leaving a factory, is in optimal condition.

I believe that for all but a tiny minority of women birth need not and should not be like this, and that to turn the process of bringing new life into the world into one in which the woman is a passive patient being delivered rather than an active birth-giver not only degrades her, but also impedes hormonal co-ordination and physiological function. It actually makes childbirth more dangerous.

I tell what I learned from my acting training, social anthropology at Oxford, and the international research that has enriched my life. For many women birth is like rape. Inspired by my daughter's work with Rape Crisis, I came to support women suffering from post-traumatic stress after birth. This gave rise to the Birth Crisis Network and my work with women prisoners.

The culture of childbirth is important for all of us because it is an expression of the significance of the coming to birth not only of a new individual but a family, and the quality of relationships between human beings.

A baby becomes a person by being loved and cared for. We have created a style of childbirth in which it is an interruption of normal life rather than an integral part of its flow. It has been taken outside the home and away from the family so that for a couple having a baby it comes as a great surprise that birth has anything to do with loving and that giving birth can be an intense and joyful psycho-sexual experience.

Traditionally around the world when a woman is transformed into a mother she gains added status, and other women, neighbours and family members, share the rituals and give comfort. This helps her over the bridge into motherhood and through the psychologically and socially difficult period in which she is 'becoming', and the demanding relationship with even the most adorable baby. In the 60s, 70s and 80s this kind of emotional support was more or less ignored. I heard doctors talk about concern for emotions in childbearing as 'the icing on the cake'. We are only now beginning to discover the long term destructive effects on human beings and families of treating women as if they were containers to be opened and relieved of their contents.

There is a good deal of discussion today about 'bonding' – providing an opportunity in the moments after birth for the mother to get to know her baby and feel it is hers. But it is not a magic chemical which can be superimposed in an alien and uncaring environment. Everything that happens after birth is the outcome of preceding events. Bonding is supported or made virtually impossible by the atmosphere in the birth room, the interaction between those in it, and the care given to the mother as a *person*, not just a body on a table.

Every culture shapes the major transitions in life and there are similarities between patterns of birth and dying. When my daughter Polly had her terrible car accident in March 2009 and was rushed to hospital to be salvaged brain-damaged and with no choice about whether or not this happened, it led to my daughters Jenny and Celia's study into how we can make informed decisions and – most importantly – informed refusals, not only when we are conscious and aware, but if we are unable to communicate at the time. Hence the campaign to promote advance decision-making, so that each of us can state how we wish to be treated.

I write about challenging the power of big, bureaucratic and often mismanaged institutions, and how to address the needs of all child-bearing women – including prisoners, asylum seekers and those who suffer post-traumatic stress after birth – sometimes only revealed many years later. I show how passionate commitment, energy, and working with other women, can create social change, and explain why that matters, the cost and benefit, and how it affects me every day.

I also talk about the set-backs and failures, sexual exploitation and abuse that I have encountered in the challenge for women's rights in childbirth, that have in my mid-eighties impelled me in a race against time. My five daughters have made a major contribution and I have worked closely with them. I share many ideals with my husband Uwe and daughters. They are an exciting family.

Though it may seem trivial to talk about my children and family adventures and crises, they are all part of the mixture. Mothers can't be single-minded. Men might be able to achieve this. Not women with children. My life is chock full of writing, lecturing and counselling, but simultaneously I run a home, am a very involved mother with five daughters and three grandchildren, and cook, paint, and since it is an 'open house', entertain at the drop of a hat. Of course sometimes I feel guilty that I have not given the children my undivided attention. When they were little I used to leave a hot meal for them in the bottom of the Aga if I was busy or had to be out when they came in from school. I thought that was pretty good going. But Polly, at age six, came into the kitchen one day and said, '*Sheila, why can't you be a proper mother?*' She meant one waiting at the school gates.

Because I do a lot of overseas lecturing I have wide experience of airports. Some people get a kick out of air travel. I hate it. It is always stressful and has demanded resilience, resourcefulness and good humour. I have been welcomed at airports by a full-scale rally of women with posters – occasionally even a choir singing jubilantly about home birth and midwifery. Sometimes I have roamed an airport, disoriented and suffering from jet lag, trying to find the person assigned to meet me, and even phoning offices of organisations to get information. Once I was not met at all, and felt I had stepped into a void, only to discover that the woman who should have picked me up had been murdered. That was Chicago in 1994.

Road transport has ranged from a limousine with a fully stocked cocktail bar to a car stuffed with kids, a trike and everything but the kitchen sink, and a harassed mother trying to fit in hospitality between supermarket shopping and school runs who was not quite sure of the way to the hotel where I was to be deposited. Or I have had to kick my heels while we waited for another plane to land carrying two other speakers, so that the three of us could be stuffed in together. That plane was all too often delayed, or everyone got lost.

I love my work. I dread the thought of sitting around on a beach roasting in the sun with nothing to do – unless there are fascinating people to watch and I have writing materials, a dictating machine or a book I am enjoying. I take enormous pleasure in exploring, learning and trying to understand human behaviour.

I also love making things – constructing pictures, shapes, patterns, producing vivid colours – changing the environment so that it makes you stop and think, presents an unusual view of objects, startles, or even shocks. The book has illustrations of some of my paintings. I have included an idea of the variety and richness that gives me zest. I would find it difficult to keep going as I do in dismal surroundings.

Neutrals and discreet shades are not for me – only as background to vivid colour. I stare disbelievingly at the make-overs on TV in which houses are turned pebble grey, beige and ash with the odd cushion to give colour accents. I like a home that is exuberant and welcoming, and that celebrates life.

Our house is a small Cotswold manor house that was modernised in 1492, when fireplaces and ceilings were put in. I like to create an orchestra of colour, strong shapes, with light glowing and sparkling, the soft shimmer of candles at night, and visual surprises. With its great black oak beams, some recycled in medieval times from ancient galleys, with holes for the oars still visible, lofty ceilings, white walls, and carvings in stone and wood, Standlake Manor is a perfect stage for vivid and striking patterns. The kitchen glows with Portuguese pottery, china intricately covered with flowers, fruit and birds, and gleaming copper pans that were once my mother's. There are tiles I have painted with birds and oranges and lemons around the sink and overhead. The table is covered with mosaics made of broken china that my daughters and I have made together, and everywhere peacocks are perched, flags poised, and boats bobbing in a sea of colour. That is where I enjoy cooking vegetarian food.

The bed where I write and dictate – I rarely work at a desk – is an oak four-poster that was designed by Uwe to echo the curve of heavy beams in the ceiling, resplendent with an Aladdin's cave of hangings, esoteric objects and birth symbols in crimson, scarlet and gold. Instead of a headboard there is an expanse of silk in a hexagonal patchwork sewn by my daughters and me when they were much younger. (Don't look at the stitching too closely. It is the impression that matters!)

I think modern furniture looks as good in it as antiques. I enjoy decorating with vivid curtains, hangings, patchwork, oriental kites, angels and dragons in bright pools of light, and objects I have made, often with the girls, in copper, silk and ceramic, together with flowery garlands, batik pictures and bold paintings. There are Polly's wall frescoes and pictures on doors, Nell's sculptures of mermaids and birthing women, and Indian and Moroccan rugs with fertility symbols spread on the dark wooden floors.

I write for pregnant women and their partners, women who have given birth in the past – with varied experiences, positive and negative – and everyone concerned about choice and control in childbirth, education for birth, home birth, and women's and children's rights.

Half a century ago men were often not with their partners in childbirth, and women had no right, or the knowledge, to make informed choices. They were subjected to routine episiotomy, a compulsory perineal shave, and often an enema, too. They were expected to lie down, be obedient, and accept the decisions of professional caregivers without question. They were merely bodies to be delivered. In Britain, and increasingly in other countries, that is now history.

I am highly critical of the ways in which antenatal classes have been taught. It changed from a training that imposed a rigid internal discipline on the mother, with strictly regulated breathing and the sounds she was allowed to make. That was how hide-bound Russian, French, and later, British and American psychoprophylaxis, was. Now we have moved from rules to spontaneity, from instruction to freedom of choice and action, from copy-cat learning to getting to understand evidence-based research, and from mere *'shopping around'* to awareness of the impact of the social context in which birth takes place.

It is easy to romanticise birth in other societies, to see it from the standpoint of our own medicalised, high-tech culture and think, *'That must be lovely – to have your mother's arms around you, sit on another woman's lap.'* But I am convinced that the challenge is to create our own woman-centred culture of childbirth. We can incorporate some practices from other traditions, yes, but the birth culture should be our own, not an imitation of something elsewhere in the world.

I open a newspaper and see myself described, yet again, as a childbirth 'guru'. I growl. That's the last thing I want to be. I don't have any mantras, creed, high priestess pronouncements or mystic incantations. My knowledge comes from personal experience, and being with women as they give birth in many countries around the world, open to their hopes and fears, and sharing the excitement and triumph of birth.

I asked Jenni Murray of BBC *Woman's Hour* not to introduce me as a 'guru'. She protested, '*But you are!*' and tells how when she went into labour she said to her husband, '*It's started*', and he announced, '*I'll go and make my sandwiches then, because Sheila Kitzinger says I may get hungry.*' That, to me, is an example of practical tips – nothing to do with inspiration or mystical insight.

This book is not only about birth, but other activities to which I am committed. We ran an aid agency from our home at the time of the Yugoslav crisis when Muslim refugees were pouring into Croatia from the massacres in Bosnia. It absorbed pretty well my whole life for two years. I tell how Tess, Uwe and I organised Lentils for Dubrovnik and describe the experience of almost being squeezed out of the house by shoe boxes piled in towers.

I describe exciting anthropological field research in the Caribbean, Australia, Fiji, South Africa, Eastern Europe, Russia, Italy, Spain, Mexico and other countries. I write about all the things that have energised me and stimulated my work: birth images and goddesses in many cultures – midwifery, birth research and activism.

The struggle for woman-centred childbirth is an uphill battle. The more we gain, the more we must reach out. There have been times when I felt I was hitting my head against a brick wall and wondered if I could go on. But then a woman rings me up out of the blue and says, '*Thank you for what you did to help me have a lovely birth experience.*' And that makes it all worthwhile.

CHAPTER ONE

AN UNCONVENTIONAL CHILDHOOD

I was born at home in Taunton, Somerset, in 1929 and weighed nine and a half pounds. Clare, my mother, gained strength during a long labour by watching a woodpecker on the tree outside her bedroom window. If that bird could continue tapping away at the hard tree trunk, she knew she could carry on, too.

She coped with a difficult labour in her pink and white bedroom – the shades of a rose garden – while my father rubbed her back, and the doctor with whom she worked, a close friend, Reggie Husbands, stood by in case he was needed. Contraction followed contraction relentlessly. I had my hand up on my head, and this slowed rotation and descent.

Clare was narrow-hipped and little. As a baby she had suffered from rickets and wore lace-up remedial boots for several years. She remembered how the baby of the family was always fed from the '*dutty pot*' that was kept permanently on the kitchen range. Tea, sugar and cereal of different kinds were mixed in it. Bad nutrition, but it stopped the crying!

In the 1920s it was taken for granted that babies were born at home. Only the very poor or destitute who had no home to go to would enter an institution. Caregivers, usually family practitioners with the nurse attached to their practice, came to the mother. They were guests in the home and the woman kept control of her own household. It was her territory.

Women could use furniture they knew well to get into different positions for comfort – a window ledge, a table, settee, a dining chair or a rocking chair. Mother looped a towel over the top corner of a door and around the handle in the second stage and pulled on it, changing her weight from one leg to the other, stooping forward, bending, or kneeling as she pulled. This was what she did for the women she attended, too. Best was a strong kitchen roller towel. You can get a good grip on that.

Mother's family were pillars of the community, bakers who lived to one side of the shop. There were seven children, five girls, two boys and my mother was the second youngest. They were staunch Unitarians and ran the debating society that met at their house. When Mother was 15 she started to work as a nurse, first with soldiers wounded in the First World War, and then with Dr Reggie and his younger brother Roland, helping women give birth and caring for them afterwards.

At 17, Alec, my father, had run off to enlist in the army as a despatch rider, disguising his age. He spent a stint guarding the Acropolis, which he told me had been a waste of time because 'it was a ruin anyway'. Then he drove into the Battle of Gallipoli in Turkey, couldn't get through because of a violent attack on a narrow pass, turned the motor cycle back the other way and sped as horses and men were slaughtered and fell into the crevasse. He was now into sports cars in a big way.

When he came out of the army he went into the family tailoring business, trading top quality tweeds from Kirkcudbright and Galloway where his family were crofters. A whole swathe of the family had come down to Somerset because the Scottish soil was poor, and they used the network of family and neighbourhood to get the best tweeds and cater for farming families. They travelled around so that customers did not have to go into Taunton to shop. My grandfather James, Alec's father, had established the business, and Alec now had two staff members and an apprentice, and was warmly welcomed by people all over the Blackdown Hills.

My father was a man of strong integrity and the farmers and their families trusted and relied on him. As he went from home to home with his tweeds and patterns and listened to the daily problems they faced, over the tea that was always poured, he was a bit like an itinerant priest going round to hear confession, or perhaps a medieval kind of psychotherapist – always there for them. Sometimes he took me with him when I was small, and I remember the welcome and warmth in their eyes.

Mother was a role model: midwife, early feminist, deeply convinced of the importance of free thought and expression who believed it was imperative to challenge racism, discrimination and violence, wherever it occurred. Striving for social equality, and against discrimination of all kinds, and for understanding between individuals, peoples and cultures was a strong theme in her – and her mother – beliefs and action, as it has been for me, for my husband Uwe, and is for our daughters.

When Mother died I found a statement in the handkerchief drawer of her dressing table. I don't think she had ever written anything before. She had certainly not been published.

It started with a description of her experiences as a girl of 14 at the start of the First World War. She was on holiday at Watchet in Somerset and the cousins with whom she was staying asked her to go to the station to fetch the morning papers. There were crowds on the tiny platform. '*Stacks of papers were thrown from the goods van and they could see the headlines: "War is Declared on Germany". Another train steamed in bringing back the Territorials from their camp at Minehead, where they had been training to fight in the war. It was tremendously exciting.*'

She returned home, and soldiers were billeted on the family. '*Many young girls got a kick out of life when they bravely presented a white feather to any young man they thought of military age who wasn't in uniform.*' She commented, '*In the majority of cases this was, I expect, innocently given, for after all, every man was expected to go to war to protect his women and children.*'

Clare longed to nurse wounded soldiers. At the age of 15 she decided to train to tend the sick, and started to nurse soldiers returning injured from the front. She described how, '*One day, two Quaker ladies called on Mother and started to talk about things which opened up a new world to me*'. They spoke about men being imprisoned for their beliefs that war was wrong. '*I was sixteen when I was shocked into listening to what war really was. The "Gentle Jesus" days of a sheltered upbringing had ended.*' A new Minister came to the Unitarian chapel who preached that war was wrong and challenged every individual to do their utmost to prevent it ever breaking out again. In spite of nationalist fervour the chapel was full of fascinated men and women listening to his preaching. '*On one occasion the Recruiting Officer appeared in our church, seating himself in the front row with several officers armed with pencils and notebooks, to hear if they could arrest our Minister on sedition. They could not. He preached on the Sermon on the Mount, and we sang "God Save the People".'*

Clare made a commitment to struggle against violence. *'Within my own family we were divided. My parents, especially my mother who lived her life befriending anyone who needed her, struggled hard to induce people to denounce war. My two eldest brothers had already gone to the war and by this time were overseas, both feeling that there was no other way.'*

Clare's mother was friendly with a young school teacher, who afterwards became her son-in-law (my Uncle Stan) when he married Liz, my mother's older sister. He was a gentle, scholarly conscientious objector arrested for refusing when called upon by the military authorities to have a medical examination, and sent to jail. *'Peace had gone from our homes and families were strained severely.'*

Imprisoned conscientious objectors had to sew rough hessian mail bags. Stan pierced a finger with a needle and it became badly infected. Nothing was done about it. The poison spread. He was discharged from the prison with septicaemia. My mother cleaned and treated it – this was before the discovery of antibiotics, of course – and he recovered.

One day in 1918, at eleven o'clock in the morning, the Armistice came. Clare wrote, *'A few days before Christmas my mother, happy and busy, was looking forward to all the family being together for Christmas. She had had a letter from her eldest son who was now in France, telling her that he would be coming.'* She was cooking in the kitchen and Clare had gone to her bedroom over the kitchen and was about to try on a new dress. *'Mother and I were alone in the house. I heard somebody come to the door, heard her answer it, and then a queer choking cry rather like the sound of an animal struggling. The low agonised cry stunned me. I can never forget it. I went downstairs to see her crouched in a chair, still wearing her cooking apron. I saw the telegram telling us that her eldest son had died in a few hours in a Canadian hospital in France. Immediately putting aside her grief, she took a taxi and hurried off to comfort his wife.*

'I was alone for the first time in my life with the shock of death. I had read about it often, and had known many friends who had died in the war, but this was our family. The whole horror of war seethed in on me.' She resolved to work against war itself. *'I saw my country no longer as patriotic songs had pictured it, but as Edith Cavell had voiced just before her death: "Patriotism is not enough. I must have no hatred or bitterness for anyone."'*

Many years later my feminist daughters gathered by Edith Cavell's memorial, off Trafalgar Square, to call for lesbian equality and to protest against injustice. They weren't aware until recently of the strong family link with the idealism of Edith Cavell through female generations.

More About My Mother

So I had a rather unusual upbringing. Mother was both a feminist, though at that time she wouldn't have called herself one, and a committed pacifist, and was always challenging powerful institutions. Father went along with what Mother believed. He loved her very dearly and admired her. It was difficult for him, because he came from a Wesleyan Methodist background. Mother's Unitarian heritage was tolerant and completely undogmatic.

As a child I absorbed this world view through practical actions and day-to-day living. It has formed the basis of my own relationships with my five daughters, and I can trace the link through three generations.

Mother started off using a child rearing method that she had read about in books expounded by Truby King, an expert in calf-rearing, which claimed to impose discipline and order on babies by strictly timed feeds and a regime regulated by the clock. Truby King's insistence on a hygienic all-white nursery with no shapes, colours or distractions to interfere with sleep and only being picked up once every four hours didn't work with me. I screamed almost non-stop for three days until she finally gave up and moved me back into the bedroom.

She later became committed to the teachings of Maria Montessori, who emphasised respect for the child, and the development of imagination and creativity, and this became the dominant influence as I grew. She had a Montessori governess for me before I went to school, and found an elementary school with a Montessori class in it. She was very interested in education that encouraged children to ask questions, not to follow a path that was laid out for them, but explore all their potential, discover themselves, and do what they wanted in life. She was convinced that I should have a career, not just marry, have children, and be content with being a mother and house wife.

Her reading was very different from the books my friends' mothers had on their shelves, *The Well of Loneliness*, for example, and Marie Stopes on birth control. I read these when I was only just into my teens and pored over her illustrated midwifery books, all describing birth as a spontaneous life event

The essence of her child-rearing philosophy was respect for the child. She aimed to develop self-confidence, and also awareness of others' needs, rather than being wrapped up in one's own concerns. It is not a matter of trimming children's natural impulses so that they will fit into polite society. The well-behaved, obedient child may turn out to be the most disturbed adult.

A baby is not a clean slate on which we etch the pattern we want. Nor a feral animal that must be tamed. We do not own our children. Withdrawal of love, or the threat of it, teaches a child that she is only valued when she conforms.

This is how I brought up my children, too. I believe that the world needs non-conformist individuals who are not afraid to challenge the system, dare to stand up to tyranny, are critical of socio-economic and political systems, and committed to constructive change. That is unlikely if we train them to obey us like pet dogs.

Then there was pacifism. Mother got to know the Reverend Dick Sheppard of St Martins in the Fields, Trafalgar Square, with whom she worked as a pacifist and activist. He was probably the greatest human being whom I encountered early in my life.

Dick Sheppard made his church a sanctuary for the distressed and destitute, and for many years the crypt was a haven for drunks. St Martin is the patron saint of drunkards and more than 6,000 indigents found a refuge there every year. It was also a sanctuary for injured soldiers returning from France who poured off the boat train at Charing Cross Station nearby and went directly to St Martins, knowing they would be welcomed and cared for.

He was a man of enormous compassion and shining vision, and I remember as a small child listening to him discussing strategy with my mother and speaking at open-air meetings she had arranged.

Some of my earliest memories are of peace marches. Mother was a passionate member of the peace movement. There were huge banners and one big rally in a park in Taunton where the central symbol was a tank captured from the Germans in the First World War. Dick Sheppard, Patrick Figgis of the Peace Pledge Union and the MP George Lansbury were among the speakers. I sat on a hard, slatted chair near the front of the crowd for what seemed like hours, as speech followed speech, and, unable to hold on any longer, to my shame, wet my knickers. I felt the piddle trickling down onto the grass, and hoped no one noticed.

One birthday was memorable. I was eight or nine years old. Mother talked to me a lot about poverty and injustice, and when she saw a long dole queue of bedraggled figures outside what we would now call a jobcentre, she invited them all back for my birthday party, including a band of street musicians. They stuffed themselves with cake, trifle and ice cream. There were balloons, crackers and live music. Birthdays don't come like that every day!

On Remembrance Sunday we honoured those in the Armed Forces who had given their lives for their country, but did not wear the usual red poppies. Instead we wore a white silk poppy which signalled that we were against all war and honoured those who strove for peace. I remember feeling proud to wear this distinctive symbol of peace. It bore a huge responsibility to work for understanding between nations and try to solve conflicts by non-violent means. The impressive Remembrance Ceremony on 11 November in Whitehall seemed to bear little relevance to Jesus's life and message, and glorified war and violence.

Mother had high ideals and fought for peace and a society in which there was equality and justice for all. She also had a keen sense of artistic presentation. I remember that Mother and Father were going to the opera. I had been put to bed and she came in to kiss me goodnight. She leant over, delicately made up, and in a cloud of Roger and Gallet perfume. Her full-length dress was ruffled black net sparkling with sequins, layers and layers of frills from the hips down. The picture is still vivid in my mind, the peachy scent, and above all, the glamour. She was the most beautiful mother in the world.

Healing

Mother was into natural healing and what we now call alternative medicine. Most of the remedies she used came from country traditions, based on herbs, onions, garlic and seaweed.

When bad colds were around I had to wear a raw, peeled garlic on a string round my neck. Certainly it kept others from coming too close! She massaged my chest and upper back with goose grease if I had a chest cold. An iodine locket was another preventative and treatment. I remember being dosed with syrup of figs for constipation, too. Every year in the spring we were given doses of 'spring medicine', a drink consisting of fresh herbs, lemon juice and a little honey.

She was ahead of her time in encouraging deep breathing and rhythmic exercise. She took me with her to Health and Beauty movement classes started in South Africa by Prunella Stack. We wore shiny satin white shirts and black shorts and exercised in unison, looking like a third rate chorus girl line up.

Mother considered creativity very important. I was sent to Greek dancing classes because she was a great admirer of Isadora Duncan, who rebelled against classical ballet, and danced bare-footed and graceful wearing a brief, thin tunic, I was supposed to float along with a scarf, act 'nature rhythms' and make myself one with the wind and the waves and flowers dancing in the breeze. But I never succeeded in being thistledown or summer clouds. With me the flowers were more likely to be lashed by a gale. I was a podgy child and not too good at imitating clouds, except angry ones. In fact, I did rather well at creating an exciting nature rhythm which depicted a rising storm, finishing with a black sky, thunder claps and pelting rain.

The Birth Control Clinic

My mother worked to establish one of the earliest free birth control clinics in the south west. Aunt Liz was proud of the first one, which she helped create with Dr Margaret Jackson in Barnstable. I used to meet Mother at the Taunton clinic sometimes after school and we'd often go out for ice cream at Maynards or a cream tea at Dellars. I stood by the door of the clinic waiting for her and saw women come out clutching small packages, embarrassed and clearly hoping no-one witnessed the surreptitious activity in which they were engaged. Contraception then was considered a taboo subject and she was very happy to do what she could to provide effective birth control to impoverished and vulnerable women who were sexually exploited by the men in their lives. Controlling their fertility was a vital element in her work to empower women. This was before the NHS existed and made it possible for all women to get contraceptives without having to pay for them.

Aunts, Uncles, Cousins

I often had short holidays with members of Mother's family. Aunt Liz the oldest sister was angular, idealistic, stern and bossy. She was married to Stan, the school-master who was also a conscientious objector, and they had an only son, Alan. He was academically brilliant and into classical music in a big way. When I stayed with them I remember musical performances with a school friend of his at the piano who later became famous as a conductor.

Aunt Nell, her youngest sister, lived close by in Bridgewater. She was warm and cuddly and I adored her. She hadn't *'married well'*. Uncle Lionel was a hard-smoking employee at Will's Cigarette Factory, who died young. I was fond of their only son, Arnold, a bit older than me, who later became a commando, and near the end of the Second World War was the only survivor of a ship sunk in the North Sea. He suffered from post-traumatic stress disorder – which in those days was called shell shock – was admitted to hospital and was like a different person from then until he died very young. I wonder now if he took his own life.

When Aunt Emily came to stay she shared my bedroom and was nervous about the gas light and heating. One fateful day she came back to check after I was asleep and switched the gas on again as she tried to turn it off, leaving gas escaping. That was when I started having asthma. I remember painful, gasping times on the hockey field as I wheezed through yet another awful game, stuck in goal because I couldn't run.

Emily lived in the middle of gorgeous woods outside Poole in Dorset in a game-keeper's cottage with her husband who was a chauffeur. Her daughter – my cousin – was 10 years older than me and involved in a passionate relationship. Their love-making was constantly interrupted by me bursting into the bedroom and saying, '*Boo!*' I thought it was funny. I don't think they did, and Aunt Emily begged me not to do it.

The most exciting family for me was the one in Somerton. Uncle Arthur, one of Mother's brothers, married a vivacious woman whom everyone called '*Bloss*', short for '*Blossom*', and they had a large family. Food and drink flowed lavishly. She was a gracious hostess. One Christmas their boys (who were well known for causing mischief) secretly removed all Blossom's artistically arranged decorations in the dining room and set-up an all white scheme that looked deceptively elegant consisting of lavatory paper rolls. When Arthur had a go at growing mushrooms and became very excited about it, they stuck ping-pong balls in the earth, carefully spaced and at first invisible, and little by little every night they pushed each up a bit. Uncle was thrilled as his mushrooms grew. Only when they eventually popped out of the soil was the subterfuge revealed.

Their home was a long, rambling Queen Anne house in the centre of the small town. Arthur was a wealthy corn merchant. One of the sons, Jack, studied pharmacy and became the local chemist. The family put on lively parties and seemed to own Somerton.

The person who was most special to me was Sis, Blossom's sister, who was an Alexandra nurse. She had a deep, full, luscious voice and performed Victorian tragic poems with dramatic intensity about death, starving widows, orphaned children, courage, desperation and love. I admired her enormously and wanted to be like her when I grew up. She died in the Second World War, nursing wounded troops in the Indian Ocean when the hospital ship was sunk by Japanese torpedoes. Her body was never recovered.

Harry, Mother's other brother, had run away underage to join the army during the First World War. The notice of his death arrived the day after Armistice in 1918.

Aunt Agnes's husband, Uncle Ernest, a loving and considerate man, was the Bridport baker. I loved staying there because at the end of an alley at the side of the house was the bakery with its exciting action and enticing smells. Making doughnuts was most fun. The balls of dough passed along a moving belt and each came to a halt beneath the jam machine. I was allowed to press the lever that deposited a squelchy blob of red jam right in the middle of the dough, which then moved on to make room for the next. As the dough continued to rise it covered the jam and ended up as a perfect doughnut. I don't think I have ever had more pleasure in cooking than as I did as a juvenile jam injector.

My Father's Family

I didn't see much of my father's family, partly because most of them lived far away. But Gran, my father Alec's mother, lived in Taunton near Weirfield School. I used to drop in on my way home from school and Gran would give me piano lessons. Aunt Edie, bejewelled, scented and plump, and married to a Birmingham jeweller, used to come regularly and stay with Gran. She was jolly

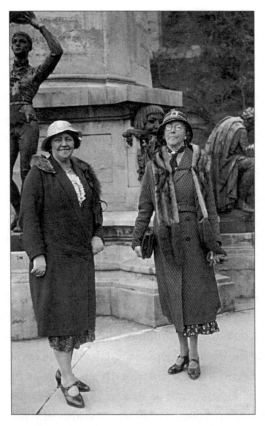

Jolly aunt Edie and straight-laced gran

and loved her food. She fancied the special cakes and desserts that Gran used to make for me. There was some competition between us over who should get the last slice or spoonful.

Ruby, Edie's daughter, stayed with us frequently. She was a journalist and Mother took her under her wing and encouraged her writing. She didn't seem to fit comfortably into that family. She published articles in the press about interior decoration and design, and Mother's design sense inspired her to write glowing rhapsodic pieces about our house – the delicate pink and grey shades of the guest room and the mingled blues of the sitting room for instance.

Gladys, Gran's niece, had a daughter Joy, slightly younger than me. I thought she was soppy. When cousin Rose became pregnant before marriage Joy didn't know how it was possible because she was not married. As all the women whispered in Gran's sitting room and we were exiled to the staircase I enlightened her and told her in detail how babies were conceived and born. I was never allowed to play with Joy again.

I revelled in stormy weather and thunder. Gran was always terrified of it and used to hide in the cupboard under the stairs. She wanted me to crouch in there with her in case the house was struck by lightning. I could never understand her fear. But I think that she believed that this is how God might punish us for our sins. While she hid in the cupboard I liked to run out and dance in the rain!

Enjoying Ourselves

At Westleigh House in Taunton, my younger brother David and I played in the street, or at any rate, since we were not supposed to, swung on the iron gate at the front of the house, until they came and took the gate and railings away to melt down to make weapons. Opposite the house were thick, tall trees in which squirrels darted. The ice-cream van visited regularly in the summer, its jingle like a pied piper's flute for the children, and stopped outside our house. The knife grinder rang the door bell and we watched as kitchen knives and garden implements were honed to razor blade sharpness against a huge grindstone.

At the far end of the street was an exciting forge, where the local blacksmith hammered horseshoes, producing a shower of sparks, and there was an enticing

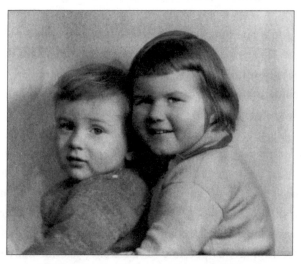

My brother and I were close as children

smell of burnt hoof as great cart horses, which pulled the brewery drays, were shod. Out of school hours there was usually a group of children standing admiring the performance. The Salvation Army gathered at the top of the street near the forge, too, wearing their smart navy uniforms with shiny buttons. They played big brass instruments and the young women shook tambourines and went round collecting pennies. When my granddaughter Laura acquired her saxophone at the age of nine and gave us her first performance – a whole scale – and the sound boomed out as we ate maple syrup pancakes for a treat in the kitchen, I suddenly felt I was a child again.

Father acquired an old rail coach and installed it in the middle of an expanse of fern at the top of the Blackdown Hills. He was very clever at woodwork and made beautiful door latches, sets of shelves, cupboards and other things. At weekends we often went to stay in 'the hut' and roamed free over the hills.

A large drain ran under the shingle road outside and it was exciting to climb down into it and wriggle our way through to the other verge. This worked well until one day I was stuck in it, too fat to get through or move backwards. David tried to pull me out, and eventually succeeded. But I never risked entering the drain again.

My parents enjoyed singing romantic duets at the grand piano: *The End of a Perfect Day*, *At the Café Continental Where a Lady Dropped Her Glove*, *Little Man, You've had a Busy Day* and *Love's Last Sweet Song*. Some of these were the ones I also heard played at Dellars, the café on Taunton bridge, where the orchestra struck up at tea-time and waitresses with frilly white aprons and little caps served fancy cakes, scones and tiny sandwiches on tiered plates. It was a special treat to be taken there, wearing our best clothes and on good behaviour. It all seemed very sophisticated.

Mr Livesey played these songs, too, as well as classical music with a lot of complicated finger-work. Mother had met him at a pacifist march and, sharing the same social ideals, and learning that he taught the piano, she engaged him to teach me as a private tutor. He was an elegant young man with tight curly hair, a dapper suit, and suave manner. I thumped away while he hovered and smiled encouragingly. When Mother came in I would climb down off the stool and he would demonstrate how it should really be done. Mother joined in, singing. I noticed that she usually wore one of her full-skirted, figure-hugging, lovely silk dresses, and smelt of roses. My lessons became shorter and shorter, the performances longer. Then suddenly Mr Livesey didn't come any more, and

I was rescued from the lessons. I think her conscience had triumphed.

She was very keen on education. She had to leave school at 14 and start earning, and was determined to give us the opportunities she was denied. She believed in developing her children's talents. As soon as I could recite a rhyme I was lifted onto the wide sitting room window-sill, my own private stage, to say a poem. Everyone had to be quiet and listen. '*I met a 'ittle e'f man once down where the 'ilies b'ow. I asked him why he was so sma' and why he didn't grow.*' Delighted with my audience, at the end of each performance I announced, '*Aw c'ap*'. Mother believed in the value of children developing skills and self-expression by every possible means. I knew the relatives who came to tea and were treated to the performances used to laugh about it afterwards: '*Clare is spoiling that child!*' I was fiercely loyal to my mother. Subsequently, I was taken to elocution lessons, and started a long series of exams in which I excelled myself. There were certificates, and later medals and silver cups, drama groups, and the Eisteddfod at Bristol. This fitted in well with taking youth services and peace services at the chapel, and being registered as a lay preacher. Meanwhile, my brother David, who had a beautiful voice, sang the spiritual, '*Were You There When They Crucified My Lord?*'

Florence, the maid, reigned in the kitchen. She was like a maid in a Victorian kitchen, long skirts, starched white apron and cap, and a will of steel. One awful day David and I invaded her territory while she was cleaning upstairs rooms, dragged a damp sheet from the laundry basket and fed it through the huge old-fashioned mangle. I turned the handle and, aged around two, David slid the sheet in. Only I mangled too vigorously and caught and squashed his fingers between the rollers. It was a dreadful thing to do to your baby brother. I still remember the horror. Florence ruled that we should never enter the kitchen again.

Mother was an expert manager. She organised the household with a deft touch. Every Thursday Mother and Father did the accounts. A green baize cloth was laid over the breakfast table, and piles of coins and notes spread on it. It was a sacrosanct occasion, and I was not allowed in. I wandered around the yard outside, bored and feeling rejected. We had a black and white terrier, and I found refuge in Toby's kennel, curling up in the straw, and often falling asleep. When Toby became old and ill and obviously in pain, my father told me, tight-lipped, that he had sent him away into the country where he would be happier with other dogs. I knew that Toby had gone forever and that Father was lying to protect me. It was my first experience of death.

The Chapel

The Unitarian Chapel in Taunton was beautiful in its simplicity. Uncle Osmond, Mother's maternal uncle, was an organ builder and we were proud that the splendid Mary Street Chapel organ had been made by him. I loved poetry and was proud that Coleridge had preached there. During the Second World War the congregation shared it with a congregation of Liberal Jews, from London, and that was the beginning of my ecumenical education.

A hymn we often sang was *'Gather us in, thou love that fillest all. Gather our rival faiths within thy fold.'* It emphasises the universal – each religion and philosophy seen as one step towards truth, since no creed or sect can encompass the wholeness of God. There is debate in place of dogma, freedom instead of life-denying rules. It is every individual's right to challenge the established order. Another hymn was, *'When wilt thou save the people? Oh God of mercy when? Not kings and lords, but nations! Not thrones and crowns but men!'*

For my brother and me when we were five or six, as we sat on narrow benches covered in baize that prickled behind our knees, in the Chapel, and I suspect for Father too, who had a bucketful of religion with his narrow Wesleyan Methodist upbringing, the services seemed long in spite of their stirring emphasis on freedom, and the idea of Jesus not as the only Son of God, but our brother in the human family. I liked the intricate wood carving on the pulpit. You used to be able to buy milk chocolate covered with darker chocolate in scrolls on the top. The pulpit was like that. When I was very little I used to imagine that I was eating it, bit by bit.

Rites

I was taken to a meet for the first – and last – time when I was about four. It seemed that anybody who was anybody was here from the county set, together with farmers and their families. At a meet of the Devonshire and Somerset stag hounds the riders were resplendent in pink, bugles were blowing, and it was a lavish and ceremonial affair. The chased deer was the sacrifice. We followed the hounds in our car from field to field and on foot across wicket gates round the country. Then suddenly, they'd got it! The dogs were excited and the riders victorious. The stag was trapped – and despatched with a shot. It lay bleeding, eyes glazing over, lifeless. It was the time for primitive celebrations. All children for whom it was the first time at a hunt must be '*blooded*'. I watched a baby of about six months carried to the corpse, the huntsman's finger dipped in the stag's hot blood and smeared over the baby's face. Another child was brought up. I cowered, frightened that they would do this to me, too. The people I had believed to be gentle and friendly became monsters, revelling in the death of an animal they had killed and forcing children to share in the glory.

Mother's Day, in March, was a very different kind of ceremony. Every Mothering Sunday people came from far and wide to climb Bunkum Hill, picked primroses and had tea in the inn at the bottom. The climb was steep and there was a thrill of achievement as we reached the top. The inn had an outdoor wooden privy with three holes, each big enough for a bottom to perch on – father, mother and the smallest for a child – and defecate into the bucket beneath. It was very cosy. But I don't think I shall ever forget the odour.

Practical lessons about social injustice

I was taken on regular visits to the Taunton workhouse, bearing comforts for the destitute women locked up in there with their small children. One woman we always met had a baby with a lolling head and tongue hanging out.

Men were separated from women and marriages and families split up. They were put to work if they were fit enough. Anyone who was ill lay in a narrow, hard bed. This woman was in bed. I think she had had a terrible birth that injured her. She was a single mother, so the baby was illegitimate, and both were stigmatised. In those days a woman who had a baby outside marriage was a '*fallen woman*'. Whenever we visited we took her Devonshire buns that she specially liked – '*chudleighs*' they were called – and it was my job to go up to the bed and hand them to her. It took some courage to do so because of the rank smell, the drooling baby, the atmosphere of despair and misery, and the way she ate, smacking her lips enthusiastically and, with her mouth open, a half masticated bun being squeezed out onto her chin. It was good discipline for a five-year-old in caring for those who were less fortunate than ourselves. Though I never wanted to eat a chudleigh again!

Rows of children, about 30 of us, sat at our wooden desks at Station Road Elementary School, listening to our teacher, Miss Mynitt, rant about bad behaviour. I was six. She was always very pleasant with me. But she hated the kids from the back streets who weren't nicely brought up and didn't catch on to reading, writing, and arithmetic. One small boy, Peter, was dressed in rags and hand-me-downs. He had blotchy, pasty, pock-marked skin, hair like straw, and legs and arms that were stick-thin. He may have been deaf. Anyway, he didn't leap to attention when she summoned him or tried to drill information into his head.

That day she ordered him to the front of the class, told him to stand up straight, and lectured him on his inattention and slovenliness. Taking her long ruler, she hit him repeatedly behind the knees until he collapsed on the floor. I was outraged at the callousness and injustice, and picking on kids who were not from my cosy, middle-class world. It was my first lesson in social injustice and gross discrimination. I can never wipe the picture from behind my eyes. Miss Mynitt taught me, in a powerful way, a lesson she had no intention of teaching. It has remained with me through life.

War

In 1936 the Spanish Civil War broke out. Looking back at this time, my mother wrote: *'Our small girl is horrified at the illustrations in the national papers and journals of bombed buildings and people lying wounded in the road. We are so grateful that our children are safe in our home and decide that we must get some of these unfortunate children from this land of war to stay with us, and so begins a realisation that a desire to mix with other nationalities can be a tremendous education.'*

We began International Friendship work in our home, although up to now we had not thought of giving it a label. No school holidays came without children from our own East End of London and some from countries overseas: a young Russian girl who had never seen Russia but had lived in Paris all her life, a Dutch student full of the most terrible hatred for the Jews – his mother was a German.

During the Second World War, the sirens went off, wailing in the night, and we trooped down to the cupboard under the stairs. Father was a senior air raid warden and on duty near the station, escorting sometimes panic-stricken people to the underground shelter, reassuring the fearful, and ensuring that no chink of light was visible through the crack of any door and thick curtains were tightly drawn. An elderly lady with violet hair, Miss Urquhart, a refugee from London who lived in the spare room, crouched in the corner of the cupboard. She smelled of patchouli and lavender, cloying and overwhelming in the narrow confines of the cupboard. Tins of biscuits and other emergency rations, and first aid boxes of bandages and iodine, were piled at the shallowest end of the cupboard in case the house collapsed around us. There was a pervading smell of leaking gas – a good thing we never tried to light matches there. David and I played snap, or tried to read, but it was difficult to concentrate. Miss Urquhart talked a lot, usually about past times. She had seen better days, and let everyone know it. Mother tried to do her needlework in the poor light.

We heard the rumble of bombers flying overhead towards Bristol, and occasionally a thud as, pursued by Spitfires, German pilots dropped their loads on Somerset towns or on the railway line – twice there were direct hits on the station less than a mile away – before turning and speeding back to the continent. Then came the shrill 'all clear', and we would go back to bed. Luckily for us, it was all just incredibly boring.

The year the war in Europe ended Mother arranged a special Christmas service with German prisoners of war from the local camp. She wrote, 'I approached the officer in command and requested that the POWs should be invited to a Christmas service, carols and a brief address given in German by my young son on the spirit of reconciliation.' When this service was arranged, she wondered if any of the men would come. 'But to our joy, thirty-eight men attended and then joined us at our house for supper afterwards. English and German voices united in "Stille Nacht, Heilige Nacht". Many of these boys had left school, joined the Hitler Youth organisation, and had never been allowed to develop their brains to think for themselves.'

Every Sunday a group of four visited us. Mother stretched the food rations to feed them, and gradually more prisoners joined them. Dieter played the violin, Dr von Schindel discussed philosophy. One winter, when snow had fallen thick, we had sledge races down the hill opposite our house. The concerts became an institution, and festivities were joined by the camp Commandant and his German wife, Gerda, who also became close friends.

It seems ludicrous looking back at it, but Mother was much criticised, and it shocked that small country town. She wrote to the prisoners' mothers, wives and sweethearts. It must have been about that time that my brother and I bought the Delius Violin Concerto with our pocket money. It expressed for me the turmoil, sorrow and striving that marked the end of the war, and the hope of a new world we were confident we were going to create. I suppose that is a contrast with most adolescents today, who are pretty sure that the world is not going to get any better.

Leadership came early for me. I was a Brownie – a Sixer of the Pixies as I recall – and much approved of by Brown Owl. But by the time I was supposed to pass on to being a Girl Guide I had decided this authoritarian role, however useful, was not what I wanted. Power corrupts. Even a sense of one's own worthiness is apt to corrupt – dangerous stuff!

Heroines

Evacuees came to stay, and refugees from Nazi Germany and occupied countries. The writer Zoe Oldenburg, who had fled from Communist Russia, shared my room and was an expert story-teller. There was usually an African or Asian university student during the vacs, and the house became an international community in miniature. This social and political education extended what I learnt at school and formed the basis of daily discussions about values and social responsibility.

I was surrounded with stories of brave heroines and women who challenged and changed society. Mother told me these stories: Grace Darling who took the lifeboat out in heavy seas and rescued everyone in a capsized ship. There was a drawing of her on my bedroom wall – hair flying in the wind, waves crashing against the rocks, the lighthouse where she lived behind her. There was Florence Nightingale, tending sick and dying soldiers at Scutari, Elizabeth Fry, sitting with women and children in prison, and Maria Montessori whose educational methods mother introduced when I could barely toddle – I remember sitting in my pram fascinated by the brightly coloured apparatus.

There were present-day heroines like Vera Brittain (mother of Shirley Williams), novelist and author of a book about her loving relationship with Winifred Holtby – and Dame Sybil Thorndike, from whom I still cherish an encouraging letter. We met them at pacifist rallies.

Later there were male heroes – above all Ghandi, a little man in a loin cloth who went to meet the rich and powerful to state universal truths and challenge the might of the British Empire through non-violent resistance: 'You *must be the change you wish to see in the world.'*

Many unusual and creative women were in and out of the house as I was growing up. One of mother's best friends Theresa Hooley, was a poet, and another, Margaret Barr, the only Unitarian missionary. She worked in Assam, had started a girls' school there, and explored the shared values in all religions. Margaret had a great influence on me. She was an intrepid adventurer, utterly committed to bringing education to the mountains of Assam, full of respect for other religions and seeing that of God in each of them. She had lived in Ghandi's ashram, appreciated Eastern cultures as a social anthropologist does, seeking out values, meanings, beliefs and ways of behaving, and told fascinating stories about what she had learned. When she stayed with us she spent hours talking to me about the teachings of the Bhagavad Gita and the Upanishads, explaining cultural norms, and describing how patterns of relationships were formed in different societies. She published a book on this subject and commissioned me – I must have been about 15 – to design its cover with strong outlines of different places of worship – mosques, temples and churches. This was the first time I used my pleasure in art for public exhibition.

Moving Into The Country

When I was 13 Father had a stroke. I came home from school to find him in bed with one side of his face slipped and unable to speak clearly. Mother nursed him devotedly and he recovered completely. She also made bold decisions: he must retire. They would sell the town house and move into the country.

Father had never been an urban dweller at heart. He was the tweedy type who smoked a pipe, and though he was a tailor he was happiest out shooting or pampering his pigs. Unusually for men of his generation, he cooked a bit – Scottish recipes handed down in his family, like the delicious potato scones on which we slathered butter when we were given some off-ration from the local farm. Mother hated cooking: *'We eat to live. We don't live to eat!'* But she made good drop scones to go with strawberry jam and clotted cream from the farm. The cream formed on top of a great pan of rich scalded milk outside the dairy, and the fat, sleepy cats lolled around waiting to be given a saucer of milk once the cream was skimmed off. Mother made a tasty squab pie too, with onions, meat, vegetables and apples.

I announced I was a vegetarian when I was nine. So squab pie was out from then on. Mother admired my decision but didn't know how she could cope with feeding me, so she served chicken, which I liked, and haddock which I adored, soon after the announcement. But the challenge was too soon. My mind was fully made up. I turned both dishes down and, having made that sacrifice, later was not going to succumb to the temptation of carnivorous tit-bits. I have not eaten meat or fish since. I got through late childhood and adolescence mainly on baked beans, apples from the orchard, and cheese when it was available.

After we moved to Little Thatch, Rumwell, Father took to a new life with relish. He loved birds, rabbits, hedgehogs, and finding the first primroses and mushrooms. He bred pigs and pampered them. When the sows were farrying he studied their diets meticulously and gave them Parrish's Food which provided supplementary iron.

Some birds he shot. I remember the rook shoot, with the bark of the trees opposite my window streaked with blood. Others he tended, mending broken wings. He shot rabbits, too. But when he found a limping baby rabbit he brought it home and nursed it to health. There was a disturbing paradox in his actions. Perhaps there is for most countrymen who breed animals and are concerned about the welfare of their animals, but who also kill them.

Mother revelled in her new home. She had space for students and refugees of many nationalities to come and stay. It offered a beautiful stage for entertaining, having poetry and musical soirees, and the peace to give counselling and succour to people who sought help – women battling with anxiety and depression, difficulties in relationships and sexual problems. There was a garden scented with lavender and roses, and she put stones with messages that had special meaning for her carved into them: 'Fear knocked at the door. Faith entered. There was no-one there.' Little Thatch was a place of healing.

One day David, with a large party taking place in the garden, was helping make the tea. A curious boy of 13, he got bored and chemically experimental. Some mothballs were in the kitchen drawer and as the kettle boiled he melted them down in the steam issuing from the spout. The silver pots of tea were carried out to the guests. I saw their surprised expressions as they sipped it. Was this a weird kind of Lapsang Souchong? Was it some other kind of exotic tea? They drank it politely. Then Mother started on her cup, and all was revealed.

The Crown Inn was next door and accidents – most of them minor – were frequent as tipsy revellers emerged from its door and were hit by cars speeding down Rumwell hill. One day there was a terrific crash. Some drunk American servicemen had run out of it and one was smashed under a lorry crowded with fellow soldiers. The scene was bedlam. Mother ran with a first aid box and I followed behind. The young soldier was lying in the road apparently dead. She started to work on him and got him breathing. I saw her deftly slip his left eyeball back in its socket. She issued instructions and got co-ordinated action from those who were standing around. She talked to him soothingly and firmly. The ambulance came and we packed up and went in to wash off the blood. At least one life had been saved.

Father's mother, Gran, wore gold-rimmed spectacles and her sight was very poor. She was knocked down by a young motorcyclist as she tried to cross the road by the cinema. Mother and Father rushed to the hospital to be with her. I waited at home. At last they came. I said, *'I'll make a cup of tea'* – an invariable English response to tragedy. As we drank it Mother told me that her death had been remarkable because of her faith. She was slipping away. Suddenly her face lit up and she exclaimed, *'Ah! Jesus!'* and died. She was with her Lord.

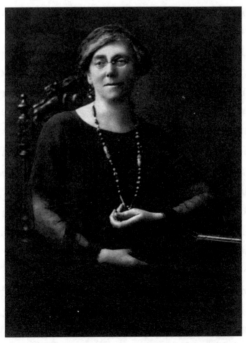

*Father's mother, Gran, had poor sight –
and died after being knocked down by a motorcycle*

Mother invited the young motorcyclist out to the cottage for tea so that he could talk about his feelings and accept forgiveness for causing Gran's death. Her sight was bad and it would have been hard for him to avoid her. Mother served home-made scones and had got hold of some contraband cream from the farm on the lane. Gran always loved clotted cream. As we put the meal together her hand drew back. She couldn't face giving him the cream. He had a bit of butter instead.

Teenage Years

Perhaps because we were a close extended family and there was so much going on, school friends were peripheral and I did not depend on them for my social life. In fact, I find it hard to remember individual friends until I was in the senior school. There was Rosemary, who was a Seventh Day Adventist, and I used to go to religious services with her, but she was not allowed to come to the Unitarian Chapel with me. Gillian was more sexually advanced and would meet boys from Taunton School Sixth Form on the other side of our hockey pitch in the lane. We knew when boys were around because you could see the prefects' sky blue velvet caps with tassels bobbing above the hedge. Pamela was a dear friend and helped run the Chapel services for peace with me. She was very musical and married Dieter, one of the prisoners of war who played the violin.

But my deepest relationship was with Pat, who was dynamic and highly intellectual. Her father was a diplomat I think, so she lived in a variety of countries and was a polymath. She was a few years older than me and a striking Dr Faustus in the school play in which I had a small part. She shared a passion for poetry and great drama. Her voice was deep and velvety, she had Hispanic colouring, and I adored her.

One day, lying in the garden at my cousin Hazel's house outside Bristol, where we were staying, she very slowly and lightly ran her fingers down the inside of my right arm. I felt a totally unexpected thrill of desire and have never forgotten that moment. It was so unexpected that I could feel like this about another woman! It was a revelation to me. That is as far as it went. But it was a great part of my education about sex and gender.

Miss Lloyd taught English at Bishop Fox's Grammar School in Taunton, Somerset. Although I became head girl, I never really enjoyed school. I didn't enjoy Miss Lloyd either – in fact, I detested her. Only later, when I was at Oxford, did I begin to realise what she had given me. She reinforced the essential stimulation to be a rebel. She'd given me the insight into myself to realise that I need not toe the line, and could dare to be different. She made me question my own values and beliefs.

She was very different herself. She had fly-away grey hair with pins falling out all over the place, wore shapeless grey cardigans and a long sagging skirt. Today a TV make-over programme would have a great time with her. She and her sister lived in a cottage round the back of the school, where they kept goats. I passed there as I walked to school. The front garden was a mud patch, and they had made a wooden bridge so the goats could go in and out of the sitting room window. There were usually two or three of them in the garden; I don't know how many more were in the house. She was very fond of animals and told me once that she preferred them to children.

Even though I disliked her because of her sarcasm and the way she humiliated girls who weren't clever, her English questions excited me. I remember her bringing advertisements into the class and we deconstructed them. We would look at them to see what they were trying to sell, how they were doing it, and the effect on us. I have since always seen advertisements, or anything people are trying to persuade me about, in the same way.

The other valuable thing she did was inspire me about English literature, and especially writers such as Jane Austen. She never managed to teach me the rules of grammar though. I was not interested and got appalling marks in exams.

I was a member of the Peace Pledge Union and wore my badge to school. One day, Miss Lloyd asked me to walk round the hockey field with her. She told me it was quite wrong to wear a PPU badge to school. She was wearing an animal welfare badge so I challenged her: *'Why do you let other girls wear animal welfare badges?'*

She fixed me with a Gorgon-like stare: *'That's quite different, because it's not political. PPU is political and you cannot make political statements at school. We must clip your wings.'*

I removed the badge, and my mother agreed that I should compromise by not wearing it at school, but continue to do so out of school. I felt bitter about it. Later, I realised that if you believe something strongly and can produce evidence for it, you need to stand your ground. I was greatly influenced by Miss Lloyd's attempt to *'clip my wings'*.

Years later my youngest daughter Jenny was asked to leave a voluntary job she was doing with a charity because she was wearing a lesbian badge. She was told it was because in counselling and helping distressed people she would be in a '*small room*' and in '*close*' proximity to them.

At Bishop Fox's we were encouraged to do part-time voluntary work to benefit the community – on Thursday afternoons and in the holidays. I worked as a nursing assistant at Taunton Hospital, at first on a men's surgical ward. I used to cut their toe-nails, often difficult because they were thick and ridged and they could not reach them themselves, so they grew into tortured, gnarled shapes. I washed them, gave them bed-pans and cleaned these out in the sluice. They were very grateful. Elderly countrymen often knew my father and sent messages back to him about how wonderful I was.

The patients found it difficult to position their penises over the urine bottles. They fumbled and pleaded that they were unable to manage and asked me if I would pop the penis in. I did as they requested. Sister noticed how delighted her patients were with me and I was moved to a women's ward.

In my teens I explored the churches, chapels and meeting houses in Taunton and was keen to learn about and understand their teachings. I also took over the youngest Sunday School class and, enthused by Herbert Read's *Education through Art*, and discovering Jung, gathered in our friend's children for self-expression on Sunday afternoons. The county psychiatrist, a friend of Mother's, was my guide, and we had art exhibitions of children's representations of God, for example, with pictures on huge pieces of paper begged from wallpaper shops. One four-year-old did a splendid scarlet painting of God as a pillar box. You pop in your requests – the prayers – and the answers come – sometimes.

Poetry, plays and comparative religion occupied most of my spare time. Shelley – '*O wild west wind, thou breath of autumn's being*' – and the luscious sensuousness of the *Ode on Melancholy*, together with the Metaphysical poets – Donne, for example – and Traherne's mystical writings, Shaw, Chekhov and Ibsen.

The beautiful Bristol Old Vic became a centre for my artistic excitement. It is one of the oldest constantly working theatres in England, was designed by a carpenter, and opened in 1766. I knew exactly where to sit and how to pay next to nothing to get a good view round a pillar when I leant slightly sideways!

I discovered that remarkable book *The Cloud of Unknowing*, the war poets like Wilfred Owen with their searing castigation of a society that had sent them to die like cattle in the Flanders mud, and later Martin Buber, struggled with Simone Weil and Kierkegaard, and revelled in Olive Schreiner and Dostoevsky.

We wanted to build a new world. It was going to have World Government, be federalist, and dedicated to peace and the eradication of poverty. There were exciting meetings in London, including the Peace Pledge Union Assembly at Friends' House, Euston, where Sybil Thorndike's voice rang out as rich as cream, yet reached the very back row with clarity in the spirit of her own St Joan.

I went to many Federal Union meetings with Mother and listened to Professor Joad, awkward, argumentative and stimulating. Sir Alfred Salter and Dick Sheppard stayed in our home when they were addressing meetings in Taunton, and other members of Parliament had all graduated from the University of Prison as conscientious objectors, and used to compare their prison experiences as other people talk about their old school. There were other lovely people like Richard St. Barbe Baker, who planted trees in the deserts.

I started to go to Friend's Meetings and preferred silence and mysticism to the structured services of Unitarianism, though I was still committed to my Unitarian heritage.

I studied voice and drama, as well as doing my school work, through all the exam grades until I got my LGSM, the teaching qualification from the Guildhall School of Music and Drama. Then I started teaching voice production and drama part-time.

As a teenager I was asked to perform at ceremonies and meetings of which poetry or drama formed a part, often alongside music. I revelled in speaking St Joan's impassioned speech to the court in Shaw's St Joan. One day I was invited to recite at a gathering of women on the estate of one of the oldest and most splendid houses in Somerset. It must have been a meeting about peace, because I chose Wilfred Owen's *Anthem for Doomed Youth*. It is a moving poem. I spoke it solemnly, clearly, with intense meaning.

> *What passing-bells for these who die as cattle?*
> *Only the monstrous anger of the guns.*
> *Only the stuttering rifles' rapid rattles*
> *Can potter out their hasty orisons.*

No mockeries now for them; nor prayers not bells;
Nor any voice of mourning save the choirs,
The shrill, demented choirs of wailing shells;
And bugles calling for them from sad shires.

What candles may be held to speed them all?
Not in the hands of boys, but in their eyes
Shall shine the holy glimmers of goodbyes.

The pallor of girls' brows shall be their pall;
Their flowers the tenderness of patient minds,
And each slow dusk a drawing-down of blinds.

I realised that some women in the audience were quietly weeping. When I finished one woman collapsed in unrestrained suffering. I was aghast. Later the titled lady whose house it was tackled us for the failure in etiquette in disturbing this guest of hers. Her lover had died in the last war. It was an unforgivable *faux pas*. We went to apologise to her and explain why I had chosen this poem. It was because the war was so terrible that we must strive to stop all war.

My First Trip Abroad

The year after the war, when I was 17, I went abroad for the first time with the YWCA to what was then Czechoslovakia. I wanted to meet girls from different countries in constructive activity to benefit society. The rail journey across Europe was long and exhausting, sitting in a carriage with an elderly lady in the far corner and a pleasant looking, balding man in a beige mackintosh who sat down next to me. He at least spoke some English. He told me he was a university lecturer and we talked. But in the dead of night, when at last I had managed to get to sleep, he shoved a hand in my knickers and started to feel me. I screamed. The lady switched the lights on and he fled up the corridor. She roused the guard, but he had disappeared.

The camp was an ordeal. The Czech girls hung together, because they couldn't speak English and I had no Czech except 'skupina' – 'squad', and remember only one girl, an Irish Catholic, with whom I could talk.

We had to build a road into a forest through which the Vltava river ran. And it was very hard work, first digging and heaving stones for the foundations, then levelling them up and finally tarmacing them.

Accommodation was in old railway stock, sleeping in bunks. We huddled round the camp fires in the evenings to sing. The culture was still Soviet, and we were controlled by rewards and punishments. The Camp Commander blew a whistle to get us out of bed, to switch squads from one task to the next, for meals – which were absolutely dreadful, especially for a vegetarian, consisting of potatoes and shredded meat – and even when we had to line up and recite the Lords Prayer.

The experience strengthened my determination to resist institutional tyranny of all kinds.

'A Matter Of Life Or Death!'

This was my first published article. My pen name was 'Hannah Torr'.

It is a little strange, when you are still at school, as I am, to be wondering if there is anything before you in life, and whether, when you dream of the future, there is going to be any future at all for you. It is difficult to face up to the possibility of slaughter and blood again, intense suffering, and then blackness and nothingness – and this happening, not in some far corner of the earth, but happening here to me.

We are waiting for something, for some tremendous event which will change peoples' hearts and minds in a flash. We may think that if we go on quietly, seeking our individual salvation in an unobtrusive way, something is bound to turn up, and everything will be all right in the end. The end – yes, that is what we are confronting, and yet we can hardly imagine it, the stopping for ever, the drop into the void, and then no existence, no breathing, no laughter, not feeling at all; and civilization crashes, and with it all art, all beauty.

Nothing will turn up. The power we are waiting for to change the world does not exist, except in ourselves. We are the people who can give humanity hope. There is no one who will come and take the burden from us, no demigod who will command us to follow him to a sure victory, and no safe haven. The eyes of the starving and fearful, of the dying and the sorrowful, look to us, as individuals who, if we wish it, can join together to struggle for life, against the blackness of war and annihilation which is sinking down upon us.

Have you ever looked into the eyes of a starving man? I did, a few weeks ago, on my way to and from Czechoslovakia. It is something not easy to forget. It is not so much the match-stick thinness of his wrists, nor the great head which seems too heavy for the bowed body, but it is the look in his eyes which turns one sick. It is the look of a hunted animal who has no strength to run further. What image is it, great God, in whose likeness we are made? Is it this tormented, suffering animal? Are You this defeated one? Or are You rather the image of the conqueror, with the blood of the children who are yellow like wax, running along the gutters.

Look into the eyes of those of all nations who have lost hope, the eyes of those who do not dare to see further than the present moment, who are spiritually stifled by their fear of the future. They are hungry too.

See those who are poisoned by their own bitterness, defiled by the cancer of hatred, whose compassion has become swamped by self-interest.

These are the physical and moral invalids of our great hospital, the earth, and we are going to have to do something about it now if it is not to become one vast mortuary.

Up against the possibility of extinction, we desperately need a plan, and the courage to fulfill it. We must not look round to see if others are agreeing with us, and doing their share of the work. We cannot afford to wait for the other nations to abolish their armaments and train the young for peace instead of war, until we do ourselves. If we are going to take as our responsibility the moral leadership of the world, and probably we are the only country which is able to, we must strike out new paths in the wilderness, and that is not done by walking round in circles. We have to decide now, life or death, glory or suicide – and there is no middle way.[1]

In my gap year before going up to Oxford I studied the Stanislavski acting method with Eileen Hartley-Hodder in her elegant eighteenth-century residence in Bristol. From this I gained a new perspective on birth and antenatal education, and devised a way to prepare for an intense and joyful experience.

There was no question of us sitting around in rows lapping up information – no room for physical jerks, either. Every class was vigorous and expressive. In two groups we used to act the parts of red ants and white ants and had battles on her elaborate Chinese decorated staircase that coiled up several floors. The ornately painted bannisters and supports shook as we charged over and clung to them at full tilt to stop hurtling down. There was no time to stop and *think* what we were doing. It was about feelings, not intellectualisation, spontaneous physical activity rather than exercises.

Our bodies knew what to do. We imagined events and social situations, interacting with other groups and individuals, drawing memories out of our personal lives, discarding propriety and social mores, and freeing our bodies to respond without question to what they were telling us to do.

I was debating whether to aim for the stage as a career, to study for the Unitarian ministry, or go to university and wait and see. I was drawn to reading psychology or social anthropology. Anthropology won.

CHAPTER TWO

OXFORD

The Conference of the Council for Education in World Citizenship in London in January 1945 was crammed with 3,000 young people. It was thrilling. We were going to change the world. No longer patriots of one nation or another, we represented the youth of a new world that would be at peace, with nations reaching out to co-operate with each other in bold ventures, and war would be no more. One eager young man on the platform inspired me with enthusiasm. I found out that his name was Uwe Kitzinger.

In those days Greek or Latin were essential to get into Oxford and Cambridge. The exam that had to be passed was *'Little-go'*. I was very bad at Latin and disliked more or less anything about Rome: its centralised power, colonisation and discrimination and exploitation of subject peoples. So I switched to Greek. I was offered a place at Girton, chose to do Greek because I thought it was a more beautiful language than Latin, found some private tutoring, and failed the exam! I had no-one to advise me. Because my school, Bishop Fox's Girls' Grammar School, Taunton, didn't reckon on getting any pupils into Oxbridge, and the staff were not interested, I hadn't a clue about the procedures, and was left high and dry. I only learned that I could have gone up to Cambridge, and taken *'Little-go'* again next term, after it was too late to sort it out.

Meyer Fortes, anthropology don at Oxford, who subsequently had the Chair

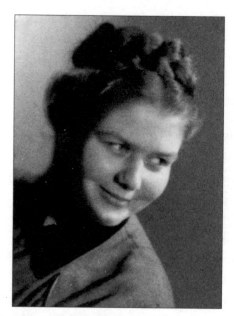

The Oxford years

at Cambridge, saved me. He interviewed me, waived the rules and accepted me at Oxford. In 1949 Ruskin College generously gave me a nominal place there until, two years later (after I got a distinction in the Diploma in Social Anthropology, which counted as a degree), I was able to do post-graduate research at St Hugh's.

I didn't read Social Anthropology at university because of feminist beliefs, but from sheer curiosity. I wanted to understand human behaviour and cultural diversity. I was hungry for anything that contributed to that – reading, travel, what social scientists call *'participant observation'*, and when doors of opportunity opened I tended to push them wider. There was no master plan. I always asked myself, *'How can I use this experience?'*

Looking For Digs

I thought the big Victorian houses in north Oxford might be the best places to find digs – one of the front rooms looking onto the Banbury or Woodstock road, or a back room with a view of the well-managed garden. So I trailed advertisements and had cards pasted up in small local shops for what would have been the maid's room. But now there were no maids. The rooms available were in the attic and very pokey. In one grand house there was a large, airy room at the front, with a big window, that seemed ideal, until my elderly and very superior hostess interviewed me in her sitting room.

My eye was caught by a curious display on the grand piano, an array of wax flowers, mostly lilies, under a glass dome like a huge cheese bell, with a bundle of something inside. 'Was it a doll?' I asked. No. It was her newborn baby who had died nearly 50 years before, and in her grief she had it mummified and stuffed so that it could be with her always. It was wearing a long, white, lacy christening gown, its cheeks plumped up and facial features delicately coloured in pastel shades. She told me she dusted it every day. I decided against moving in.

Later, when I was doing post-graduate research at St Hugh's, and moved out of college, I found a large basement flat in Park Town, near College, the shops, and the Institute of Social Anthropology. My brother David had rented it before and was comfortable there. He was at Ruskin but had now gone to Amsterdam to be Secretary of the World Student Federalists. What appealed to me was the lovely pattern of flourishing ivy across the ceiling, where water was seeping in and providing the right habitat for green, growing things. Not every flat has its own indoor garden!

I started at Oxford in effect without a college and social contacts developed through university organisations. There was Professor Radakrishnan's Society for the Study of Eastern Religions, the small group that met in his rooms at All Souls. It included a Jain, a Jew, a Buddhist, a Hindu, a Muslim, a Quaker and a few others. We went regularly to All Souls to meet with Professor Radakrishnan, explore holy writings and beliefs, and learn how they related to individual lives and social organisation. There was another society for the study of religious thinking based on Manchester College, the Unitarian College. There were Quaker meetings. There was the Oxford University Labour Club, too, where Michael Summerskill was a leading figure, and, of course, a mixed bag of social anthropologists, including select Sudanese and other students from Africa who had been hand picked by lecturers (some of whom were having hectic affairs with them). One of my closest friends doing the diploma with me was a lovely Ghanaian (though then it was still the Gold Coast) who became chief minister of the Ashanti Kingdom.

Needing to earn some money, I stuck up a notice in the local post office advertising myself as a babysitter, and this led to caring for three children while their academic parents were lecturing and tutoring. The Wheares were a high-powered couple. One lovely summer day Joan asked me to take the children to the University Parks. I set off with the baby in the pram, the toddler in a seat near the handlebars, the older boy, Tom, with his bat and ball and a supply of play things. Then I saw a large group from the Institute of Social Anthropology sitting on the grass with what turned out to be an impromptu seminar with Professor Lloyd Warner, author of *Black Metropolis,* the first study of urban Afro-American culture. This was too good to miss! They beckoned me over and I joined them with the little ones, while Tom went off to play. I was engrossed. But suddenly a shout went up! *'Child in the river!'* I looked round and Tom was nowhere near. He had fallen in. By the time I had raced across the grass someone had fished him out. I piled the babies up in the pram again – it had tipped up – and took a dripping wet child home. No one was there. I washed his clothes, and hung his shoes, shorts and shirt on the line to dry.

Professor Wheare was the first to return. I told him, *'I'm very sorry – I let Tom fall in the river!'* There was a pause while he considered this carefully. Then, as an afterthought, he asked, *'Did you get him out again?'* I nodded, and he commented, *'Good'.* Tom later became Headmaster of Bryanston.

At Oxford I discovered sex, too, a mix of philosophy, religion and physical excitement in, of all settings, the Society for the Study of Eastern Religions.

Yatti was a Buddhist from Sri Lanka (then Ceylon) and I first met him when he came to stay with Mother as a guest of the Victoria League which arranged international student visits in English homes. We had sex and curry in his digs on the corner of St John's Street. With stars in my eyes, I never thought about contraception and trusted he would pull out in time. Though there was physical intimacy I don't think we ever achieved any emotional closeness or understanding. We didn't really talk – just bounced around together while curry was heating up on the gas ring.

A Jewish member of the Group for the Study of Eastern Religions, Vernon, was aware of the affair and tried to protect me and rein me in. He was very sweet and caring, but I thought he was being stuffy. It was partly because he criticised my clothes, too. I had bought a bright pink skirt and waistcoat in the softest wool and wore it over a dark green jumper. He told me I looked '*like a shop girl*'.

When I discovered I was pregnant I took it for granted that Yatti would stick by me, and that we would marry. He didn't. His Brahmin high caste family would disapprove and reject me as grossly inferior. His loyalty to the family was paramount, and he cold-shouldered me.

I returned home at the end of term to tell Mother. My fantasy was that I would go off and live in a caravan in the middle of a field with my baby and somehow get my life together. We discussed this realistically and she sorted out an abortion that was performed with skill, tact and understanding in my own bedroom by an obstetrician friend of hers who was the father of one of my close friends at school. It was at that time a criminal offence and I owe a lot to him. Father assisted him, and I shall never forget the look on his face when the doctor introduced the cannula to drain amniotic fluid and I started to bleed. I felt incredibly guilty at what I had done to my parents.

Yatti was very snooty about it all. He took a part-time job with the railway, and every time I bought a ticket to London I confronted him through the booking office hatch. It wasn't a plate glass thing – more like a hole in a hen coop, and you had to bend down to communicate. We never spoke again, except about tickets. I later learned that he returned to Sri Lanka and married an obstetrician who was part of the island's elite.

I thought of that child, and what he would have looked like, for years afterwards, especially on his birthday. It felt as if the sperm had wiggled its way into my uterus and stayed there. I carried a burden of guilt and there was no-one I could talk to about it. Years later when Celia was born and I lifted her into my arms I was surprised that she was light-skinned.

Social anthropology sharpened my sense of gender injustice, as I confronted scholarly men who perceived women as marginal, relevant only in terms of kinship, economic and political systems. I wanted to learn more about women's lives cross-culturally, and Margaret Mead, who came from the United States to run seminars at Oxford, encouraged me to explore the subject of birth, while my B.Litt thesis grew out of research into the experiences of African and Asian students at British universities.

I joined the Society of Friends, found a front room in Fairacres Road near the river, and had a Quaker landlady, Mrs Weatherhead, who took in strays. She was a generous woman. I once found her making cakes with her breastmilk. She was milking her breasts very efficiently straight into the mixing bowl, and told me she had plenty and didn't want to waste it. They tasted *very* sweet.

I remember keenly one night in Fairacres Road when something extraordinary happened. It was around 2 or 3 a.m. – and there was activity on the other side of the road, with lights on upstairs and down. I was woken by a car that had stopped opposite, somebody bustled out with a bag, the bell rang, the door opened and shut, and the figure disappeared. Another light was switched on upstairs. I could just hear music. Then everything was still.

Half an hour – perhaps an hour – went by. There was the light steadily burning on the first floor, and now and again human outlines were etched against the curtains – walking, bending, stretching out, leaning over, walking again. The music changed. They put a fresh record on, a Brahms lullaby. Then all was still again.

The night was dark – no moon, a thick, heavy, brooding night. Then suddenly the quiet cracked open and a sound pierced the darkness. It was like a lamb's bleat, a shrill wail that summoned instant attention – a human cry. A baby greeted life for the first time. I had eavesdropped on the miracle of birth. I shall never forget it.

One of Mrs Weatherhead's guests was a young woman who had run away from home, and in her turn had befriended some prostitutes. There was a taxi service in Gloucester Green and the drivers acted as pimps for the American service-men in the camps around Oxford. They would get a group of teenage girls and take them out towards the camps, introduce them to the airmen, and sex took place in the taxis. Then they ran them back again. I got to know these girls and became fascinated by the social set-up, finding out why they were doing it, the relationships between them, and the very different relationships between this group and other prostitutes who came regularly from London on pay day. These were the '*Piccadilly Queens*'. They had much more money and swept into Oxford on the train from Paddington. There was great rivalry.

My tutor, John Peristiany, encouraged me to study this, use anthropological concepts and methods of enquiry, and learn how to interview by exploring their lives with these women. It was a great education for me! I became friendly with them and was able to help them a bit. In this way I began to learn how to do qualitative feminist research, which is different from studying people as if you could stand aside and be coolly objective about what you are doing, filling in boxed numbers on questionnaires and adding them up. I tried to understand them as women. Most had deprived lives. Many had been sexually abused by fathers, step-fathers or uncles, and it was not surprising that they had run away from home. It was the pattern of their lives – disadvantage, even if they weren't financially disadvantaged, the kind of society in which they grew up, inter-personal stresses in the family, and the powerlessness they experienced, that drove them into sex work. Statistics are important, but quantitative studies need to be balanced with in-depth qualitative analysis.

The thesis for my research degree was on race relations in British universities. You can't discuss Oxford without talking about inside and outside, the people who are accepted and those who are marginal. In those days these were Pakistanis, Indians and Caribbeans. I looked at the social groups they formed to cope with this experience of being marginalised, and attitudes and behaviour towards them. A friend at Trinity smuggled out the JCR book for me to see a particular entry after an Indian came up: *'A black man in Trinity! Gentlemen, what are we coming to?'* It was signed by a member of a well-known brewing family.

St Hugh's

When I started post-graduate work I moved into College for a few terms. At that time St Hugh's was stuck between an old fashioned boarding school for girls and an Oxford College which permitted certain freedoms, expected students to have a vigorous social life, and which provided a comfortable background for learning. I think the Fellows did not quite know what to do with us or how to treat us.

Only two of us were vegetarians, Maura and me. The kitchens hadn't a clue, gave up, and served cold baked beans straight out of the tin meal after meal.

Men were allowed to visit the undergraduate rooms, but only in the afternoons before 7 p.m. So many liaisons were surreptitious, and that added to the thrill. The custom was that if a man was successful in his aims he took a bath tap as a trophy. It was a bit like hunters who display moose heads on the walls. John, who had been at school with my brother David, apparently made it with a woman in a room along my corridor and went off with *both* bath taps from the nearest bathroom. He subsequently became the distinguished head of an Oxford college. I don't know what he did with the bath taps.

The rooms were so pokey that it was difficult to know how to decorate them. Mirrors helped. I chose the colour orange and hung orange velvet curtains, and had the same colour bedcovers and rug on the floor. Every day in cold weather the scout would come in to clear and lay the coal fire, and, presumably, to check there was no man there. He was supposed to be the only male on the premises.

My Brother David

The *Guardian* described him as a '*BBC producer with a media mogul's flair. With his knowledge and contacts, he was almost ambassadorial.*'[2]

As a child David was a cub. He didn't go on to be a boy scout. He liked independence and the chance to think for himself. He was sent to Taunton School, a public school that, like many others, put great emphasis on games, the Officer's Training Corps and corporal punishment administered by prefects. David had an independent spirit. He dared to go to a film he wanted to see at the Odeon wearing his school uniform. The consequence was that he was summoned for trial by the prefects and subjected to a flogging. The method they used was to make a boy kneel over a stool with his head under a table. Then the prefects took turns at caning him, trying to outdo each other and cause most pain. It not only produced wounds to the buttocks but battered the boys' heads, too. One of the prefects who caned David later became my husband's best friend at Oxford. He was a committed Christian. I never could feel close to him.

What the school had not realised was that breaking school rules and going to the local cinema was a vital part of David's development as an investigative journalist with media flair working with colleagues in high places, including governments on both sides of the Atlantic.

Mother's protests against violence of all kinds and her work for peace was continued by David, expressed in his refusal to serve in the armed forces when he was called up, after the war, for National Service and his conscientious objection.

It was a simple matter for members of the Society of Friends who produced evidence of religious membership and joined the Friends' Ambulance Service to justify their conscientious objection. Though the media described him as a Quaker, he was an agnostic and it was harder for him – he faced the threat of being sent to prison. He needed a good lawyer. He was represented at his tribunal by an African barrister who was a close friend. He was excused from military service and directed into alternative work as a porter at Great Ormond Street Hospital. But he really wanted to get to the continent and help set up an organisation that meant that nations would never resort to war again.

David was offered the job of Chair of World Student Federalists in Paris. So he sent a letter to the Minister responsible for National Service, informing him that he felt his alternative services as a CO would be of more value if he went to work in Paris instead of sweeping floors and changing bandages in London. He left without having any answer. There was the risk that if he returned to England he would be put in jail, and we were anxious for him. In the event, he did not come back until conscription had been abolished.

In Paris David shared an apartment with the African-American novelist Richard Wright. Whilst there he became friends with the Abbé Pierre – a revolutionary priest, champion of the homeless and founder of the Emmaus Community, who lived in poverty and slept on David's desk – which was always a big one! David had very little money himself and with not much food, became very thin.

He worked in Paris for two years, first with WFS and later also as Director of the World Movement for World Federal Government.

Then he moved to Amsterdam as Secretary General of the World Student Federalists, in charge of the Amsterdam office. Lucy Law, National Student Chairman of the United World Federalists, regularly wrote to him as she was fascinated by the photograph of David that was used for publicising World Student Federalists. It was taken in the bathtub of a Count who was a friend of WSF and depicted him at his leanest when he was poor and hungry in Paris. Lucy, who later became his wife, tells me that she was disappointed when she first met him in person, because he was a good deal plumper by then and didn't look like the publicity photo.

When in Amsterdam David lived in the Red Light district and had loads of friends, famous and infamous. It was exciting to visit him there and feel the sense of community. Amsterdam life was swinging – philosophers, writers, revolutionaries, sex workers, artists – the lot!

It struck me at the time that the women on show behind the windows had better lives than prostitutes in London who roamed the streets. They had their own territory and the drug scene was relaxed. I didn't examine it more closely and find out who, if anyone, was exploiting them – questions I would certainly ask today.

David had loads of friends among these young women on exhibition. The relationships were free and easy and I think he didn't analyse this set-up in political terms. Maybe Amsterdam was not the lovely place it set out to be.

He spent a year at Ruskin College, Oxford, and then became a journalist with the BBC, first a Production Assistant with *Panorama* in 1959, and its Editor in 1967. The *Guardian* commented on its '*authoritative journalism and good storytelling*'. He was immensely loyal to the BBC and convinced of its importance in national and international affairs. In seeking information and comments from corporations and foreign ministries he always by-passed press officers and went straight to the top.

Lucy wrote to me, '*I remember very clearly David's departure for Dallas after President Kennedy was shot. He came racing down our hill on his moped and rushed into the house to pack before a car picked him up to go to the airport. Our son, Daniel asked, 'Is Daddy going to save Mr Kennedy?'*'

At *Panorama* he worked closely with Richard Dimbleby and together they made programmes after the terrible earthquake at Skopje. He also made programmes in Vietnam and visited many overseas countries.

In the 1970s he became the BBC's Director of Public Affairs and was on the Board of Management, and then BBC Director in the United States. During this time he and Lucy divorced.

Subsequently he created the Transatlantic Dialogues on Broadcasting, an international organisation to train journalists of ex-communist and other countries and show them how they could resist coercion from government and organisations that abused power. He was strongly supported by his son Daniel, who took over as David's health deteriorated.

David had type 2 diabetes, breast cancer – unusual for a man – and heart failure. All his interests were based in the United States, especially on the political scene in Washington DC. We were pretty much out of touch. He phoned occasionally, but always to ask for Uwe because of their shared interests in developing democratic media in ex-communist countries, and never wanted

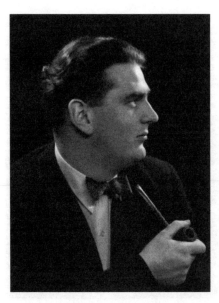

David as the BBC's director of Public Affairs

to talk to me or find out what I was doing. Yet our radical upbringing led us both to taking political action on an international stage and challenging powerful institutions.

In the words of the *Times* obituary after he died in Washington DC in the summer of 2003, *'In everything he did he sought influence, not power.'*

How I Met Uwe

Uwe and I met in July 1950 on a plane going to the United States, a week after the Korean War broke out. It was at the end of my first year at Oxford. He was up at Oxford, too, and had a shining career there, becoming President of the Union. We each had a student research fellowship with a Quaker-based action organisation, International Fellowships for Students Overseas, run by Phil Ruopp, an American at Oxford. Phil and his wife Frankie were friends of Mother's and often visited Little Thatch. This was one way in which they put their religion into practice. We were to spend the long vac working in the United States, and there were choices between social and community work, teaching and journalism.

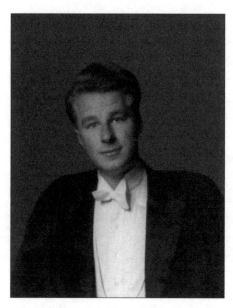

Uwe

I had to go to London for my visa and in the hall at the US embassy I noticed that the same young man I had seen on the platform five years before was sitting waiting for his visa, too. He spent the time moving between dozens of people whom he obviously knew, and I watched him. He was eager, outgoing, and very active at getting people involved in the exploits he was planning. I couldn't hear what they were arranging, but he generated terrific enthusiasm.

Uwe was going to Washington DC, working in politics, and I was going to Chicago to look at race relations in what was then called the *'Black Belt'* and to work with under-privileged black children in a community centre. The task was to give them an enriching and stimulating break from poverty and race discrimination.

We were flying in the same plane to Chicago, an old rattling Flying Tiger from the Second World War and it was the first time I had flown. We were free to sit wherever we liked so I found a window seat and settled down. I was reading the safety instructions and looked up to see someone sliding into the seat beside me. It was Uwe Kitzinger. He told me he'd done Classics at school, and was now at New College reading PPE (Philosophy, Politics and Economics) and had a sister at Somerville. He struck me as a visionary and someone who was determined to make the world a better place. He also had delightful manners.

The flight took about 20 hours. We stopped in Shannon, then Gander, in Newfoundland, and chased the sunset across the Atlantic, that glowed red right through our journey. The plane seemed to climb upstairs laboriously and then fall down repetitively. I was writing 'purple prose' about how marvellous this was in a long letter to my mother. Then Uwe started to feel sick, grabbed a sick bag, and vomited off and on until we reached New York. All the same, he did a pretty good job of relaxed wooing. He was obviously very good at it. He said he particularly admired the way I wrote and how I described the view and the whole adventure. Fortunately he did vomit fairly quietly.

We parted when we reached Chicago. Uwe went to join the Senate Press Gallery and lunched with the notorious Senator Joe McCarthy, the man who thought Communists lurked everywhere, wanted all suspects imprisoned, and who led the American people to spend a lot of time looking for Reds under the beds. Then he was off to New York to stay up the Hudson in the castle of the president of a well-known cosmetics firm. I went on to a very different way of life in Chicago.

Chicago

When I attended a church in the '*Black Belt*' I was always asked to speak, and each invitation led to another, and often young people's conventions.

In a letter to my parents I wrote: '*I met Father Divine, alias George Baker, a black preacher and founder of the Faith Eternal cult who sways a large congregation. He was never born in the normal way, but combusted at the corner of 134th Street and 7th Avenue, New York, around 1900. He provides free chicken dinners (all you can eat, everybody welcome!), set up a communal household and his followers give up everything to him. So he has become fabulously rich and married a white woman.*'

I started work at the International Trade Fair alongside another young woman, whom in a letter to my parents I said was '*rather smug ... as so many English women abroad are*'. Enquiring where the ladies' room was at a large hotel, the porteress directed me 11 floors up, adding '*We have one on this floor but it's not very nice. The coloured use it, and I have to use it too.*' I said quietly, '*Oh, I wouldn't mind a bit.*'

Day after day I feel trapped in extreme racial prejudice. I asked the driver of the bus provided by the Fair to drop me off at the Parkway. He said, 'Oh, you can't go there. It's coloured!' He needed quite a bit of persuading before he allowed me to get off the bus and I was late for my appointment.

3rd September
'*I have discovered this about my self – that I am not interested in the abstract, but in the actual, and that it is necessary for me always to be doing things with my hands if I am to be reasonably contented. You'd never believe how really practical and earth-bound I am, with all my ideals. To think of life's vast problems in a vacuum frustrates me, but I am tremendously exhilarated when I can work from hand to hand or from heart to heart. I am much happier teaching children than arguing about the world's educational problems. I like intellectual discussion, but the proof of it is down here on the earth, I think. It is in the home and the church and the community as a whole. And all problems can only be resolved eventually in this context, in a rather unspectacular way.*'[3]

I was staying with a couple who were psychologists at Chicago University and baby-sat several times a week. But I needed cash for day-to-day expenses and Carl, a university student who was also at the community centre, suggested I sell my blood at the hospital, so that is what I did.

The African-American Way Of Death

Carl lived in his uncle's funeral home and was doing a course in social science while also working part-time as a volunteer at the community centre. He liked the funeral home because it was a peaceful place to study. He invited me back there so I could write up my research report. There is no place more conducive to quiet study than a room in a funeral home when it is not open to viewing. I got quite a lot of work done there. I can recommend it. He also showed me how the morticians worked and I learnt about the ceremonies surrounding death, the laying out, viewing the body, and the mingled sorrow and rejoicing.

I watched his uncle at work draining fluids from the body, packing it with scented stuffing, and rejuvenating it with carefully applied cosmetics. He was very proud of his corpses. They were creations of art.

However poor the deceased had been, there had to be a lavish send-off. The room for the ritual viewing was splendid with great vases of gladioli at the head and foot of the deceased, many coloured flower offerings filling every available space, with written messages from those who knew him, and solemn music played from a mechanical organ. Since then I always associate gladioli with death, and seeing them I can still smell the scent of mortuary unguents: an overpowering odour of violets mixed with lavender, lime and rose, like a strong toilet deodorant. On the wall above the open coffin, which was resplendent with cedar wood, shiny brass and purple velvet cushions, was a thorn-crowned glass statue of Christ with strobe lighting twinkling like the lights on a Christmas tree so that blood appeared to be continuously streaming from his head and wounds.

The moment the doors were flung open and the mourners surged into the funeral home it took on the spirit of a festival. Each member of the crowd, old and young, signed the attendance book. Little children gaped in fascination at the technicoloured spectacle. I was the only white face and at first felt awkward and out of place. But people seemed to accept that my involvement was a mark of respect for the dead. Far from being a voyeur, I became one of the mourners.

This experience fed my interest in the values surrounding the human journey into life and out of it and the ceremonies that give pattern to these major transitions.

The West Indian Society

I think I knew all the West Indians and most of the Africans at Oxford – not very many. I was a member of the West Indian Society, which was great fun. They discussed openly with me how it felt to be 'marginal men' in Oxford, and what they did to try to be accepted. These men (for there were no women) were to become politicians, take up appointments in the higher echelons of the administrative and social services, be top administrators and academics and sometimes prime ministers of their islands. They were under social pressure to define their identity as distinct from dark skinned people who manned buses and the underground in London, and when outside Oxford their standard dress included a college tie or scarf and a rolled umbrella. This was a conscious and carefully thought through decision to express their social status.

One of my closest friends was a Trinidadian, Max Ifill, who later married an English woman, and whose son, Richard, was sent to boarding school when they returned to Trinidad. He spent some school holidays with us, got on well with our girls, and became a proxy brother.

Uwe Again

By chance Uwe and I met again in Oxford next term, and he invited me out for dinner at the Taj Mahal in the Turl. Apparently I spoke so enthusiastically about my experiences in Chicago, waving my arms about, that the waiters stopped waiting, and hovered, keen not to miss one bit, and he was hooked! I was hooked, too!

He had the nicest smile I have ever seen. Uwe was that rare person, an intellectual who was inherently sociable, highly political, fascinated by ethical issues and world problems, skilled at speaking and campaigning, charming, and delighting in female company. He is a very different kind of person from me, but we think alike. His ideals about society, especially at that time after the war, were very similar to mine. We were both working with the Council for Education in World Citizenship, believed in federalism, and in overcoming national and cultural barriers.

Then I bumped into him again outside Marks and Spencers. We strolled along together a bit and he invited me to a debate at the Union at which he was speaking. I felt privileged.

I sat up in the front row of the balcony overlooking crowds of eager undergraduates who had flocked to hear the debate of the year. There was Uwe! He looked very striking and authoritative in the scene below as people crowded round him. I smiled at the woman sitting next to me. She asked, 'Are you a friend of Uwe's? He invited me as well.' I turned to the one on my right and offered a tentative smile, 'Are you a friend of Uwe's, too?' she said. Eventually I discovered that every woman in the front row was a guest of Uwe's. It looked as if each of this retinue was a girl friend.

We talked about politics, social anthropology, religion and our ideals. He told me about his tutors whom he much admired – Isiah Berlin, Peter Wiles, Alan Bullock and Herbert Hart. He had a wide circle of friends that included other Oxford luminaries – Tony Benn, Ken Tynan, William Rees-Mogg, Godfrey Smith, Robin Day, Jeremy Thorpe, Vera Brittain's daughter Shirley

Williams (though that was before her marriage to Bernard, a philosopher), and just about everybody who was going into politics and the media. Later I learned that you couldn't walk along the High without meeting the well-known people who greeted him.

Uwe was compassionate, too. When one of the young women who was camping at Mrs Weatherhead's had nightmares and flashbacks and needed to be able to contact me in the night he came and fixed up a bell so that she knew she could get me quickly if she wanted to.

I invited him to my home for Easter 1951. Mother was startled when he stepped forward, bowed, and blonde hair flopping over his high brow, with great elegance, kissed her hand. He gushed his pleasure at being invited to this beautiful house. His manners were impeccable, but overwhelming. When I went to the kitchen to carry the teatray Mother stared at me with horror and whispered, '*Sheila, what* have *you brought home?*'

Falling In Love

The months at Oxford after I met Uwe were days of wine and roses. We walked along the Isis and made nests in the long grass. We spent a heavenly summer with butterflies, flowers, delicious scents of hay, puffy little clouds in a blue sky, birds singing, and exploring the finer arts of petting.

Then he invited me to meet his parents. It was important that we got on well. They lived in a small upstairs flat near St Albans. I was a little nervous, but they seemed to take it for granted that he and I should talk in his bedroom. Of course, we did more than talk.

The doorbell rang, and a neighbour called in. We were asked to meet him and drank coffee. As Uwe's mother went to the kitchen to replenish the cups he muttered an aside. Apparently the floor acted as what he called a '*baffle board*' and he could hear more or less everything we were doing, saying and exclaiming. He thought we ought to know.

I don't think I made a good impression on Uwe's parents. They thought he could do better and counselled him against me. Before lunch, Uwe's mother described the main meat course she had cooked. I said I was a vegetarian. She said, '*Never mind, I can give you sausages.*' My response: '*Mrs Kitzinger, I do not eat mashed up corpses!*'

* * *

On taking his First Uwe was offered a diplomatic post in Strasbourg and we wrote to each other all winter.

In the spring I met Uwe off the train from London and told him to get straight back on and we went for a weekend in the Cotswolds, to the Old Mill, in Shipston-on-Stour, where we had separate rooms but met, very quietly, in the dead of night. We found a restaurant on the river, the Bull, that had the very latest post-rationing food delicacies – frozen peas and an omelette with '*real shell eggs*'! The menu stated that with pride – six years after the war.

In early summer 1952 we went to a conference on world development and poverty in the Netherlands, a very flat country. It was at Wageningen, about the flattest place there. The trouble was that there was nowhere where we could kiss and caress that wasn't visible to everyone else attending the conference – except behind the gas works, the largest building in the town. So that was where we slipped away whenever there was a gap in the conference programme.

Years later at another conference we met a lady who said that we have never been introduced before but she felt she knew us because she had seen us in Wageningen. Long pause. She added significantly, '*I live opposite the gas works*'. We hastened to tell her, '*We are married now!*' '*Oh, that's all right then!*' She said with evident relief. End of conversation.

At Wageningen we decided to get married in October that year. I returned to Oxford, notified College, and gave them the details. I was summoned to her study by Miss Proctor, the principal. She was a tall, angular, steel-grey haired lady, a theologian, who didn't find it easy to talk to students, but who had a keen sense of duty, I entered, sat opposite her at her wide, highly polished mahogany desk, and she addressed me, '*Miss Webster, do you understand the significance of marriage?*' '*Oh yes, Miss Proctor, I do*', I replied expecting a conversation to develop. She stood up to shake my hand, '*Good*', she said, '*Goodbye*'.

A Long Distance Marriage

We married on 4 October 1952 at the Quaker Meeting House in St Giles. I wore a silk broderie anglaise dress the colour of clotted cream with a nipped in waist, which entailed wearing a waist corselet like a wide belt. It had a full, flared skirt and the hem was just above the ankles, like the dresses worn by Celia Johnson in *Brief Encounter*. It was the Dior New Look, launched way back in 1947 when Dior was the first haute couture Parisian to sell his designs to the retail market. We found the dress in Taunton at Mr Dodd's boutique, the only high style dress shop in the town. After rationing and clothes coupons there was much criticism of the amount of fabric these New Look clothes involved and they were often denounced as wasteful. It cost more than any other dress I ever had. I used Mother's Elizabeth Arden clover pink lipstick and powder, and dabbed lily of the valley scent behind my ears, but in those days it was not *de rigueur* to have a bridal make-up session, and anyway, I preferred to look natural. There were no bridesmaids or pages, and I didn't even carry a bouquet. There was a bunch of flowers in a pot.

I had researched different methods of contraception and decided that the diaphragm would be best for me. I didn't want to go on the Pill because it might muck up my hormones by introducing other chemicals into my blood stream, and I didn't know the long-term effects. So I went to a gynaecologist to discuss this with her and get fitted. On the second visit she showed me how to fit the rubber cap over my cervix. I thought we were all sorted.

But then she said I couldn't have it yet as I wasn't married and I was to go to her the morning of the wedding day to collect it. Since meeting for worship was at 11 a.m., I should turn up around 10 a.m. and I could pop it in my handbag and take it. She was a formidable woman – not to be argued with.

I dressed in my wedding finery and Father drove me into Oxford. I walked the length of Holywell, and picked it up, and went straight to the wedding. A busy morning!

Our wedding seemed very special at the time and I did have a new dress, but it was not intended to shock, thrill and amaze, but to be a gathering in which we pledged ourselves to each other and shared our joy with close friends, colleagues and family. The Society of Friends doesn't stage weddings. A marriage is recorded at the Registry Office after Meeting.

Some of those who attended didn't have any idea what Quakers were about. The mother of one of Uwe's girlfriends, in the silence of Meeting, in a loud and ringing voice proclaimed, as she addressed Norman Marrow, Uwe's Classics teacher at school, '*I know him, but don't know anything about her. Is she* all right?'

After about half an hour's silence we stood up and, holding hands, I said, '*I take this my friend Uwe Kitzinger to be my husband and promise, so long as we both on earth shall live, to be unto him a loving and faithful wife.*' Uwe made the same promise and we were married! We didn't exchange wedding rings and I have never worn a ring – I suppose because it holds a hint of bondage, and it seems to me that if you are indissolubly linked with another human being it is not necessary to demonstrate it formally. But today, our eldest daughter, Celia, holds a different view, and believes that when she and her partner Sue wear their rings they make a statement about equal marriage rights. They slipped the rings on in their marriage ceremony in Canada, and took them off whenever they were in a country which did not acknowledge marriage between two women.

After the Meeting for worship we had a small, relaxed and happy lunch at The Feathers in Woodstock when our friends could get to know each other. We spent our first night in Dorchester, and then stayed in Little Thatch, my home in Somerset. A complete absence of ceremony, yet a blossoming of our relationship.

Father's Family

Shortly after our marriage Uwe and I drove up to Wigtownshire in the South West of Scotland to explore my father's family history.

The Websters of Wigtownshire lived, worked and married within five miles of each other. They were crofters who leased land in return for work on the landowner's farm. John (1814–1901) had 12 children and outlived all his siblings. He died at the age of 93 as he walked through Black Loch Plantation one night in a snowstorm, after having a wee dram too many to help him on his way. The *Wigtown Free Press* reported the discovery of his body three weeks later as the snow melted. The story is that a boy in the woods shouted to his father that he could smell mushrooms. '*The body was in an advanced state of decomposition and sadly disfigured by vermin.*'

Willie, John's son, and his wife Isabella had triplets – born at home of course. One died at birth, but Martha and Mary survived.

Willie's sister, Hannah, had a daughter outside marriage, Grace. On the birth certificate the father is named as '*Hugh Love*'. There was an agricultural labourer of that name at a nearby farm. He would have been about 15 when the baby was conceived. Hannah married Robert Lauderdale before the baby was two years old and went on to have eight more children.

The Aunt Hannah I knew, Father's aunt, was very tall and handsome, and wore her hair in thick plaits across her head. She was a dairy farmer at Mochrum. One day, when shopping with us, she tripped and fell over my brother David, who was two then. I remember that mother was very frightened for him, but after a good cry he was fine. It seems to have been a characteristic of the Webster family that they were sturdy and bonny, with wide shoulders. As we were exploring the family history we met an elderly man who had known Willie Webster and pointed to Uwe's new Mercedes and said to me, *'I could tell you were one of them, because they all had shoulders on them like the front of yon car.'*

Reality And Imagination

Uwe was in the Diplomatic Service, Secretary to the Economic Committee of the Council of Europe, and went back to Strasbourg, and I returned to Edinburgh where I was doing research in race relations for an Oxford Research Degree. I commuted and at the end of every term travelled to Strasbourg, became a diplomatic wife, made love intensively and had *'honeymoon cystitis'* for a year!

In the summer after we were married we went out to the Rose Revived, a sixteenth-century coaching inn at Newbridge, near Witney, and swam in the river. I wore a new gold satin stretch bathing costume. The water sparkled, leaves glistened in the sunlight.

I have never been a great party-goer but Uwe enjoys social occasions of every kind, loves meeting new people, and has high expectations. In 1953 the Oxford Group, otherwise known as the Buchmanites, invited me to visit their international HQ at Caux, outside Geneva. It came about through a fellow undergraduate, Louis Ozanne, who, like me, was active in the Society for the Study of Eastern Religions. Uwe thought we should grasp the opportunity. The Buchmanite movement developed in Nazi Germany, but by this time had embraced ideals of charity and peace.

We found ourselves enveloped in a *'holier than thou'* atmosphere where devotees held the leader not only in great respect, but in reverence – and we were terribly bored. Uwe's thoughts were that we should escape and he had the idea of visiting one of the Geneva nightclubs as an antidote.

We skipped off feeling like naughty children, only to encounter a dismal scene in which an overweight, ageing erotic striptease artiste manipulated a huge python round her body and limbs, sticking it between her thighs, kissing and stroking it, and doing just about everything which she might do with a penis. It went on and on – tedious, predictable, crude and unappealing. Uwe muttered under his breath that this was dreadful and though we couldn't draw attention to ourselves by getting up and leaving at this point, we should escape at the first opportunity. But we were trapped, and had to put up with it.

I whispered that he ought to take off his glasses, leaving something to the imagination. It was an amazing and instant success! Everything went fuzzy and the erotic dancer became glamorous in that moment. This is an important lesson – imagination is the essence of pleasure. If you want to enjoy yourself, make space for fantasy!

A Miscarriage

Writing to a friend in December 1954: '*We leave Strasbourg this coming week-end for England – first to Garston, then all of us to Taunton for the actual Christmas, and then back to Garston for the New Year. I think I am more excited about Christmas this year than ever before because although Toby (or Anna) isn't born yet I look at all the gay Christmas shop windows, the bright lights and the twinkling decorations as if through his eyes, and it all seems very wonderful and new, as if I had never seen it so sparkling or colourful before.*'

There were only two drops at first, and I persuaded myself that some bleeding was common in early pregnancy. But then there were more – and more. A French gynaecologist examined me, said the fetus had a beating heart, and prescribed hormone supplements to keep the pregnancy going. I was reassured – wrongly as it turned out. I took them assiduously. Then one day blood started to pour out. Obviously I wasn't going to have this baby. I had thought I was 24 or 25 weeks pregnant. I even believed I felt movements. But the baby had died much earlier.

The only thing was to accept it and let my body do its work of emptying and cleaning out the uterus. We were on holiday with my parents in Northern Italy and I took to bed, nestled in an impressive and very comfortable four poster, with detective stories, and marvellous, lavish meals sent up on ornate trays.

That's where I discovered white truffles. My memories are of sitting in bed in luxury in a beautiful room eating the best food there is in the world while losing a baby. It was sad, but at the same time this was self-indulgent gourmandising and an intense sensory experience.

Mother once wrote to Uwe, '*Father looks after his pigs when they are pregnant better than you do Sheila.*' I had no complaints! I didn't seek cossetting when pregnant. The important thing to me was freedom.

Uwe and I travelled a lot and also lived abroad because of his job at various times. He was often off to other countries leaving me wherever I was based, too, and the relationship was kept fresh. We were never a couple to '*settle down*'. I was lecturing around the world and usually extended the engagement to do research in other cultures – a condition I made when I accepted a booking. He usually moved in superior circles and saw more picturesque or impressive aspects of a country than I did – parliamentarians, colleagues at Harvard University, or working with all the big wigs in Brussels, for example, whereas I was with the poorest of the poor.

So we had a complex and colourful view of societies around the world but our frequent absences produced some confusion among our daughters. They weren't certain where we were or what we were doing. Tess, in her mid-teens, answered Uwe's phone since he was abroad. '*And who shall I say called?*' she asked. '*Winston Churchill,*' came the reply. She snorted and said '*And I'm Florence Nightingale!*' It was Winston Churchill's grandson.

CHAPTER THREE

HOW BIRTH WAS FOR ME

The first time she has a baby, it is difficult for any woman to know what to expect or how she will feel. A large question mark hangs over the whole experience of birth: *'Is it possible that I can give birth to a normal baby?' 'Shall I really be able to manage without drugs for pain relief?' 'Will I make a fool of myself?' 'Is my body capable of giving birth?'* For many of us, that first birth is viewed in terms of how well we cope personally and whether or not everything turns out *'all right'*. Political awareness and social action usually come later. That is how it was for me.

When our first daughter was born in October 1956, we were living in Strasbourg, France, where Uwe was Secretary to the Economic Commission of the Council of Europe and in the Diplomatic Corps. As a *'diplomatic wife'* in Strasbourg, I felt under pressure to conform and not draw attention to myself by challenging behaviour or stepping out of line in any way. It applied to how I had my first baby, too. There was a choice of two private maternity hospitals, one Catholic and one Jewish, and it was simply a matter of deciding which.

So when I was pregnant I went to look around each. I was horrified to see the delivery rooms in the Catholic home with a high, flat delivery table opposite an enormous painting of Christ on the cross, blood pouring out of wounds in his chest, side, arms and legs. The message for the mother was *'you are suffering incredible pain, but Christ was in greater agony. Endure your pain in a Christ-like spirit. There is no escape. This is your cross.'*

I attended a birth in that hospital and was shocked when a nun determined to get the baby latched on the breast correctly stood at the door with one in her arms and shouted, '*Brace yourself, mother!*' and then ran full tilt, the baby's startled mouth gaping, and clamped it onto the breast.

Another diplomatic wife, Pat Beesley – a close friend – recommended the Jewish hospital where she had given birth. When I researched that I discovered that it was highly prescriptive, and mothers had to follow instructions and accept whatever intervention was proposed.

Either way, I realised that I was handing my body over to be managed by an institution that imposed a concept of birth very different to mine. I was determined to avoid this. The answer I decided was to give birth at home with a midwife who knew how to help women labour as naturally and spontaneously as possible. In France that was called '*accouchement sans douleur*'. My best bet was to get one who had some training in what was then newly introduced as a method of conducting childbirth, psychoprophylaxis.

My baby was *my* baby, and I wanted to get to know my child from the earliest moment on. I felt that I could trust my body. I realised that my choices seemed to be in very bad taste and friends told me that I was behaving 'like a peasant'.

Although a doctor was in the background and saw me for several prenatal visits, I was looked after during my pregnancy by a young midwife who had attended a course in psychoprophylaxis run by Lamaze in Paris. I told her about Grantly Dick-Read's teaching and the pioneering work of Kathleen Vaughan in India; we discussed books I had read, especially those by Minnie Randall and the physiotherapist Helen Heardman. We agreed to see if we could combine the best aspects of each of these approaches. We didn't exactly see eye-to-eye but it seemed the neatest solution. I read everything I could find about birth – anthropology (in which detailed accounts of birth were few and far between), my mother's books, and any other literature that could give me some understanding of the birth experience.

I wanted it to be as natural as possible and was absolutely convinced that I could birth in my own way, in my own time. Uwe shared my confidence and gave me strong emotional support. I loved being pregnant, exercised, breathed, relaxed, and was in peak physical and emotional condition. I could not wait for labour to start!

One evening when the Council of Europe was in session we attended a gala dinner. The wines and food were splendid. When I climbed into bed that night,

I said, *'I hope the baby doesn't come tonight; I've eaten too much!'* Two hours later I woke with a delicious, warm sensation, and as I drifted out of sleep, I had the satisfying feeling of having wet the bed. The waters had broken.

This occurred long before the vogue for water births. Nevertheless, I made for the bath and soaked in warm water, breathing at first slowly and fully, and then lightly and quickly, over the waves of the contractions, revelling in the swelling power of my uterus. Lying there, I started to time the contractions and realised that they were coming every three to four minutes. I was in the full swing of labour. I was exultant! It was like jumping into a river and finding that I could swim after all. I could do it! There was nothing unfamiliar, nothing that I could not handle myself. The pain was a by-product of the work my uterus was doing so efficiently, but it was pain with a glorious purpose, pain at which I marvelled because it was quite different from the pain of injury.

Once out of the bath, I helped Uwe get the room ready for birth, made the bed, boiled the water, and rang the midwife. We wanted to tape-record the sounds of birth and our baby's first cry and intended to borrow equipment from a friend, but I suddenly realised I was feeling low pressure and said to Uwe, *'I don't want you to leave me.'* I bent my knees and went down spontaneously, holding on to the big, bulbous leg of a heavy table in the study. Every two minutes, with each contraction, I squatted on the floor. I still remember the garish yellow, black and purple stripes of paint I had applied to this ugly Victorian secondhand furniture. I rocked and tilted my hips as each contraction built up, climaxed and faded.

I had never been any good at games at school and was put in goal in the hockey team because with my bulk I might at least stop the ball in a more or less stationary position. But even that didn't happen often, as other girls darted round the pitch. Not me. Sports were a misery and I felt a complete failure. Yet working with my body in childbirth I was able to dance my way through labour. It was amazing! I suddenly thought, *'Wow! This is a sport I can do!'*

The midwife came in, assessed the situation quickly, examined me, and said, *'You can push now'*. Push? Push? I did not want to push. I told her so and said I would rather wait until my body told me to push. My body seemed to be telling me to relax and let the baby's head slide out gently. She looked worried: *'Lie on your back. Push or I'll cut you.'* I was really frightened of having an episiotomy, or being surgically mutilated, so I took a deep breath and pushed, and after a second stage of only 10 minutes, I felt the prickling sensation of the baby's head crowning. Like a pea popping out of a pod, a head slipped out, and then I felt a warm, amazingly strong baby kicking between my legs. This was what it was all about – a baby! She was *gorgeous*. I put her to my breast immediately, and she suckled as if this were all she had been waiting for. The birth had been three hours from start to finish.

Meanwhile, the midwife examined me and said that I had a second-degree tear and that she would call the doctor to come and suture my perineum. He came in, slapped a cloth soaked in ether over my face, and tried to suture me while I was moving restlessly about. As I returned to consciousness, I heard him announcing that his handiwork was not good enough: *'Bring her to the hospital, and I'll redo it under proper anaesthesia.'*

We spent the next two hours enjoying the baby, called to tell English parliamentary friends that we had a daughter, and then drove to the hospital. It was there that the obstetrician, after injecting me with a general anaesthetic, dared to ask my husband (man to man), *'How tight do you want her?'* Uwe did not know what to answer. I was duly sutured and then handed back to him with these words: *'I've sewn her up good and tight.'* I was furious. He had given me the French equivalent of the American obstetrician's *'husband's stitch'*.

A couple of days later, I determined to go for a long walk in the woods so that I could work the stitches loose. It turned out quite an eventful outing. We set off in the car to the Black Forest, I got out and walked. It was snowing and I did rather more than walk, since the car stuck in a snowdrift and I had to push it out. I lifted the carry cot out of the car in case it slid forward over the edge of the mountain, got a grip and shoved and heaved. It wouldn't budge at first, and then – triumph! It moved and the wheels shifted. For six months, I felt quite sore and did not enjoy intercourse; however, when my English GP examined me later, she commented, *'I wouldn't have known that you had a tear.'* I don't recommend pushing cars out of snowdrifts on a mountainside, but it worked for me!

That was the beginning of my commitment to understand the spontaneous and unforced rhythms of the second stage, to learn how women could give birth without fighting their bodies or putting on a performance – could open up and deliver without injury. My experience sowed the seeds for my interest in the psycho-sexual aspects of childbirth, my concern about the unnecessary and mutilating surgery performed in both obstetrics and gynaecology, and my determination to challenge women's powerlessness and victimisation by a male-dominated medical system.

Childbirth Education

When Celia was about nine weeks old the Health Visitor called with forms to be filled in to fit me into the health system. Pen poised over the questionnaire, she asked me, '*What are you feeding her?*' '*Breast milk*', I said. '*Aren't you giving her anything else?*' I said I wasn't. '*You need to give her mashed brains.*' I told her I was a vegetarian. She was horrified and delivered the authoritative judgement, '*If you don't give her any brains she won't develop any.*'

I had just come back to England from France two months after giving birth and wanted to use the experience so that I could reach out and help other women enjoy their birth-giving too. The Natural Childbirth Association, founded by Prunella Briance earlier that year to promote the teaching of Grantly Dick-Read, had launched an appeal to find women willing to train to become birth educators.

Well into the 60s birth was considered '*private, undignified and disgusting*', as my daughter Jenny illustrated in a chapter she wrote for a book *The Politics of Maternity Care*.[4]

Readers responded to birth photographs in the *Sun* in 1965 with shock and outrage. One woman asked in the Letters page '*How many men were put off their breakfast?*'

My colleague Gwen Rankin recalls that one man threatened legal action against the Natural Childbirth Association because he had been shown photographs depicting birth that he claimed had made him impotent.

One of the flaws in all methods of training for childbirth, is that they have tended towards salvationism, which does not take into account differences between women. This was the problem with the Natural Childbirth Association, the organisation which started it all off in this country, and though it was valuable as a protest movement of mothers against the failure of medical services to provide adequate antenatal education for women who wanted to know what was going on and how they could actively help themselves and even enjoy their babies' births, it didn't take into account that different women have different needs.

There was the woman who insisted that the midwife leave the bedroom door open so that her husband, downstairs having his tea, should hear her screams and realise what she was going through. Or one who decided to wash her hair when she felt the first faint contractions, and had to be delivered with her head swathed in towels and rivulets dripping down the back of her neck. Or the West Indian peasant women who call on Jesus with each contraction and are obviously obtaining satisfaction from the religious context of their suffering. There are women in Italian hospitals where they are fitted with earphones and press a button as a pain starts to be assailed by white noise – a cacophonous din like a thousand waterfalls, so loud that they hardly notice the contraction.

In England instruction was at first based on the teachings of Grantly Dick-Read, the forerunner of all education for childbirth, who believed that fear caused a great deal of the pain that many women felt in labour. Through the centuries they had grown up to expect pain. The instant they felt uterine contractions they tensed up and resisted them, which resulted in more pain, which made them more afraid, and they reacted to this by getting more and more tense, which produced yet more severe pain. This he called *'the fear-tension-pain syndrome'*. The basis of re-education of the mother was to give her accurate information about what was going on in her body, reassurance and self-confidence and teach the art of complete relaxation. Many women benefitted enormously from this teaching. To others the reality of labour still came as a shock and they felt let down and deceived.

Dick-Read intrigued Russian obstetricians already working in Pavlovian psychology founded on the conviction that pregnant women could be *'de-conditioned'* from their environmental influences and *'re-conditioned'* in such a way that they could adapt themselves to the stresses of labour. They aimed at setting up a series of conditioned reflexes both to verbal stimuli and to those coming direct from the dilating cervix, so that a woman could respond with behaviour which *'blocked'* pain and she did not notice it.

Lamaze, a French obstetrician in a Communist trade union clinic in Paris, visited the Soviet Union and was impressed by the quietness of maternity hospitals practicing these methods and the calm of the labouring women. He invented techniques by which the woman could adjust herself to labour – notably the *'panting like a dog'* method of riding over contractions. Labour was transformed into an athletic activity for which one trained as if for a race

In Britain meanwhile, the Natural Childbirth Association, together with the first obstetric physiotherapists and a handful of midwives, had been influencing more women; they met much opposition along the way, but persevered.

Organisers and helpers used to have cups of coffee with nervous expectant mothers, reassure them and show them simple breathing techniques (breath-holding for bearing-down and quick panting for delivery) and relaxation '*until you feel you are floating on clouds*'. Some midwives and obstetricians, pleased with the results, became interested and started to send patients for help – but on the whole were tongue-in-cheek. Gradually hospitals began their own classes, gave morale-boosting talks, instruction in the use of the gas-and-air machine, and encouraged women to lie on the floor and relax while the midwives made a refreshing cup of tea. But the results of this hospital based training were unimpressive.

The Natural Childbirth Association

I had got to know Dick-Read towards the end of the 1950s and invited him to speak at a meeting. He came with Jess, his elegant and adoring wife, to stay at our cottage Toby House in Freeland, Oxfordshire, where we'd moved in 1956.

It was tricky organising all the children, the publicity, the meeting, looking after my guests and still taking the opportunity to learn something from him. At breakfast time, with the children playing around, we were discussing the side-effects of birth on the mother's self-confidence and interaction with her baby. I suggested that it would be interesting to do research on this. He paused in slicing the top off his egg, looked at me sternly and said, '*Research? I have done all the research that is necessary.*'

We discussed natural childbirth, of course, and he told me about his experiences with women in the East End of London and during the Second World War. He was never an elitist and praised women's courage and confidence. He had watched them working with their bodies giving birth in the slums or outside in the fields. He died in 1959 and I spoke about this on *Woman's Hour*.

'*He didn't believe for one moment that you shouldn't use pain-relieving drugs in birth, but thought they were often used in place of good, emotional, loving support. When Dick-Read died he was very bitter and isolated. It was a time when technology was being introduced in a big way into British obstetrics. Dick-Read was way ahead of his time, but it isn't so much that we've gone back to his ideas, as drawn on the wealth of his experience, the way he listened to women and respected them and considered birth a celebration of life.*'

Dick-Read, like many other gurus, saw those who supported him, as well as those who questioned his teachings, as hangers-on, and if they advocated research he might even regard them as traitors. As far as he was concerned he had revealed the truth. Their role was to accept it uncritically and enthusiastically and propagate his message.

In 1959 the Natural Childbirth Association, seeking to broaden its base, changed itself into the National Childbirth Trust (NCT), not just advocating one method of preparation but becoming a sort of consumers' council of childbirth. One year it elected as its chairman a specialist in hypnosis; another year a consultant who believed that previous instruction about what to expect often led women to behave unnaturally and to interfere with physiological processes which ought to be smooth and unstrained. The Trust started to vet its teachers more carefully. Many were midwives, physiotherapists, school teachers or social workers who brought special skills into their work and the sympathetic understanding without which obstetric information, however detailed, is never enough.

With the fresh stimulus coming from the Continent – under the name of '*psychoprophylaxis*' – antenatal education in Britain changed dramatically. At first claims made for the '*new*' method were excessive and a woman who felt pain was made to feel as if there were something wrong with her and one who needed the help of a forceps delivery or a Caesarean section suffered desperate feelings of failure.

While Prunella Briance was in the United States in 1959 and the Natural Childbirth Association became the National Childbirth Trust, the organisation changed its objectives and eradicated any mention of Dick-Read. Lamaze was substituted as the method of childbirth – the system he had based on Russian psychoprophylaxis. This reflected bitter conflict in the childbirth movement.

I started to run groups (the first '*couples*' classes) in our cottage outside Oxford, with discussion about emotions and changing relationships. From my background in social anthropology, I wanted to look at the values in our birth culture. I never did believe in just doing breathing and relaxation exercises – or, at least, I didn't think that was sufficient to make birth joyful. These groups became very popular. People went to great efforts to attend. I remember one man bringing his very pregnant partner wheeled in a huge retro pram, trundling it five miles from a neighbouring village. He took a liking to another very attractive woman in the class. I don't know whether it came to anything after their babies were born. But there were rumours of him being seen sitting on a ladder below her bedroom window when her partner was away one night – climbing up to help with changing a nappy perhaps!

I had good friends in the NCT – remarkable women like Gwen Rankin, a tower of strength and wisdom, Philippa Micklethwait, peacemaker extraordinaire, who became President, the lively Joan Gibson who made us all mind our Ps and Qs, Ruth Forbes, who introduced a mix of yoga and encounter groups, and Betty Parsons who taught duchesses, and became antenatal teacher to Princess Diana and Prince Charles. These women brought a range of skills and distinctive personalities.

I was increasingly fascinated by emotional aspects of birth. I was more interested in minds than muscles and in personal experience than exercises.

Central to this was a woman's relationship with the unborn baby growing inside her. The uterus isn't a dark, soft cave, a retreat from sensation. Or a piece of anatomical equipment we might be just as well without. It is the place where the fetus has its first sensations, the environment for a person who is coming into being. The baby hears the throbbing of the mother's aorta and other blood vessels magnified by the amniotic fluid in which it floats. The uterus isn't a secluded, silent place, after all.

When I started to work in childbirth doctors tended to refer to emotions as if they were merely trimmings, gilt on the gingerbread of reproductive physiology, and the obstetric manoeuvres they conducted. Things have changed. We are beginning to learn that mind and body are inseparable. In childbirth education, too, labour used to be talked about as if it were an athletic event for which a woman trained as if for the 100 metres, or an ordeal for which she had to be brainwashed so that though it hurt, she didn't *realise* it hurt.

Giving birth is a psycho-sexual experience. Many women are swept up in these rhythms in spite of themselves, and regardless of techniques taught in antenatal classes. Each contraction follows on another like the waves of the sea, and every one brings nearer the birth of the baby.

A midwife friend who loves doing home births rang me after a birth in which the mother had music during labour that they had selected together – Brahms' *String Sextet No.1 in B-Flat Major*. And this midwife, called by one of her mothers 'the shepherdess of birth', exclaimed, 'Oh, it was lovely! The baby was born at just the right point in the music!'

* * *

This was a great time in the NCT because we were developing teacher training. With Ann Proctor, I devised an educational programme based on the Oxford tutorial system: individuals and small groups meeting with a tutor in a one-to-one continuing relationship. I was a tutor and taught study days and workshops as well as antenatal classes at the NCT office in Bayswater, London.

For many of us the NCT served as a source for canalising energy, exploring ideas with other women and working for change. For me, it was never about coffee mornings. It was about women striving to reclaim childbirth as an exultant personal experience, rather than a medical event – and, in the process, creating a social revolution! Childbirth is a political issue.

In my work as an NCT Tutor some remarkable students shared my enthusiasm. One was Janet Balaskas, who created the Active Birth Movement and has trained teachers from all over the UK and in other countries. Another was Janette Brandt, who started the Swedish Childbirth Association. Like me, Jan had Stanislavski drama training and took to the teaching methods I was developing like a duck to water.

Many of these students went to live and work in other countries – Australia, New Zealand, the United States and Eastern Europe. It has been exciting to have had close contact with these adventurous women and be invited to lecture in places around the world in which I worked with them to develop a new kind of birth education. Others became writers, midwives, childbirth researchers and university teachers. I gained a great deal from those I have taught and am grateful to them.

Birth Classes Were Fun

Running classes was an opportunity to meet a wide range of fascinating people from all kinds of backgrounds: actresses, academics, artists and authors, dress designers, doctors and film directors, potters, poets, policewomen, priests and TV presenters. There was a group of Muslim women who came *en famille* – aunts, cousins and sisters – to support a young pregnant woman in their traditional style, and who contributed a lot about their cultural traditions in childbirth. There were lesbian couples following self-insemination. I remember one couple for whom it was very hard for a partner to support the other, because she had recently miscarried, and had to work through the grief she was feeling while at the same time rejoicing for the pregnant woman. There was a surrogate mother and the woman who was going to be the social mother who came to this group together to be as close as possible through the experience of pregnancy. An elegant model was on a strict diet – and effectively starved herself – to keep her figure. She was concerned that the bedroom into which she was going to take her new baby was painted completely black, with black hangings round the bed, and that this was going to be bad for the baby. Her partner was a well known photographer – obviously with a great sense of style – and their baby is now an artist. Ronnie Laing, the psychoanalyst, came with Jutta, and we discussed the significance of birth for the baby as well as the mother, and the ideas he had developed about how birth ought to be.

One of the loveliest people was Felicity Kendal who attended with her husband, the theatre director, Michael Rudman. She was very like the character in her role in *The Good Life*, excited, bright-eyed and shining, and wanted birth to be as natural as possible. She was a committed member of the group, and missed only one meeting when she was on holiday. I loved having her there. In fact, at the end of her pregnancy, she switched from her private specialist obstetrician when she couldn't get answers to her searching questions, and was told she would not be allowed to move freely in labour or use water, and opted for midwife care. She had a joyful and triumphant birth, in her own space, able to be upright and do whatever she felt like doing. Later she helped me launch my book *Freedom and Choice in Childbirth*.[5] Many years later, in an interview for the *Independent*, she said that my writing had changed her life; '*She gave me the courage to do what I wanted to do, in the face of doctors trying to shout me down.*'

In every class there was a buzz of conversation, laughter, and sometimes – as at the best parties – debate, but always vitality, reflection, honesty and celebration of pregnancy. Occasionally there were tears. If a woman was traumatised because an experience cast its shadow onto this birth there was always someone there to reach out. If she was deaf or disabled in some way, or didn't have much English, others were ready and eager to help. The groups were lively and exciting because of this vital mix. They certainly didn't just sit and listen or get down to a lot of exercises. They swapped ideas, explored feelings, shared experiences in ways that were much more stimulating for them than if I had only been advising and teaching. It was in dramatic contrast to antenatal classes that were mainly about acquiring information and being instructed. I described this in one of my early books, *Education and Counselling for Childbirth*, the one I wrote sitting beside my mother's bed as she was dying.

Psychoprophylaxis developed still more exercises based on the Pavlovian discovery of conditioning and deconditioning in experimental animals. In France practitioners of psychoprophylaxis talked about *'verbal asepsis'* in childbirth. That is not surprising given what they inherited from Russian psychoprophylaxis. Velvosky, who introduced the method, opened one of his lectures with the announcement: *'If you make a sagittal section of the corpse of a woman who died in childbirth you will see …'*[6] He warned women, *'Your vagina, which will have been greatly stretched during the birth, will never again return to its prebirth dimension'* and advised against having baths at the end of pregnancy *'as this may damage the vagina'.* They called relaxation by a new name – *'decontraction'* – and invented new types of breathing rates and levels for different phases of labour. Under the impact of psychoprophylaxis breathing exercises proliferated, so that wherever classes were taught there seemed to be some new variation or complication of exercises, and as I travelled on lecture tours across the United States, Canada and the UK, I was often asked if I taught, *'huff and puff', 'slump and blow', 'choo-choo breathing', 'the sigh', 'levels A,B,C and D', 'H out, H out Hoo-hoo', 'SSSS', 'tune-tapping'* or whatever. I do not know if the mothers were as confused as I was. Certainly it all tended to be very noisy, and labour wards hummed with activity as women busily breathed their way through contractions, often to the consternation and dismay of midwives, who sometimes saw these exercises as rites which were exhausting for mothers and midwives alike.

That teaching method and the way of talking about bodies and birth was quite different from my approach. For one thing, I explored feelings in a way that some of my colleagues in the NCT found disturbing. One told me that she didn't need to discuss feelings because *'All my girls are normal!'*

I talked about how strong emotions can overtake you at different phases of pregnancy, too. Between six and four weeks before the birth a woman often has a sudden failure of nerve, focused for example either on labour or on being a good-enough mother. Around half the women in classes said that they lay awake in the night thinking like this. One woman said, *'Tom doesn't want to be at the birth.'* So I asked, *'Why not?' 'Because of the blood.'* Tom said, *'No, it's not blood.'*

She said aggressively, *'You wouldn't want to see a road accident!'* Tom turned to me and said, *'I am desperately disappointed that she doesn't want me there'*, and at last Sarah could say quite simply, *'I am awfully scared!'* Another couple were discussing breastfeeding, and the woman said, *'He has always advocated breastfeeding. It is a passion of his. He would make a much better mother than me!'* A pregnant woman is like an actress before the curtain goes up on the opening night, and may be afraid that she will forget all she has learned. It is, in one woman's words, *'an abrupt breakthrough of cold reality. It is like living in a warm, cosily lit house where a door is blown open onto the dark night outside. Suddenly the bump is à baby – a baby which, somehow, someday, has to get born. Whether by the birth canal or a Caesarean, whether it lives or dies, it is in and must come out.'* For each woman pregnancy has its private meaning.

Muslim Birth Culture

It was one of the most imposing houses near Buckingham Palace. I had been summoned to teach a young pregnant woman from one of the Gulf States about childbirth. She was not allowed to attend classes, so it had to be one-to-one and I was expected to do it in a single meeting. She spoke no English. It all had to be enacted with my flexible baby doll, plastic pelvis and foam rubber vagina and a dramatic performance by me. I breathed my way through contractions, sighed, relaxed, tackled a difficult late first stage with a torrent of powerful contractions, pushed, groaned, breathed, gasped, pushed, panted, and – gently, gently – smiling and shiny-eyed, gave birth to a gorgeous baby whom I lifted straight to my breast. But the only thing the older woman – her mother-in-law, or a senior wife (I never found out which) – who was in charge of the proceedings was concerned about was that I should show her young pupil how to push, long and hard. That was what she had to be taught. The mother was a little slip of a girl and the older woman feared she wouldn't have the stamina or will-power to do it.

After that, I always invited women to bring all the female members of the family to classes if they wished. A one-to-one relationship helped a great deal, but drawing on the sisterly relationship of Muslim women in the extended family was even better. A group of four or five accompanied one woman to my classes – sisters-in-law, a cousin, and an aunt I think they were. They were enthusiastic participants and when we got down to acting through different kinds of birth, massage, holding, supported positions and movements, joined in with relish, drawing on their own experience. Seeing the lively companionship and shared female knowledge in that group may have made the male-female couples in the class feel rather deprived. The emphasis on the isolated husband-wife relationship in North American and European industrial birth culture misses out on the emotional support and life experience that women can bring each other. Having a group of women from one culture infuses confidence and gives realism in a class. There is a case for making women-only classes available. These may appeal especially to Muslim women and others from minority religious and cultural groups where involvement of men in pregnancy and childbirth is considered inappropriate. It is worse than useless to try to prepare a devout Muslim woman for childbirth without taking into account the religious convictions in her community. This entails, wherever possible, drawing in other significant women in their lives, learning from them and approaching childbirth together, instead of teaching a pregnant woman in isolation. Birth education is not just about techniques. It should also involve discussion of memories of birth in the family, social and personal values, and may entail exploring deeply held religious beliefs.

The Five Pillars of Islam are the oneness of God (*kalmia*), prayer five times a day (*salat*), giving alms (*zakaat*), fasting during Ramadan (*sawm*) and making a pilgrimage to Mecca (*hajj*). Concepts of modesty (*hiya*) and seclusion (*purda*) are central, and wearing a head scarf or completely covering the head (*hijab*) is the visual symbol of modesty. *Hiya* is important for Muslim men too, and entails respecting women's space, and not intruding on it. Food allowed under Islamic Law is called *halal*. When a Muslim woman is in hospital she wants to keep her modesty and privacy, eat only *halal* food, and have a quiet place in which to pray regularly. A Muslim midwife bathes herself before attending a birth and prays to the Creator. If the birth is complicated she recites a special chapter from the Koran.

I learned that every child has the right to be breastfed, ideally for two years. There are symbolic rites around birth. It may be important for Muslim parents to enact these in privacy. The father, or a respected member of the family, whispers a prayer, the *adhan*, into the baby's ear as soon as possible after birth. It includes the pronouncement: '*There is no God but Allah and Muhammad is the Messenger of Allah.*' A member of the family, often the father, places a small piece of date or a spot of honey in the baby's mouth. If other family members are not allowed in the birth room this ceremony cannot be performed at the right time. It symbolises introducing the baby to the sweet things of life. Muslims on the Indian sub-continent tie with black string a small pouch containing a prayer to the baby's wrist or neck, as protection against illness. This should always be handled with respect.

I have always used masses of verbal imagery and visual demonstrations of organs and physical functions in childbirth. My body is the canvas for this expression. Rather than issuing instructions to make the rib cage expand and force the diaphragm up to inhale and down to breathe out, for example, I suggested imagining it as like a jellyfish that could surge and spread out and downwards, allowing the lungs to fill with air. A rather odd image perhaps, but it works!

This all came from Stanislavski acting training. Our senses are important aids to understanding how we might feel in pregnancy, labour, and afterwards, too. I thought there was great danger in intellectualising birth and turning it into something our brains try to analyse and manage, but which is really an overwhelming experience when it comes to be lived, and surrender to the ocean and the roaring tempest. After a birth in which a woman has struggled to keep her brain in control and found it impossible, she is likely to feel an utter failure.

Some Stanislavski exercises I invented included squeezing stiff egg white through a syringe to make meringues, carrying a heavy tray, ironing, putting on a bra two sizes too small, struggling into jeans two sizes too small; driving – about to overtake – and a car coming in the opposite direction sweeps round the corner at speed, making a cake in the kitchen and a visitor comes in and asks if she can help, buttering toast and suddenly seeing that the milk is about to boil over; lying in bed at night feeling very unhappy and trying not to cry or to let your partner see you are crying, waiting at the station booking office for a ticket with the train just about to leave – it is desperately important that you catch it – the doors are being closed, people are saying goodbye and the clerk *still* hasn't given you the ticket, and then recreating in your imagination an actual situation that has caused you great distress personally. Each exercise was followed by complete relaxation and a few minutes peace before embarking on the next so that residual tension was not carried over from one to another.

If I had gone straight from school to university and slotted smoothly into the higher education system I couldn't have had my acting training and got to know Stanislavski's method. Failing a Greek exam opened the door for me to create a way of approaching relaxation and body awareness to help women prepare for birth. What at the time seemed a set-back turned out to be a success.

I took failures and used them constructively. My Stanislavski-based exercises made a bridge with real-life situations. There might be a simple task based, for example, on domestic or office activities – then more complicated ones done under some pressure. Finally there were situations involving great stress, both general ones which could be shared, and other personal and private ones, which might be the subject of recurrent fears or dreams – things that the woman herself knew worried her.

She began to understand what happened to her body when she reacted to stress with tension, and found that she could let it slip away with active relaxation, a skill useful for stress situations in everyday life as well as for birth.

I found that it was a good idea to get members of the group to act and move. Then they learnt that static muscle contractions could re-enact these events in the same way without entailing movement. It is these static muscle contractions which encase our bodies and form each individual's own *'body armour'*.

Instead of saying to yourself, *'I must relax!'*, *'I must release all muscle tension'*, or, as in psychoprophylaxis training, *'I must hold the muscles in one arm tight when relaxing those in my left arm'*, the contact from a partner's hand gave the message of release, and eventually just thinking about it could stimulate instant relaxation. Then, when labour started, the pressure of contractions themselves inspired the same response.

I wanted to present the experience of birth vividly and prepare women for the intense physical sensations and turmoil of often conflicting emotions they might feel. Birth is psycho-sexual. I acted the thrilling and irresistible sensation of the urge to push building up in a powerful wave-like orgasm. My breathing speeded up, my eyes shone, and at the peak of desire I held my breath and opened up. Then I could breathe again and a second and a third wave of longing came.

When I did this journalists sometimes described it as *'faking orgasm'*. Far from it. It was a way of expressing the passion and fulfilment of spontaneous action in the second stage of labour. I wanted to convey the thrill of childbirth, contraction following contraction like waves in a mounting storm, the energy that pours through your body, pressure building up to the next roller-coaster, and the peace of the blessed lull between contractions.

When beautiful births are described or photographed, however placid the mother looks, and though there is a tranquil atmosphere, for her the earth is moving. I thought it was important to capture the passion of birth-giving.

I acted birth-giving and the different phases of pregnancy and labour. My torso became the uterus, my arms fallopian tubes, and fingers the sea-weed-like tentacles that hover over the ovaries to catch a ripe egg and sweep it into the tube.

I invented a foam-rubber vagina – a hollow plastic kitchen container big enough for a birthday cake with two layers of soft sponge and a slit in the middle to represent the pelvic outlet and the perineum, and used a flexible baby doll that looked as nearly as possible like a real baby to act giving birth energetically. The baby's head rotated and crowned, slid through the opening folds of tissue, the shoulders turned, I pushed in response to a passionate urge to do so, waited with a relaxed, open mouth and breathed gently, gave another little push, breathed rapidly, paused and pressed down once more, and when the baby's body slipped out, reached down to lift the newborn up into my arms.

Instead of the language of text books and chunks of information from them, I combined vivid visual images with gestures and movement. To understand the uterus at conception, for example: *'It's a muscle about this size,'* and I'd clench a fist in front of me as I said this, *'a bit like an avocado pear – only hollow, the baby floating inside in its own warm amniotic fluid, protected from bumps and bangs, with sound passing easily through the liquid.*

'As pregnancy progresses the walls of the uterus stretch, and grow new tissues as well. The cervix projects like the stem end of the pear or the neck of a bottle (I let my thumb stick out from the fist). That's the bit that opens up in labour to let the baby out. A plug of mucus, like the cork in a bottle, seals it from the outside world, and from infection, and slips out before labour really gets going. At the end of pregnancy hormones soften your cervix, more blood flows through it, it gets puffy and begins to be drawn up into the uterus, so it's shorter. That's called "effacement", and it's a good sign. If you squat over a magnifying mirror with legs apart, you can see your cervix when the baby is pressing down against it. Part your labia and feel and look between the fleshy folds.

'It's like a plump Victorian button cushion with the mucus plug the button in the middle. When your cervix is ready for labour it is said to be "ripe".'

Though it helps to know obstetric terms and a woman can ask, for example, how many centimetres her cervix is dilated, and realise what the answer meant, the vital thing was to visualise what was happening to her body.

Small boys experiment with controlling and cutting off the flow of urine, and use their pelvic floor muscles to do so. Small girls don't seem to have any kind of game like this. But children often know that they can play with their pelvic floor muscles in one way or another. As one of my own daughters said, *'Us can talk wiv our bottoms.'*

Pelvic floor exercises were all the vogue in the 70s – rigidly tightening pelvic muscles to tone them. They were called '*Kegels*', and still are in the United States. Dr Kegel was an obstetrician who directed attention to the importance of strengthening these muscles after childbirth, and even before, because of the strain that would be put on them. As a result women religiously practised '*Kegels*' and stuck notices to their fridge doors reminding them to exercise. They bashed away at them – attacked them actually – and felt good about doing them, and bad when they couldn't be bothered.

I preferred a more subtle approach, using the imagination. I suggested thinking of a circle of muscle halfway up inside the vagina that was like a lift in a five storey building. Get into the lift. The doors close. Now gradually tighten the muscle as you move from the ground to the next floor – pause – go higher – and so on till you reach the top. Then slowly, carefully, descend one floor at a time, and when you finish, go up one floor again. That way you keep the muscles springy and firm. This exercise has become standard in much antenatal teaching now.

But there is another way of thinking about it too. It is a kiss inside when making love. Then the exercise becomes sensual and intimate.

As an unintended goddess of pelvic floor exercises I must have made a lot of women feel guilty and inadequate. Journalist Deborah Ross interviewed Pam Ayres and wrote a poem in her style, '*Oh, I Wish I'd Looked After Me Pelvic Floor*'.

Oh, I wish I'd looked after me pelvic floor
And done them post-natal work-outs
I wish I'd been wise and I wish I had said:
    'I'll do 'em, and do 'em times four!
Oh, I wish I'd looked after me pelvic floor,
But what did I do? I did snicker
So now when I sneeze, or laugh quite hard,
I wet a bit of me knicker.

The Twins

When Celia was nine months old, I discovered I was pregnant again, sooner than planned and I intended to have another home birth with a midwife. One day, six weeks before my baby was due, my GP was carefully palpating my abdomen and commented, '*I think I feel two heads.*' My first thought was that I was having a two-headed baby, but then I realised what she was saying. I definitely did not want twins. It took a week or so to get over the shock and begin to look forward to them. Now, of course, I would have to visit the big teaching hospital, and not be allowed to give birth at home. Or would I? This was my body, my birth, my babies. I was already teaching childbirth classes for what later became the National Childbirth Trust. If I did not organise my own setting for birth, how could I expect other women to do so?

The antenatal clinic at the teaching hospital was like a cattle market. Women were sitting on rows of chairs and waiting hour after hour, holding their bottles of urine. Each woman, as she was called, went into a boxlike cubicle where a notice exhorted: '*Take off all your clothes and put on the cotton gown.*' The air was thick with sweat and the smell of fear. Through the flimsy door I could hear everything the doctor was saying to the woman before me as well as the glup-glop of his gloved fingers as he stuck them into her vagina, probed, and then withdrew them with a plop.

I climbed onto the examining table, lay down, and realised that this was a three-sided cubicle. At my feet was an open hall where the obstetrician, registrars and students walked about, talking to one another, as they stared at each woman's perineum, gave the bulging abdomen a quick shove, and then passed on to the next woman. We were laid out in rows like carcasses of meat.

At my next visit, Margaret, a friend who was studying medicine happened to walk by as I was waiting. She had given birth to twins in that hospital and they had not survived. '*My God, you're not coming here!*' she exclaimed. That decided me. I was not going to have my babies there if I could help it. I continued my antenatal clinic visits, however, because I wanted to know that my babies were a good size, their hearts were beating strongly, and their heads were presenting. They were. After one pelvic exam, when I came home and found myself bleeding, I made up my mind not to return. The babies were almost due.

* * *

Nuffield College, Oxford, where Uwe was a don, was planning its Charter ceremony the day before my due date; the ball was to be attended by the Duke of Edinburgh. I bought an attractive midnight blue dress speckled with bright Botticelli-type flowers, put a towel in the car, and danced all evening. Later that night, I woke from a dream in which I was having a period on a double-decker London bus. While wondering what the dream meant, I got up, walked out of the room, and suddenly realised that the balloon of unruptured membranes was hanging down between my legs. I poked it, swung it to one side, tucked it back in, and waddled back to the bedroom. As we got things ready, I became aware of easy, rhythmic tightenings like ocean waves.

We called the local midwife, who came and told me to go back to sleep. Uwe persuaded her to examine me, whereupon she exclaimed, 'Oh, a head!' I opened up, pressed down, and let out the first baby. She caught her in a roll of cotton wool, as she did not have time to get out her maternity pack. I lifted the baby straight to my breast. Then I felt a thud in the small of my back as the next baby dropped down. I asked the midwife to hold the first baby while I had the second, and with one push the second twin was born, inside the unruptured membranes. Their fused placentas came with her. It had been an hour and a half since I had woken up.

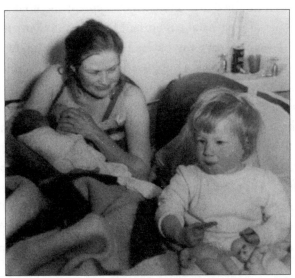

Me with my new twins and Ceila with her twin dolls

If I had attempted to get to hospital the babies would probably have been born in a lay-by on the A40. Uwe photographed everything: me dancing (on a table for some reason) before it all started, smiling down as a head was born, and babies suckling – this at a time when women in birth photographs were commonly shown with their faces blacked out, or wearing masks.

Celia, our firstborn, came in and was presented with twin dolls. In a party atmosphere, we ate chocolate, laughed and cuddled. I did not tear and had minimal bleeding. Both babies suckled enthusiastically.

The twins, Tess and Nell were born on a Sunday, and on Thursday my class turned up to find the bump gone and two babies waiting to greet them! I joined the NCT national committee and used to travel by train to London with the babies head-to-toe in one carry-cot.

'The Experience Of Childbirth' – My First Book

Two years later Polly was born, another home birth. It was January, my room was full of hyacinths in bloom, and this flower still symbolises for me the heady scent of birth. Polly's was a painful, tumultuous, triumphant 40-minute labour. I dilated gently during the week or two before birth, so that the actual labour was the final flourish to a process that had been going on quietly beforehand. The other children tumbled in to share the excitement and hold their new sister.

I was in a state of post-natal euphoria. I hadn't wanted my mother around because I didn't want to have my babies in the way she might have hoped. I wanted to do my own thing – I suppose I was still going though adolescent rebellion, a bit late in the day! Afterwards she said to me, 'Darling, I knew you must be in labour. I felt every pain you had', and I said – it was very cruel – 'That's odd, Mother, because I didn't have any pain.' I wish I hadn't said that.

I decided I wanted to write about the joy of birth, being able to work with my body and feeling the great waves of contractions sweep through me. Though painful, they are exciting; like surf riding. I thought, Why can't all other women feel this exhilaration too? Why do many think of birth as like a surgical operation? Why do they approach it as if it were a road accident? As if they can't make decisions about their bodies and their babies and other people must make them for them?

Six weeks later I began writing The Experience of Childbirth. Polly was waking at 5.30 a.m. in the morning to breastfeed, and it was an ideal opportunity to write before everybody else woke up. Writing early in that precious time in the morning, in the first light of dawn, has stayed a habit – a quiet, peaceful time when my mind is still rich with waking thoughts, ideas and phrases. That first draft took me six weeks. Then I read it through aloud (that was important, I think, because I wanted to speak to women in my own voice, not to harangue them, and not to be literary) and amended it over another few weeks.

The challenge I faced was to create a language to convey the multi-faceted sensations of labour and birth, physical and emotional, to find words for the rush of energy as contractions welled up and squeezed the uterus, and the power that builds mountains was released in your body, for the feeling as the baby's head crowned as if in a ring of fire, and the birth passion. I have been criticised for discussing giving birth in terms of sex, as if I were imposing on women a kind of sexual performance, birth with orgasm. But for me birth was an intense psycho-sexual experience. This is not surprising, since both childbirth and lactation involve the same hormones as in sexual arousal, and both are an expression of what is going on in the mind, not just the body.

Nothing like this had ever been published before. Grantly Dick-Read had written *Childbirth Without Fear*.[7] But that was from a kindly male doctor's point of view. He couldn't describe the amazing energy that poured through a woman's body. He taught that birth 'shouldn't hurt' if the mother relaxed. But of course it did! Though the pain was a side-effect of the creative process, of muscles tightening and stretching as the baby's head pressed down to be born – positive pain, pain with a purpose. He had photographs, too, but the women's faces were all stamped with black rectangles so that they couldn't possibly be recognised. They looked like brick-headed robots.

In France, psychoprophylaxis was the latest fashion. An American, Marjorie Karmel, wrote *Thank You, Dr Lamaze*[8] – to my mind a sycophantic book extolling the benefits of his method of strict training in breathing and relaxation. It was an enthusiastic instruction manual. If a woman obeyed his teachings she 'should' have no pain. If she did feel pain, however, it was evidence that she had not obeyed the obstetrician's instructions, conformed to the 'correct' number of huffs and puffs, or did not hold her breath long enough when pushing, failed to practice assiduously, and lacked commitment. In his book *Painless Childbirth*,[9] for example, Lamaze discussed the second stage of labour as taking place 'under the command of the obstetrician-in-charge. One parturient has defined this very well: "The obstetrician was the conductor; I was the first violin." And went on to say, 'The woman, having settled down to her delivery, will inform the obstetrician each time she has a contraction. He will then direct her thus: "Breathe in, blow out"; then, "Breathe in, hold it, pull on the bars, bring your chest out and push well down."' This was nothing to do with what I believed, or my experience. I was fed up with women being blamed for everything that happened to them.

I had no agent, but knew that the firm of Victor Gollancz was innovative and idealistic. Gollancz published detective stories with bright yellow covers and radical sociology and politics. I sent the manuscript off to him, with several photographs taken by Uwe of me giving birth, breathing my way through contractions, smiling as I reached down to stroke the top of a glistening head that was just emerging, and holding a naked baby against my breasts. My brother-in-law, Hilary Rubinstein, who was married to Uwe's younger sister Helge, worked at Gollancz. Victor called him to his office and said, apparently with shocked disbelief, 'I have photographs of your sister-in-law's private parts on my desk.'

I am grateful to them for their courage. They decided to go ahead and publish. It was clear sailing from then on. The editor suggested a few minor adjustments. Otherwise the book was published in 1962 exactly as I wrote it in that post-birth milky, glowing 'babymoon'.

The *Observer* serialised three chapters, the first extract taking up the whole front page of the supplement. With four children under five, I had no spare time. Any career as a social anthropologist was certainly on hold. But I was a writer! *The Experience of Childbirth* was subsequently sold to Penguin and went through 23 impressions with them. It has been published in many languages, and sold well over a million copies. It is still in print, now with Orion. The whole experience was astonishing. The only thing that compares with having your first baby is having your first book.

Jenny's Birth

Jenny's birth at home in March 1963 was really do-it-yourself. My waters started leaking, and I had backache for five hours or so during the night. I thought

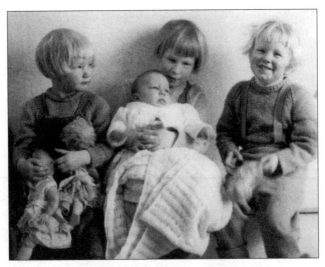

I had four children under five in 1961

labour was probably about to start, slept fitfully, and was suddenly awakened by hefty contractions. We just had time to get ready before they came thick and fast. It was daybreak, and the birds were singing outside the open window.

I did not want to call the midwife too soon, as my own midwife was on holiday and I did not know her replacement. We decided to wait until we were absolutely sure that the second stage was about to start. By then it was too late. I felt my body opening like a rose. Uwe was filming and saying, *'Smile, darling.'* I did, and opened more. I put my hands down and stroked Jenny's head in my vagina. She gave birth to herself, emerging like a swimmer doing the crawl, and then crept over my thigh and up my body, knowing perfectly well what to do and the way to my breasts. It was the perfect birth!

The labour had been 40 minutes of action. The other four children came in wearing new flower-sprigged night-dresses especially bought for the occasion. They helped me wash and dress Jenny. And then we remembered to call the midwife.

Birth has been empowering for me. I do not believe that childbirth is the *only* way that women can find fulfilment, but for me it has been a peak experience, one that has liberated the energy to strive for better birthing conditions for *all* women.

For many other women, what began as an experience that we wanted to ensure was intimate, part of the ebb and flow of life – the birth of a child *from* love *into* love – opened the way into a deeper political awareness. For in childbirth,

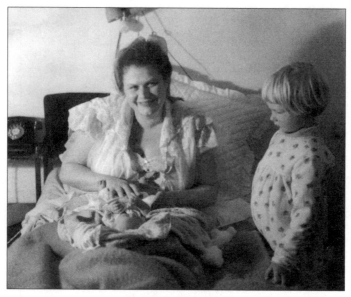

Jenny's first day

as in other aspects of women's lives, the personal *is* the political. When we acknowledge this, we create the conditions that make it possible to liberate women from the degradation, senseless mutilation, and violence imposed on them by medical systems everywhere. We start to reclaim our bodies in joy, drawing strength from our shared experiences as women.

Me As A Mother

Now I had five little girls under seven! With intermittent help from an au pair, it wasn't the easiest way of mothering. But I carried on combining teaching with lecturing.

Motherhood is never what you expect. It is an incredible adventure. You discover a lot about yourself. I don't think it can be for any woman exactly what she thinks it is going to be. I thought I would be in control somehow in bringing up my children, whereas, in fact, you find that they bring *you* up. Motherhood is a magical mystery tour and you soar to the heights of elation and swoop into depths of despair. It is one of the best forms of education there is if you are prepared to learn from it, and you learn along with your children.

I made up my mind to have my babies close to me to be able to respond lovingly when they needed me. This was when they were hungry, of course, when they needed a nappy changed, were too hot or too cold, but also when they couldn't reach, or manipulate, something that attracted them, manage to do something they wanted, or were bored and sought stimulation.

Mattresses are for bouncing. Water is for pouring. Sand is for scattering. Walls are for drawing. Paper is for cutting. Those were my five maxims for happy living with five children.

Sleep training methods that were given scientific justification by the Behaviourists in the 1920s have made a come-back and become popular today. They can be highly successful at producing a compliant child. For many parents there is no doubt that they work. In a 1928 edition of *Enquire Within Upon Everything*, a book of general household advice, the author, a man, wrote that if a mother responded to crying by immediately feeding her baby it would demand milk '*at improper times and without necessity.*' Cuddling and carrying a baby around exposed it to infection. The right place for a baby was in its cot. He explained that a baby used crying to exert power over parents and also needed to cry to strengthen its lungs. A nurse or mother who tried to stop it crying was harming it. Crying was almost the only form of exercise a baby got. It caused blood to circulate, helped digestion, and promoted growth.

Today, once again, methods of '*controlled crying*' and rigid time-tables are ways in which mothers are taught that they must exercise discipline if they are to gain the upper hand and avoid being manipulated by their babies. This approach is popular with parents who want a quick fix for sleeping problems, do not understand the separation distress experienced by babies, and who fail to consider that if we do not respond to babies we risk them learning to give up and becoming emotionally detached. They may grow into people who are despairing and depressed, find it difficult to form social relationships, and sometimes are in a more or less permanent state of resentment and hostility.

I enjoyed breastfeeding. With the twins it was easy, too. I did not introduce tastes of solids till they were six months old, fed Tess for over nine months, and Nell, the smaller one, for a year. She was usually ready for a feed about half an hour before Tess, so I had time to concentrate on each one separately. Polly, number four, usually woke for a breastfeed at about 5.30 a.m. She suckled energetically, and then lay happily on my bed while I worked on the first edition of *The Experience of Childbirth*. I was excited by birth and words came pouring out on a wave of energy.

This has remained my general pattern for the day: get down to putting ideas together and do some solid writing before the pressures of the rest of the day are upon me. I know that there is a fashion to train babies not to wake until 7 a.m. on the grounds that the mother's life will be chaotic otherwise and she will get exhausted, but it didn't work like that with me. Polly's early waking gave me an opportunity for my own time, as well as time to share with her. That is how I started writing books.

I believe that children should have a lot of space to experiment, play, interact and learn from each other. As a result I have never wanted to feel '*in charge*'. When I was writing a book and they were small the playpen became maternal territory, and I sat inside it with my papers and reference materials so that they could roam the house. They could see exactly what I was doing and I was there if they wanted me, but I was in no way dominating or directing them, and far from being isolated in my study, with the kids in the nursery, we lived in the same world.

Mothers often talk in terms of phases. We say, '*When he can find his thumb to suck he won't cry so much*'; '*It'll be easier when she can crawl ... or walk ...*' or '*no longer wakes at night*'. It is as if a woman thinks, '*Once we are over this I can be a good mother. I shall be able to cope.*' She is really saying something about herself, of course, about the goals for which she strives, and how she is going to meet those standards in the future. Gradually it dawns on her that she is face to face with an individual with a personality of incredible strength, and that motherhood is never going to be easy.

Some mothers never enjoy their toddlers for this reason. They get caught up in a constant battle of wills as an imperious little creature commands, resists and dares. They see antisocial – even potentially criminal – tendencies in this arrogant, egotistical selfhood, and believe it is the result of their own failure as mothers.

In the Toby House surfaces in the children's rooms – furniture, walls and floors were washable. The floors were of rubber composition and in their playroom it was of black and white tiles on which they could play a variety of games, traditional and personally invented ones. One whole wall in the playroom was a gigantic blackboard – and because children delight in scribbling everywhere, walls and beds were covered with specially treated hardboard which could be cleaned with a damp cloth. Over the years I have found providing children with anything but the essentials is a waste. Toys, for instance – they never played with any of them, but if I threw out a piece of paper or a length of string and they knew about it, they would be frantically annoyed. The toy cupboard was crammed with boxes, paper, string, scissors and paste, crayons, paint and pencils – that's all they wanted.

One important thing I have learned in mothering five daughters, now grown up, is that this self-confidence, this assertiveness to be able to say 'No!', is basic to an individual's ability to take responsibility, resist glib explanations and meaningless rules, and challenge prejudice and injustice. What I have enjoyed is witnessing and sharing in the excitement of children's growth to independence and the development of strong, courageous personalities.

After we had moved to the Manor House in 1966 with fields at the back, the girls used to run round the track encircling the paddock fighting. '*We fought with laundry basket shields, saucepans and brooms. You just closed the door.*' Jenny says, '*We grew up fearless*'.

Native American warrior tribes always valued these qualities in their children. But in our society there is a legacy of heavy emphasis on obedience and conformity to rules. When we come up against the chilling facts of child abuse, violence within the family, and the exploitation of women, we may stop and consider whether we should instead aim to rear warrior children.

Yet we can't hand on beliefs to children. All we can do is lend them ours for a while. They must then forge their own. They have magic ways of making light of our cherished convictions and creating their own space in a world geared to adults. There were Sundays, for example, when we all trooped to Oxford Quaker meetings – five blonde little girls, washed and brushed and on their best behaviour. Among the rows of silent Friends, each seeking inner light, there is something deeply satisfying that even a two-year-old can feel: no sounds but birdsong outside and the hum of traffic in the distance. I felt sure that the children were aware of the spirituality of the meetings – until I learned about the game they had invented, which kept them in rapt concentration. One child thought of a food and mimed eating it, and the others tried to guess what it was. When one of them caught on, she mimed eating the same food – until they were all doing it, and then the one who first found the solution switched to another food. In the quiet of Quaker Meeting my daughters made their way through imaginary bowls of steaming soup and corn-on-the-cob with butter running down to their elbows. They licked ice-cream cornets and peeled oranges, apples and bananas. Then one day, hearing suppressed giggles and noticing an amused elder on the bench facing us, I turned and saw the full drama as they wound long strands of spaghetti around invisible forks, let them uncoil into their gaping mouths, and then wiped tomato sauce from their chins. Thinking about it afterwards, I realised it was evidence of their resourcefulness, creativity, co-operation and skill in communicating ideas, even though the results were embarrassing! But it did mean that I had to stop taking them to adult meetings.

As the girls grew older, I found that I was learning a lot from them. Though domestic guerilla warfare and angry arguments at mealtimes were hard to tolerate, and I often yelled at them, I enjoyed the conflicts and confrontations of adolescence. There were long discussions about how society should be changed. They questioned things it was easy to take for granted, challenged my assumptions, always with a keen ethical sense and the courage to take a difficult path if they thought it was the right one to follow.

The theory is that togetherness and sitting around a table eating in a civilised way and making conversation form the heart of family life. This is when parents and children gather to enjoy each other. It is when the foundations of society are laid. Politicians, experts in nutrition, psychology, education, social science, religion and ethics, and pundits representing just about every branch of human knowledge, tell us that we should draw around the dining table in harmony. Otherwise we have a sub-standard family. Mum provides the right food, beautifully fresh, properly cooked, bursting with vitamins and minerals, and then the family will flourish and each child will develop emotionally, intellectually and socially.

I can only say that it didn't work like that for us. I tried. One thing we always did was to hold hands in a Quaker silence at the beginning of each meal. The children called it 'sniffing the food'. Meals were often the trigger for disagreements, violent arguments and sometimes outright rows that broke into physical attacks. Seven strong personalities close to and sitting facing each other are a recipe for confrontation and conflict. Now I think back to it, it is just possible that those exercises in mutual confrontation were highly character forming.

The pleasures of motherhood come from being flexible enough to retain a spirit of adventure, and being able to grow through the mother-child relationship into adult friendship. For that to happen, it is futile to try and train our children into obedience or impose on them our own beliefs. They should not have to live their lives on someone else's terms. None of our children live in the world in which we grew up. They must face new problems, new dangers, but also have new opportunities. The really important thing is to give them self-confidence together with the courage to explore, challenge, and strive for the good as they see it. Then they can become their own free people.

We believed in encouraging independence in the children – Uwe often even more than me. Maternal protectiveness sometimes won. He has had a very strong influence on me – offering intellectual rigour and a challenge. Very often when the children got up in the morning he said to them, *'Now, what are you going to achieve today?'* At the end of the day he would ask, *'What have you achieved today?'* This became a great joke in the family. *'Your mother has already written ten pages before breakfast.'*

CHAPTER FOUR

JAMAICA

The comparative sociology of childbirth fascinated me and I wanted to do anthropological field work. The opportunity came in 1964 when Uwe decided to spend his sabbatical from Oxford as visiting Professor at the University of the West Indies. The idea was that I could do research into pregnancy, childbirth and mothering among Jamaican peasant women if I had help with the children. Our youngest daughter was two and the whole family and Sandra, our Scottish mother's help, went to Jamaica for nine months.

My experiences in Jamaica were utterly absorbing. I was fascinated by the birth practices and women's beliefs, behaviour and relationships. Far from studying as if at a lab bench, I became an actor in the drama myself.

Yes, a research thesis demands objectivity. Yet in this section of my book I also record vivid personal experiences and emotions that drew me into these women's lives.

We rented a rambling wooden house on the campus at Mona, and I applied to the Medical Research Council which was doing research there into nutrition and mother and child health, to see if they could offer me a base at their centre. They very generously provided an office, a secretary – the wife of the Chief Justice – all equipment and services, transport into the hills and back-up. I could do whatever I liked, and Professor Ashcroft was lovely to work with.

I worked up in the hills and in the poorest parts of Kingston – in Rastafarian camps and in the public maternity hospital – where patients were often two to a bed, and the only pillows in the delivery room were used to hold over the faces of labouring women to stop them screaming!

At six each morning I climbed into a jeep going up in the hills to Laurence

Tavern. The GP who drove me held a clinic there and the home nurses and midwives agreed to take me on their visits so that I could be introduced to peasant women, traditional midwives – *nanas* – and professional caregivers, school teachers and postmistresses.

In every Jamaican village there was a female triumvirate of the midwife, the teacher and the postmistress. All community news went through them. Every important decision was guided by them. They had to be the key players in any research into women's lives. There were opportunities to record group interviews – what we would now call informal focus groups – in clinics, churches, at the river where the women did their laundry, and while they cooked meals and tended their children. I talked to mothers, grandmothers and aunties – the last two vital in running family life.

At 3 p.m. I was home again when my older children came out of school in the next hour. So we had a good part of the day together. The three older ones went to school and Polly was cross and bored because she could not go, too. She longed for her Grandfather, my father Alec, with whom she shared a love of the natural world. She decided she wanted to get on a plane and fly back to England to be with him. So that is exactly what she did! We saw a gallant and determined four-year-old with a tag around her neck hurry over the tarmac and climb the steps to the plane with utter confidence. She didn't look back or wave. She was accompanied by Uwe's mother. The next thing we heard was that she had enjoyed the flight and was rapturous about being with her beloved Grandfather again. She said later that it served as an illustration of the sort of parent I was. I took that as criticism, but she protested: *'No, you treated each of us as an individual and listened to us. That was what I wanted, and you made it happen for me.'*

Culture Shock

My time in Jamaica was an amazing experience – a culture shock – and opened my eyes to how life was for women who don't have my privileged existence.

I wrote: *'Living in squalor, I'm surprised that these people have the same emotions, the tenderness and love, the devotion of a mother to her children, the trust a small child has in its parents, the pride a father in his baby, that we know in our own clean, suburban, polished-knocker society, with its trim hedges and milk on the doorstep, sprung prams, full shopping trolleys and Italian shoes. The sweetness of being human in spite of the dirt, constant hunger, the misery of malnutrition, wasting away not only of body but of mind, that results from serious deficiency diseases.*

'*A woman stands, her body swollen with many pregnancies, legs ulcerated with yaws, while her baby grips her tightly, head cradled in her arm in exactly the same way that an English child nestles against her mother, clinging to her for protection in the face of these strangers who have invaded the home. The older brother pokes a straw through holes in a tin can to amuse the toddler, who is too weak to toddle, but leans in the crook of his loving arm.*

'*This child has kwashiorkor, abdomen swollen with oedema, hair discoloured. His limbs are flabby and his eyes dull. Two older boys, lumps of ringworm crowning their curly heads, sit in the dust playing and laughing merrily. Animals live a sort of symbiotic existence with them, pigs lying in the baking sun on the threshold, hens darting under our feet, kids gambolling on the mud patch surrounding the hut.*

'*I feel ashamed that other human beings should have to live like this while I live in comfort and luxury. The concern I have that my children grow up healthy and strong is the same as this mother's concern. Only she is forced by the circumstance of birth to accept her fate.*

'*What do these babies in the dirt have in common with my clean, shampooed English child? In spite of filth and disease I am linked to them by virtue of our common humanity. Here are my brothers and sisters – my children.*'

Discovering Feminist Research

In the 50s feminist research had not yet been invented. Anthropologists undertook research along the lines of the masters of anthropology who either brought powerful philosophical theory to the discipline, as did Lévi-Strauss in France, or, intense observation of a dramatically alien society, like Malinowski working in the Trobriand Islands, or, like anthropologists in Oxford, they sliced up society and systems – economic, political, kinship and so on, demonstrating how the pieces interlocked, like a complicated Lego construction.

This was almost exclusively about men's lives and men's power. Nobody was trying to see society through women's eyes except a handful of cultural anthropologists, like Ruth Benedict, much scorned in British academic circles, and Margaret Mead. They were perceived in Oxford as story-tellers, frivolous as only women could be. Now extracts from their writing are in every anthropological and psychological anthology, but then they were marginal.

I felt very alone. The questions I was asking were about women's lives, values and relationships. The word '*bonding*' was not yet current, but they were to do with bonding between women – and how this affected the way society worked. The method was called '*participant observation*'. So I was approaching my research in a way that I think seemed reckless and shallow to most male colleagues and mentors.

There were other differences, too. Instead of concentrating on one informant at a time, I became involved in dynamic interaction in groups, women talking as they did their laundry, prepared food, cared for children or laid out a dead body. I noted agreement and disagreement, harmony and conflict between women facing problems and issues that mattered to them. This preceded focus group research – the kind in which my daughter Jenny became a specialist in the 90s.

My research was also rooted in observation of women's bodies, how they were used, and the physiological processes that found expression in religious ritual and the life transition of becoming a mother. So I recorded in detail gestures and movements, posture and breathing.

At the time I did not realise that what I was doing was unique. Only later, discussing it with women sociologists, can I understand its significance in feminist research.

Women provided a grapevine of communication through which I could get to know *nanas*. These traditional midwives often worked surreptitiously, though they were vitally needed, and offered their time and skills either free or in an elaborate system of barter. No woman would ever be left unattended in or after birth. *Nanas* didn't just care for mothers and babies. They wove the community together and held its history. Grandmothers, mothers, daughters, granddaughters and families spread out; the women stayed put and the men came and went. The expression used about a man was that he had '*run*'. The most common time to run was following the birth of a baby. The children had aunties, too, some blood-related, others not. That is the way women would sort out child care. They all brought up their children in much the same way, so it usually seemed to be a smooth process, and every woman in the community kept an eye on them.

I didn't have to seek out anyone to interview. Relationships flowed and developed. There was always someone happy to talk about children and birth.

Girls got pregnant in their teens, though that first relationship was unlikely to last. When I was at the clinic which specialised in reproductive health I met 17 year olds who had not yet become pregnant and were desperately worried that they must be '*mules*'. Though having a period was called '*seeing your health*', knowing that you could get pregnant was just as surely seeing your health, and if you weren't certain this was possible, it was almost obligatory to try.

Jamaica Talk

My field work lasted nine months. I remained slightly surprised that I could make contact with most of the women I was interviewing, and that we had a good deal in common, although our backgrounds were so different. In fact, they were eager to talk, explain their problems and gain a sympathetic listening ear. But I needed to understand the subtleties of Jamaican Creole.

'*Jamaica talk*' is more than a dialect of English and less than another language. Socially mobile people tended not to let it be known that they spoke it and often made great attempts to speak '*polite*' English.

The negative '*no*' could, for example, be used to emphasise a statement and so draw an expression of surprise from the listener, or to assert something that seemed unlikely – '*mi waak*' meaning '*I walked*' and '*mi no waak*' meaning not '*I did not walk*' but that '*I walked contrary to expectation*'; '*no fient me en fient*' meaning '*I fainted*', the repetition serving to stress the extraordinary nature of the occurrence, and '*no mango dem gan luk*' – '*it's mangoes they have gone to look for*'.

I had to learn a new language of gesture, facial expression and even monosyllabic utterance, which at first bypassed me completely.

But apart from difficulties in language, accurate information – especially any which involves dates and ages, was hard to come by, and I had to constantly check and re-check what I was told. Facts might approximate to ideal rather than actual behaviour, the socially praiseworthy rather than correct. This was partly from sheer lack of concern with anything involving figures and measurement of time – '*plenty-plenty*' fills most needs – and partly from delight in outwitting by talk. I had to be able to sit and listen without looking at a watch (in fact I never carried one). It also involved willingness to give as well as seek information; I found myself talking about my own children for instance.

Anyone doing field work in Jamaica would do well to bear in mind Louise Bennett's poem about the census:

> *Ah laugh soh tell ah cry*
> *Me dis dun tell de census man*
> *A whole tun-load a lie ...*
> *Him doan fine out one ting bout me,*
> *For fe me y'eye soh dry,*
> *Me stare right eena census face*
> *An tell him bans a lie.*
>
> *Me tell him sey, dat all me parents*
> *Dem is still alive*
> *But me mada she dead twelve 'ears*
> *An me fada him dead five.*

But it is not necessarily with intention to deceive that someone gives inaccurate information. The questions one psychologist, J C Flugel, suggests that the interviewer should ask – '*How do you feel your own ideas on how to run a family are like those of people you know / are different from them?*' – is hopelessly involved for Jamaican peasants to answer. I asked very simple, yet far-reaching, questions: '*What is a good mother? What is a good father? What is a rude child? When you trouble, where you go?*' Even the addition of a single word – '*like*' – '*What is your mother like?*' for example, confused the issue, and the reply might well be, '*Me mada she like paw-paw.*'

There were no fashions in child care. As she grew up, a girl coped with babies casually and unreflectively. Unlike the English or American baby in its cot, a Jamaican baby was handled constantly, petted, stroked, kissed and nuzzled by mother, sisters, brothers, grandmothers, aunties, and all the children and young girls in the neighbourhood. They patted his lips and combed his curly hair. They helped bath him in cold water (containing washing blue to keep away the '*duppies*'). He was alternately breastfed and had bush tea (tea made from any bush, leaf or root) or tit-bits from grown-ups' plates pushed in his mouth. He was jostled and shifted over to make room for others, flung up and down by the menfolk, cuddled and playfully cuffed, held upside down and right way up, head lolling or dangling – then hugged warmly and wrapped up in an old dress of his mother's and put in the shade while she prepared a meal. He might be placed in a tub on the mud clearing in front of the hut, and other members of the household nonchalantly brushed flies off him when they happened to pass. There were chickens squawking, dogs barking, pigs grunting, and children playing '*dutty pot*' (making mud pies), a goat or two, lizards darting about, women shrilly arguing, and a transistor radio turned on full. All this was extremely worrying for the nurses and health workers, whom I saw correcting and training mothers in clinic waiting rooms whenever there was an opportunity. The mother complied with the nurse's wishes while she was watching, and then went on as she did before.

Her main task revolved around provision of food for the family. Children went on a food '*binge*' in the mango season, and their health improved a lot once mangoes were freely available. Adolescent girls told me that their mothers worried if the children were still hungry at the end of a meal and try to '*hush*' them, though one said, '*Me maada say I'm too craveful*' (wants to eat too much). There was a nutritional crisis when breastfeeding was finished, some time between one and two years of age. They stopped growing and might develop kwashiorkor with fatty filtration of the liver, oedema, apathy, and the colour of their skin and hair might fade. Other children were marasmic – wasted, and short – but without oedema or depigmentation.

A good mother gave her child enough food. She '*see them go tidy, send them to school regular*' (there was an average 60 per cent attendance at primary school on any day, and this dropped further on Fridays when, by tradition, parents had the right to use a child's labour), had patience and tried to '*grow them in the right and proper way*.' A mother '*is like a piece of gold to the sight of her children.*'

Woman's lot was hard, every woman told me. The concept of leisure was non-existent. Cooking and washing filled the whole day. Cooking was never considered a recreation, but washing was, often because women met together and gossiped. If I asked a woman what she did in her '*spare time*' she often said '*washing*'. With few clothes and high standards of cleanliness for Sunday dress, garments were repeatedly boiled and washed. A woman met her friends at the river after tidying her hut and brewing up bush tea in the morning and spent several hours there. Washing and plaiting straw or '*hatta*' (weaving straw belts and in some part of the island hats or baskets for profit) were communal activities.

Social interaction depended on the weather. In the rainy season women and children stayed indoors as much as possible, since they believed it was dangerous to get one's hair wet.

At night an unweaned child lay beside its mother. Other children might be tucked in at the end of the bed, and some even under it. Mothers aimed at having another bed for the older children, even if it had to be erected specially every night. Far from indulging in nightly orgies – a stereotype about peasants often held by the Jamaican middle class – intercourse was hasty, conducted so as not to wake the children, and, according to many women who talked to me, unsatisfactory.

Whenever there was illness or trouble in the family a woman, if on good terms with her mother, sent her children back to her. In late pregnancy children were often sent to the grandmother's. If her mother lived near she might have a number sleeping with her who go home for meals during the day. A baby who was weaned at about a year to 18 months was often sent to the maternal grandmother, who if she was no longer lactating herself, took him into her bed and gave him bush tea if he cried.

When I asked women, '*If you need help, where you go?*' (the only way in which the question can be formulated for quick understanding) they usually named their mother, and an older female relative (frequently the mother's sister) or a sister. Sisters clung close if they were still living near each other. Women went to their mothers for advice, and often too, to their partner's or ex-partner's mother. Sometimes a woman mothered a child of a partnership which had failed, and this built a bond between the two women. They were united in shaking their heads at man's lack of responsibility and infidelity.

Active members of the church asked the pastor for help, but only when motherly and sisterly assistance had failed. Women sought assistance from the *Obeah man* (witch doctor) too, especially if there was discord between partners, or if repeated illness or accident made them feel that evil had been set on them. Many of the Zionist and other evangelist churches helped their congregation with shoes, for instance, and with feasting and ritual sharing of food.

Women rarely asked doctors, nurses or social workers for advice or help.

They supported each other in times of trouble, and there was a network of reciprocal obligation.

Getting The Spirit

I went up into the hills to attend revivalist services – and was often invited to preach as well! And I talked to women about how they guarded against harm from the '*duppies*' (ancestor spirits).

In the home it was each woman's responsibility to protect her family against the duppies and to live and organise her household so that she attracted good angels. From the moment of a child's birth, and even in pregnancy, the mother's primary ritual responsibility towards the child was to guard it from the hands of the ancestor spirits – mainly those in the maternal line, who would come and take it away. She was the only one who can keep the family from harm.

Women were also responsible for all community rites. Men could not be relied on to do these things. They were called on to perform minor manual tasks, such as the weaving of palm leaves to cover the roof of a booth in which a dead body was laid out, or when a wedding party took place. But the woman had final responsibility to see that it was all done properly.

For all peasant women the main, and often only, recreations were sex and religion. Since sex proved hazardous, and came to be used for the most part to get support for children, a woman had to rely largely upon religion, and found expression in spirit possession for her creative outpourings, reaching beyond the routines of ordinary living. In revivalism she could leap away from the dreary self she knew and the cares of every day. '*Life is hard*', but when she got the spirit it was transfused with glory.

Women formed the core of revivalist worship, and ran the church. Although a man was the main leader, and in different congregations was known as '*Daddy*', '*Father*' or '*Pupa*', he was dependent upon women assistants who supported him, counselled members of the congregation, were responsible for church organisation and the distribution of charity, or occasionally, as in some Pocomania groups, the pooling of resources, and led worship. They were known as '*shepherdesses*', '*governesses*', '*queens*', '*queen doves*' or '*sisters*' and often wore special dress, called '*uniforms*'. They propelled the worshippers into a state of ecstasy. The congregation was dependent on them to lead them into the experience of religious rapture through dance, song, *'groaning'*, *'labouring'* and *'trumping'* – testimony and speaking with tongues. Though most of the congregation might never reach the same heights, they got vicarious satisfaction from mystic union effected with the other world which sisters had entered on their behalf. Unity with the past as well as among the living was sought in spirit possession. They were the primary mediators between the divine and the human, the past and the present.

The process of *'getting the Spirit'* – which was accepted by everyone as being very exhausting – implied a good deal more than prayer, hymn singing and testimony. It entailed physical participation in worship which could result in a transformation which was in complete contrast to the individual's usual stance and gait. In extreme cases, as for example in the spirit possession which took the form of identification with a particular animal in Pocomania, physical ills were forgotten and the old and arthritic glided along like snakes.

This metamorphosis was triggered by dancing, hand clapping and adjustments in the rate, rhythm and level of breathing. These, in turn, were regulated by the reiterated beat of drums, *'shake-shakes'* and other musical instruments and repetitive singing with a pronounced and simple rhythm, by a senior woman worshipper.

Ecstasy was above all a group activity. When cult leaders described solitary conversion, as did a revivalist father who told me the story of the sudden blinding flash of revelation that came to him in his youth when he realised that he must dedicate his life to God, they described a command from on high, an absolute certainty concerning the right course of action to be taken. This was quite different from spirit possession, which did not involve personal decisions and was essentially communal.

Only a few were possessed at any one time, and some women quickly became ecstatic. Others were spectators, and others active participants in the sense that they reinforced the rhythmic background of song, dance and music and other stimuli so that those possessed became more and more taken over by the spirit claiming them. As worshippers tired or attention wandered they dropped out of the ceremony, strolled to the outskirts of the group or outside the meeting house, had a drink of water or a bite to eat, suckled a baby, or dozed off, and came back with renewed energy. Exit from and entry into the ritual was casual, inconsequential and unregulated, and this informality enabled small children to enter the drama.

The dancing took place in a circle around ritual symbols on the floor and extended as others were drawn in. Round and round the worshippers went in the same direction. This led to giddiness and loss of balance.

The dance was exaggerated pelvic rocking, as in the *ska*, with alternating contractions of the abdominal and buttock muscles, extension and flexion of the lower spine, and probably also contraction and release of the pelvic floor muscles. This was accompanied by arm movements; arms were often raised, and fluttered as ecstasy became more pronounced, with deeper breathing. As the experience became further intensified the woman's spine was spasmodically flexed and extended in convulsive-like movements, her head thrown back, and jaw dropped. At the same time the breath was forced in with great gasps through her open mouth, and out with a heavy grunt or deep sigh, or a cry of 'Jesus!', 'Lahd!' or 'Saviour!'

As the beat of music and the rhythm of dance speeded up, she panted rapidly. Her arms extended, her rib cage was raised, her mouth opened, and deep chest breathing was reinforced not only by the rocking, swaying trunk movements, but abdominal pressure as she breathed out (like an opera singer holding onto a prolonged note). There was a rhythm involving rapid, heavy panting and her back arched. This quickly led to hyperventilation.

Talking About Sex

Sex is tumultuous. Just as the wind blows and the rains pour down, the mango bears ripe fruits and the hibiscus its blossom, the power of sex sweeps through human life, causing torment, joy, pain, but in whatever form it comes and whatever it brings, it is unavoidable and overpowering.

Jamaican vocabulary was rich in sexual terms. I learned that reality was often otherwise. Though spontaneity was uninhibited in early adolescence and may continue to be for men, for women it was soon modified by the cares of childbearing and rearing and the crowded conditions of peasant life.

Jamaican peasant women often told me that they get no pleasure in sex and could not *feel sweet*'. It is all summed up as '*him trouble me plenty-plenty*'. As one woman said when I asked her about sex. '*Whenever him feel that way.*' Whenever *he* feels? What about when *you* feel like it? She laughed, '*Whenever you feel or not!*'

Occasionally women told me they felt sorry for their men because they no longer enjoyed their '*exercise*' as they once did, and sometimes they asked me how they could get excited again. So discussion often turned to the conditions of existence, the problems of too many children, sleeping not only in the same room, but often under or at the end of the same bed. Children who were still being given the breast at night – up to two years of age – slept next to the mother. Women sometimes said that they could not even turn over in bed without risking waking a child. Is it any wonder, they asked, that their men sought '*outside*' women to '*satisfy their nature?*'

But it was not only the one, two or three room peasant hut or urban shack that was the problem. A woman was often very tired after her day's work with inadequate protein in her diet, consisting as it did in lean times of '*rice and peas*', a dish of polished rice and a form of dried bean (like a small haricot bean) mixed with scraps of mutton or salt fish. But it was the man of the household who was given the choice pieces of meat, if there were any, and if there was no man there was often no money to buy meat. This was eked out with bush teas and a spoonful of sweetened condensed milk. Fresh milk was rarely drunk.

Water was scarce in the dry season, and women had to walk long distances to get it from the nearest standpipe or spring. It often involved an uphill climb. Clothes were washed in cold water at the spring, in a creek or in a tin by the standpipe, and rubbed hard against large stones to remove the dirt. Standards of cleanliness in clothing, at any rate for Sunday best, for adults and children alike, were much higher for Jamaicans than they were for many Europeans. Fuel had also to be carried from the bush for all cooking operations, and women did this with great bundles on their heads.

It was not surprising that a woman with a family to rear was exhausted at dusk. So the man '*broke fence*' – if he ever '*responsed*' for the woman at all, and probably '*ran*' (left her) sooner or later. She then, finding life '*hard*', sought another man for whom she could bear a child, on the understanding that he would offer some support in return for her services. If a woman was to '*call the name of a man*' as the father and persuade him to '*obligate himself*' for the maintenance of the child, she must be prepared to continue a sexual relationship with him as witness to the obligation. That is, by '*obligating*', in the words of one woman, meant '*to come for the money so he could have sex dealings*'.

The man often agreed to pay the midwife's fee but no more, or might give a few shillings cash down but refused to continue payments. Sex was something she engaged in for and on behalf of her children, a necessary duty if she was to feed, clothe and educate them.

When A Daughter Gets Pregnant: The Ritual Quarrel

On finding that her daughter was pregnant, a mother would start the ritual quarrel and ask 'Who trouble you then?' or 'Who bother you?' and question her to find out whose stomach it is. She would call the boy to visit her, or went off to him if he could be found and lived locally, saying she cannot hold up her head for shame at what has happened, and asks whether he will 'stand manly' and marry her. There is a public row, involving neighbours, acquaintances and relatives. She, for her part, will point at the girl and say that, far from bothering her, she has been bothering him and she can't be responsible. The ritualised exchange is crystallised in a calypso:

> Keep your daughter inside Miss Miriam,
> That girl child looking for trouble.
> If my boy child trouble your girl child
> Doan' hold me resp-ons-ab-le.

The girl would often be flogged by her mother or father or the mother's partner with a strap. She was turned out of the house overnight. This was always described as 'a quarrel'. Sometimes there was a quarrel but the girl was not turned out – 'me maada still bear'. At this point other female relatives on the maternal side were also involved; the girl goes to her auntie's or seeks the sympathy of middle aged friends or other relatives of her mother's. After a few days the mother takes the outcast daughter back in the house again and there would be reconciliation.

When I asked what she would do if her daughter was pregnant, one married mother of 12, pregnant with her thirteenth child, got very excited, and the words tumbled out as she told me, 'If you had been showing her right from wrong and you keep warning her, as soon as she get pregnant she have to leave. We must stiffen our necks, harden our hearts. You can't go sympathising with everything that is wrong, but if she should get pregnant for a fellow that I don't know about, then I would pardon her.' That is, it was her responsibility to approve her daughter's boyfriends and watch over her behaviour.

Most mothers I talked to told me that there was no point in quarrelling with a pregnant daughter, and the girls reported that their mothers were '*happy*' when they conceived. One woman said – '*Try to give her a good education so that she may not go as you. If you have a child and you do not married, you do not want she to come as you. I say, "Winsome (the name of her daughter) you see what you maada is going through. Please do not do as she. You maada is trying her best, please take you lessons". But if she decided to do what you do – to take you footsteps – nothing stop her'*. Another said '*I would tell her that she is wrong but I would still have to keep her'*.

The most badly hit was the socially mobile mother who was concerned to give her daughter opportunities that she herself was denied. Then the ritual rejection might have been enacted in bitter earnest. For example, a woman who was proud to see her daughter at commercial college discovered her pregnancy and to hide her shame immediately sent her away to her sister who was a nurse. She kept the girl indoors for six months, behind lock and key, until she went into labour. She took her once to the doctor, on her arrival, and after examining her, the doctor warned the pregnant girl that she had a gonorrheal discharge and needed treatment. However, nothing was done, since this would stamp more shame on the family, and she arrived at the public hospital in the early first stage of labour in a state of terror. Doctors could not examine her as she was trembling violently, screaming and on the point of collapse. I sat and talked soothingly to her and discovered that she was afraid the baby would be born blind. (The baby was fine.)

Taboos In Pregnancy

Taboos guarded the dangerous passage through pregnancy. A pregnant woman was in a state of ritual danger.

One of the most important prohibitions was that she must not look at a dead body. She could not be present when a body was laid out in '*the booth*' at a '*set-up*' for the dead, but must not look at it.

I was at a set-up one day and asked a pregnant woman why. '*A reason is in it. There is a way*', she told me. '*Yes! If you're old perhaps you may get over because if you are young doan' worry, because that child may not live.*' (The '*doan worry*' means '*whatever you do to avoid it*'). '*As well as, perhaps you may happen to lose your life because – what happen? Your body get cold. Energy leave you in bringing forth that child.*' There is a correct temperature for the body and any loss of heat and chilling is dangerous. Looking at the face of a corpse reduces the body's natural warmth. This a healthy person can survive, but anyone sickly, facing childbirth, or liable to get chilled just after giving birth, may die.

Pregnant women must drink with discretion because water can drown the baby. They must not make too much preparation ahead of time or the baby will be still-born. They must not lift heavy weights nor carry another child because '*it generally lean the baby to one side according to how you hold it.*' They must not drink soursop juice (from the fruit of the soursop tree) or they will have pain, nor stretch their hands above their head '*because the baby's neck will scorch. It will be stretched and when it come back it will get scorched.*' Don't sleep too often. '*Plenty of exercise and walk plenty, will have the baby quicker*' and an easier labour. A woman must be careful *how* she moved, too. It was particularly dangerous to double your foot under when sitting. She must avoid '*much bending*' and stooping. A treadle sewing machine was especially risky, and women who must use one to do dressmaking and support the family told me that continued sitting at the machine caused backache. A pregnant woman must not eat coconuts '*because it will develop the baby too fast*', '*drink out of bottles or coconut or baby will have cast eyes*', '*climb a tree, or the baby will slip from the womb*', nor '*walk over soap water or it will give you a bad stomach.*' She must not step over a rope – for example, one that tethers the donkey – or a broom, or the birth may be overdue. She must avoid getting upset. A woman told me, '*When I'm pregnant I don't like to look on anything that is out of order. People say that your child if you look on anything and sorrow for it – that's you know out of order – that your child will come the very same. Suppose you went to Kingston now and see an old lady who have half a foot (leg) or half a face, and you sorrow for it, or in any way deformed, people say that your child generally come that way. Or if you killing a fowl and you sorrow for that fowl your children come with some part of the looks belonging to the fowl.*' So this woman never killed chickens when pregnant.

Heartburn, as in the folklore of England and France, was supposed to be caused by the baby's hair; the longer the hair the more the heartburn. I met one expectant mother who was anxious that her child had no hair because she didn't have any heartburn.

Duppies attacked pregnant women. Eclampsia was spirit possession. The *duppies* had come and taken over the soul of the sick person. So many eclamptic and pre-eclamptic patients had seen duppies haunting their ward in the maternity hospital in Kingston that it had to be moved to another floor of the building. (Among Hindus in India, too, eclampsia was seen as spirit possession and, as it was more common in the rainy season, it was believed that spirits seeking re-incarnation wandered abroad then and slipped into the bodies of pregnant women. In fact, their health probably does deteriorate during the rainy season. This also happens in Nigeria where this annual period of food shortage when crops can't be gathered and the family only eats what is left around is also a peak time for eclampsia).

Positive advice was less clear. It was good to take '*bitters*' (any bitter herb) particularly the plant cerasee in the form of bush tea. '*Although it bitter you have plenty of mothers that love it. It help to make the child healthy; it keep the blood bitter.*' Cerasee is one of the most well known bush teas and used to treat hypertension. Expectant mothers should eat oranges, okra to make the baby slip out, and callaloo, a leafy vegetable dish, to '*help the blood*'.

How To Grow A Baby Right

Women talked to me about how the baby grows from a stalk. Its feet are embedded in the small of the mother's back, like a statue modelled out of clay which is ripped out at birth, leaving a wound where it was torn off. The baby is curled round so that the head, too, is normally in the small of the back, above the level of its feet. It breathes inside her, and gets either milk through the '*soft spot*' or anterior fontanelle, '*the mole*', or – other women told me – blood from the mother through its mouth. The great danger was that a baby may '*come up in the chest*' and to avoid this, and ensure that it did not grow too big, the mother wore a tight string below her breasts. Modern girls in the towns simply did up their bras very tight to prevent this happening. Women feared that if the baby went '*up*' it may never come '*down*', and in labour could choke them.

The baby's sex could be foretold. A boy lies on the left side. When '*the belly round it is a girl, but if it have a point, it is a boy*'. Fetal movements could also foretell sex: '*To the movement of the child I know whether it is a boy or a girl. The boy doan' move as often as the girl, bit it move more stronger than the girl*'. And from Claribel, pregnant with her twelfth child: '*I cannot keep up my urine every time I having a girl child cause my urine pass thin, and it is more like down there (touching her pubis) and the boy he doan' give me any pain like what the girl give me, but this one I can hardly sit down'.*

The womb should be nourished by sex so that the birth canal is kept open and delivery easy. Maud said she told her man that she '*didn't want to feel much pains to bring the baby into the world*', and if he loved her '*he must continue nourishing the womb by constant sex dealings*'.

One woman told me that when she gave birth to her first baby the midwife remarked that she had not had enough sex during pregnancy, so the vagina was closed. She was careful with the second baby to '*have sex up to the last minute*'.

Midwives And Mothers

Birth was not a dramatic event. Pregnancy, labour, breastfeeding, sex, were part of the inevitable and rhythmic flow of life, and bearing or feeding a baby was a normal state of existence. The abnormal would be to stop for any prolonged period.

A woman got up a few hours after giving birth to cook the family porridge or do other household tasks. She carried on with jobs like these as long as she could during the first stage, too, and reckoned the length of labour from when she took to her bed. Usually it merged imperceptibly with pregnancy. She was not used to thinking in terms of set times and routines and rationing out her daily existence, so would be hard put to say when labour started. Her attitude to the start of labour was usually unhurried, casual and almost nonchalant.

Midwives were skilled at adapting simple equipment. They made do with one or two jugs of boiled water, might work by the light of burning wood, candles, or a Tilley lamp if they had one, and used newspapers for sheets, boiled rags for swabs and lemonade bottles for glass utensils. Boiled empty condensed milk tins were used for sterilising scissors and hypodermic syringes. The main hygienic equipment was a bar of soap and a small bottle of Dettol. Sanitary pads were hemmed rags, boiled and ironed, since commercial products were too expensive.

Like the *Obeah* man or woman and the religious cult leaders, a good midwife was a counsellor, both in practical, economic terms and in spiritual matters.

She reprimanded a man for wife-beating, arranged to go to see the employer of another for failing to support his wife and 13 children so that the money could be docked at source, gave advice on morality and child psychology, and exchanged banter with those calling to her in the street. She may have been the only social worker in the area, and was the agency through whom the people communicated with bureaucracy – government offices, and welfare and health departments.

I went with district midwives on home visits. The front of the houses gave a deceptive appearance of respectability to the district. But behind almost every one was a mud yard in which the occupiers had built perhaps a handful, perhaps several dozen, one room shacks, constructed of packing cases and tin sheets. There was no drainage, no equipment, other than old oil drums, for storing water, nothing but minimal privacy for anyone, young or old, ill or healthy, dying, making love, or in childbirth. Small children were for the most part unclothed, and played 'dutty potty' with old cans in mud or danced to the blaring music or half a dozen radios all going at once turned on full. Enormous lizards scuttled like small battleships fighting and chasing each other, starving dogs, bitches and puppies nosed among the huge piles of rubbish and excreta, women scrubbed clothes in the hot sun, and in every alley-way, walled by tightly knotted dusty cactus, littered with broken bottles, shit, cigarette cartons and other waste, squatted groups of unemployed young men playing cards or dominoes for money, sometimes smoking *ganja* at the same time.

Taking place in the one-room hut, birth could not be allowed to disrupt the day-to-day life of the family. Children still had to be fed and washed and the rent paid. They might sleep in the same bed as the mother. If they could not be sent across the yard or out to play, they were separated from her by a strip of cloth hung over a clothes line suspended vertically down the length of the bed. The midwife would tell them to lie still and be good children and soon they would have a new brother or sister, and they would lie in breathless silence, sharing in their mother's labour, listening to the midwife's instructions and encouragement, hearing the first cry of the newborn baby, and seeing it as it was lifted damp from its mother's body.

Hospital Birth

In the hospital there were two eight-bedded first stage rooms which were not only for those in the first stage, but also women well advanced in the second stage and those who had been returned to this ward shortly after delivery. Babies were frequently born in the first stage rooms, sometimes in the lavatories, or were dropped as the woman rushed into the delivery room. Thirty-five to forty patients gave birth in each of these wards every twenty-four hours.

The midwives had a very different and much more limited function from that filled by those working on the district. It was mainly concerned with efficiency and speed of delivery or the patient, cleanliness, hospital routines relating to hygiene and orderliness, and the control and limitation of emotional factors in labour and the first 48 postpartum hours so that the greatest number of patients could be effectively treated in the shortest possible time without disruption of hospital organisation.

They confronted almost insuperable obstacles. Equipment was always in short supply, even basic things like cotton wool, which was allowed to run out before it was re-ordered. The clock on one delivery room wall had not been repaired for two months, the emergency lighting supply had been out of order for one month, and for six months there was no tape for tying name labels on babies' wrists, so that midwives had to spend time cutting up gauze. Sterilisation of swabs took 48 hours, liquid soap containers had been broken and not replaced so that everyone had to wash with odd bits of soap. There was no hot water after early morning, and midwives had to walk across the length of the delivery room to get water in chipped enamel jugs from the sluice. There was no isolation ward. And with no staff meetings or suggestion boxes, or any means of regularly and effectively communicating up the staff hierarchy, the midwives were dissatisfied and frustrated.

Women came long distances to the hospital to give birth. To avoid delivering on the way it was the custom to balance a brick or other heavy weight on the head. This was said to have the effect of pressing on the baby and preventing its birth. The mechanism of this brick technique is probably fairly simple. The first effect is psychosomatic; the mother does not become anxious that the baby may be born on the way to the hospital, so continues to breathe rhythmically and does not hold her breath and bear down. The second effect is postural. To balance a weight on the head, the pelvis is tilted forward and the pelvic floor musculature has the effect of delaying delivery. Some women removed the brick on reaching the hospital and promptly delivered in the admission room.

It was in keeping with the mood of the labour wards that someone stuck up at the entrance of the hospital a card bearing the words – *'Death is sure. Sin the cause. Christ the cure'.*

Birth in hospital was completely different from home birth. In hospital, it was a dramatic, physical experience, and the cries coming from the labour wards are those of pain and fear. At first sight the drama of suffering is almost overwhelming, and it was only as I observed the behaviour of women individually that a pattern emerged of women going through the same physiological experience, who were led by a few who were specially active, moving with repetitive cries.

These women tended to have large families. Young first time mothers watched them in spellbound fascination, a fact which midwives frequently deplored. Throughout labour they danced and uttered cries which were typical of behaviour in revivalist cult groups, particularly that of spirit possession. They sparked off similar reactions in newcomers to the ward, and kept each other at high tension all the time.

This might be reinforced by the administration of the *'Jubilee cocktail'*, an analgesic and sedative mixture which, called *'knock-out drops'* or a *'Mickey Finn'*, is well known in the underworld. Thirty grains of chloral hydrate were given in one ounce or more of rum and shaken up with an ounce of sugar syrup.

Listening to my tape recordings of Zionist church services with dance, prayer, chanting and cries to Jesus – and the largest proportion of worshippers and the most fervent are women – and comparing these with tapes of women in labour in this hospital, it was not easy to determine which was which.

Hospital midwives told me that a woman cried, *'Jesus! Jesus! Jesus!'* throughout contractions of the first stage, and they knew when she was in the second stage because it changed to, *'Jesus Christ! Jesus Christ! Jesus Christ!'*

There was close physical contact between women. They bled over each other. Their waters broke over one another. They had contractions leaning against each other, flinging out their arms to hold on to the next body, and shared in a common sense of salvation when they were delivered. I did not meet one woman who said anything which suggested that she felt that she was being denied privacy in the hospital. Even when two women were on one delivery table, neither flinched from the mingled blood, urine, faeces and liquor of the other.

* * *

Immediately after the birth hospitalised Jamaican mothers were in a state of emotional withdrawal, in spite of the fact that they had quick and easy second stages. This contrasted strongly with the woman's delighted bonding with the baby when born at home. They seemed to leave the matter of the child's life or death, health or ill-health to people who know better, resigned themselves to the hands of experts and often lay back wearily moaning, apparently too exhausted to look at their babies. Often too, the arrival of the baby forced home to them their economic condition and after the efforts of labour they felt unable to cope with the sheer problems of survival, of feeding, clothing and caring for their now enlarged family. The custom of showing only the baby's sex to the mother, and not its face, and of rapidly moving the baby away before the she had had a chance to handle her baby, emphasised this trauma. At home the midwife rested the baby in the mother's arms while she prepared to wash the child. The number of knots in the umbilical cord indicated the number of children the mother still had to bear. Many women took this very seriously, and trained midwives sometimes did this, if only in fun. If a hospital midwife commented on the number her verdict was accepted in all earnestness, since given the added mystique of hospital routines her every word had special significance.

This counting of knots comes from West African placental divination. Sometimes I saw a mother's satisfaction at birth turn to despair on seeing these 'knots', but, I have seen a mother beam with delight after I explained that they were just bumps, not knots, that she had had her 'lot', and suggested that she should now register with the birth control clinic.

Babies And The Breast

Jamaican babies were breastfed as a matter of course. Probably few would have survived if bottle feeding had been the norm.

In the 50s the Government introduced dried milk (Semilko) for distribution from welfare clinics. Till then feeding on cow's milk meant a teaspoon of condensed milk in a large jug of hot water; in lean times the milk was stretched further. When I was there new cheap (or if need be free) dried milk could be obtained, and in the towns much advertised American dried milks, some of them expensive, but all containing the same ingredients, had become very popular. Women skimped on protein for the older children so that the baby could be give SMA, Lactogen or Ostermilk.

Babies were fed on demand, and it usually worked out at around two-hourly intervals. A sleeping baby was never wakened. After night feeds, and there may have been three or four at first, mother and baby fell asleep with the breast still available to the baby, often with the nipple still in its mouth. Night feeds continued for as long as the baby wanted them.

The pattern of night feeding was based on a system evolved under slavery. While mothers worked in the fields during the day their babies stayed with an old woman who fed them on a pap of bread flour and water. So most breast feeds were given at night.

A woman carried on doing domestic work, combing the toddler's hair, or eating, and other things while she fed.

Since there was no embarrassment about exposing breasts, nipples dried in warm air. Women rarely wore bras and when worn they were invariably of cotton. This meant that air circulated easily around the nipple. The mother did not mind if her dress or blouse was wet with milk, and made no attempt to wash it off, and never wore pads, so her nipples did not lie in a container of stale, congealed milk. Sore and cracked nipples were rare.

Every mother expected to be able to breastfeed, and did not anticipate difficulty. I only met two women who failed to breastfeed satisfactorily out of approximately 200 with whom I discussed the subject. One was in the hills and one in Kingston. One woman persisted for three months, using complementary bottle feeds. She told me with evident surprise that her baby was flourishing and said she knew a mother who did not want to breastfeed in Kingston. The baby was '*fat and well nourished*' in spite of being on a bottle.

A Jamaican baby was fed casually – its head was not always supported – without concentration of purpose or attention, and without anxiety. An English mother would often try to prop the baby into exactly the right position, to feed for the set number of minutes, and for only so long at each breast. She was often in a quandary about not only how she could get the baby on to the breast if it was unwilling when the clock said it was time, but how to get if off again, once its jaws were clamped round the nipple, since the book said she should get its wind up at this point, or terminate the feed.

I watched mothers breastfeeding, sitting in the shade of a tree or house and chatting to everyone who passed by. Other women broke off doing their washing, husking coffee beans, or plaiting straw, to stroll over and join her. Far from being a solitary activity, it was a social occasion in which gossip and local news could be exchanged.

A mother had no idea of the time spent at the breast, or how long it was since the last feed. The baby usually fell asleep at the breast and when it dropped off she continued to chat, moving her whole body in a gentle rocking motion, then put the baby down on some rags indoors, or in the shade outside in the yard.

When I asked when they stopped giving the baby a feed – and how they knew when to stop – mothers looked at me with amazement and I added, *'Mothers do different things in different parts of the world'*. They then said, *'When I put it into her mouth and she draw back'*. *'When him leave the breast; he just sleeps.' 'When him take enough him spit out the breast out of him mouth.' 'When him seem bellyful, him burps and stops.'*

A baby wore little clothing – only a short cotton vest and a cotton napkin; or buttocks could be left bare and the baby be put lying on some rags. Frequently the only bedding the mother had for her baby was her own best dress, which, carefully washed and ironed, was put down as a sheet for it to lie on. Arms and legs were left unrestricted and the baby's movements were free. Its life alternated between periods of marked freedom when it could wave its arms and legs about and periods of restraint provided by the close juxtaposition of other bodies as they crowded together for the night. The physical boundary the baby was meeting was not one of fabric or plastic, wood or shawl, but the flesh of another member of the family, most often that of his mother.

At the breast the baby was held loosely. This freedom of movement and freedom for exploration was in marked contrast to the cocoon-like shawl or blanket-enveloped European baby, and it was encouraged to touch the mother's breast and stroke and squeeze her.

When I asked them what their babies did after feeds they all said, *'Him sleep'*, as if this were a surprising question. Asked what they did when their babies cried, mothers explained that this was when the baby was hungry or wanted a bit of *'hushing'* (to hush a baby a mother takes her in her arms and rocks her, meanwhile talking or singing): *'When this baby cries I know that the baby is hungry,'* but (this mother added) mostly because he was hungry, and then of course she fed him. *'I take him up and feed him, but sometimes him want a little bit handling.'*

But when I was talking to women in the presence of a nurse, they were often apologetic and said things like – '*I can't stand crying*' to explain why they picked the baby up.

When a baby at the breast had a bowel motion or passes urine a mother simply parted her legs.

Volunteer assistants from the local high school, who hoped to become nurses, attended the infant welfare clinics to help out. These girls of 15 or 16, in blue and white school uniform, copied the nurses in everything, including their manner of dealing with patients, and were sometimes addressed as '*nurse*' though it was well known that they came from local families. The way in which these girls tapped a mother on the shoulder and commented curtly, '*Come!*' or lifted a protesting baby as if it were a sack of potatoes, without speaking or attempting to soothe it, faces impassive, hands strong, firm and unyielding, was almost a caricature of the nurses' way of dealing with patients.

In contrast, the mothers' behaviour was all tenderness. The babies sat on their laps, thumb sucking, stroked, petted and caressed. Occasionally a child would slip its hand down inside its mother's dress to lift out her breast, at which she would laugh. If babies could speak, the mothers vied with each other at producing baby talk – '*Mama*' and '*Papa*' even if '*Papa*' was not a permanent feature of the household and changed his identity rather often. But if a nurse had her eye on a baby a mother might quickly take the thumb out of its mouth and say lightly, '*You suck you thumb too much*'.

The nurse's task was to train ignorant mothers in correct baby care. The mothers always agreed with everything the nurse said. For the nurses, work was tedious and rewards few. In the rainy season they had to walk miles in mud, slush and driving rain. In fine weather the sun beat down as they covered vast distances to reach recalcitrant mothers who failed to attend clinic appointments. The surroundings were dirty, flies, mosquitoes and other insects abounded, and they had none of the equipment they would expect in a hospital or clinic in town.

Much of the advice the nurse gave was negative: '*Stop feeding him at night.*' '*Stop feeding him so many times in the day.*' '*Stop feeding him whenever he cries.*' '*Don't give the porridge in a bottle. Thicken it and give it to the baby in a spoon.*' But under the stress of family living in overcrowded conditions it was obvious that mothers were going to give the baby what it liked rather than obey the teachings of an expert.

To all these mothers, the nurses, doctors and other medical personnel, teachers, social workers and enquirers from University and the Government are 'Them' – members of that other world of the middle class who lived in undreamed-of luxury. Colour was secondary to this, and it did not really matter much what a person's colour was; white or black, a member of the middle class who patronised the poor and gave them advice and tried to help them, who criticised their behaviour and the ways in which they reared and fed their children, who asked 'What did you give him for his meal?' and 'Why don't you come to the clinic?' and said 'Don't give the baby condensed milk' when that was what the baby liked best - whatever her colour, she was one of 'Them'.

Discipline

From the age of about four a child was progressively and sometimes sternly disciplined. He was expected to be bowel and bladder trained, and might be smacked or 'slashed' with a belt if he made a mess. Until now he had just been left 'to dirty him baggy'.

The boisterous, rebellious child was 'rude'. He whistled behind his teeth or sucked in his breath, pulled the little girls' pigtails, answered back and is 'facety' (impudent) and precocious, wanting to 'turn man' or 'turn woman before time'. Bad children 'lick one another', and the treatment for this was to 'catch them and flog them with a strap'.

A girl was 'easier' than a boy, and mothers often said they preferred to have daughters for this reason. When I told them I had five daughters they often told me how they envied me.

After a seven or eight-year-old boy first joined the gang of neighbourhood children his contact with home was minimal, except on Sundays. He picked up food as best he could, stole with members of his gang, and took his luck.

The mythological folk hero for these children was Anansi, the little spider man, crafty, cunning, thoroughly amoral, and triumphing over the strong by his wit and wiles. He was really the same hero as Brer Rabbit or the 'signifying monkey' of Afro-American and Akan-Ashanti origin. Anansi represents the poor and powerless who win by deceit. The girls and I were often treated to a spell-binding array of these folk tales when Carmen Manley, the Prime Minister's sister, used to drop by in the early evenings introducing us to the fables and songs of her own childhood.

The nine months in Jamaica were in extraordinary contrast to life in an Oxfordshire village. I valued the warmth and vitality of the friends I made and the sheer *joie de vivre* of the carnival. I also met poverty face to face for the first time in my life, and was struck by the dignity and generosity of women who struggled against terrible odds to bring up their children and give them a life worth living. I got to know Rastafarian brethren who took me to their camp and let me take part in their religious services and listen to the drums saying, *'Death to the white oppressor and his black allies!'* I once asked them why they welcomed me and discussed ideas with me. The reply came: *'You have a white skin, but a black heart.'*

CHAPTER FIVE

OUR HOUSE

Back from Jamaica in 1966, we felt that the Toby House in Freeland was too small for seven people and fell in love with the Manor House at Standlake. It was perhaps foolhardy to pay four times Uwe's salary, but we have never regretted it; we are still here, feeding the great fireplaces with logs from trees we planted 45 or more years ago.

The village is set in the flood meadows of the upper Thames. It has its roots in the Iron Age, and in the Roman occupation was used as a base for waste disposal. When I mentioned that I lived in Standlake, Uwe's friend George Forrest, the Wykeham Professor of Ancient History, remarked, *'Ah yes!*

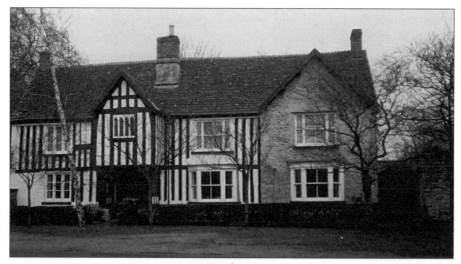

Our home

Standlake, the midden of the Roman army!'

A lofty medieval mud and straw one-room hall with a thatched roof, a hole in the roof for the smoke to go through – beams in the attic are blackened by smoke – and a rush-strewn oak floor. Cotswold stone, Plantagenet timber, wattle and daub, Stonesfield roof slates – they all come from the people who lived in the house. But people are shaped by houses, too.

Standlake flowered briefly in the thirteenth Century when it was described as a town. The Lady of the Manor, Eva de Grey, daughter of the Lord of the Isle of Wight, who survived four husbands, secured the right to a Friday market and a fair every year in honour of the parish church's patron saint, St Giles. This made trade for the village. She also had a licence to hold a court in the Manor. Over the years, four families descended from her husbands took it in turn to provide the living for the priest, and had to prove their right to install a new rector.

During the Reformation the Lords of the Manor provided hiding places for priests. The wall at the side of the great stone fireplace in our bedroom is hollow. It was probably a priest's hole. There is just enough space to hide a man.

When I show American guests round they usually exclaim, '*Wow! Before Columbus!'*, because this is the most significant event in their time. The world didn't exist before.

No-one knows exactly when the Manor House was built but it was extensively modernised in 1492–1495. An upper floor was put into the old open hall and the fireplaces and first floor porch were added by Edmund Yate, who left his punning heraldic badge – a gate – on one of the beams. A timber porch was installed with a small room above it, which is now part of my bedroom.

Decorative symbols were also carved in the stone fireplace in the sitting room: the Tudor rose of Henry VII and his crown, the cross keys of the Abbey of Gloucester, and the ragged staff in bend sinister of the Boyes family. Boyes is derived from Bois, indicating that the family was Norman. It was later anglicised to '*Wood*'. The '*ragged staff in bend sinister*' shows that this branch of the family came from the wrong side of the sheets. The Lord was having it off with a serving maid who became pregnant. He acknowledged paternity so that the descendants could carry the emblem of the family, but it was adapted to slant the other way.

Thomas Cromwell, Earl of Essex, bought the Manor in 1537. After he had advised Henry VIII to marry Anne of Cleves, he was executed in 1540 for high treason and the house was confiscated by the Crown. But not for long.

Henry VIII was shocked when he met his fourth bride, Anne of Cleves, to find that she didn't look anything like Holbein's painting with which he had been presented. She was rather toothy, and he called her *'the Flemish Mare'*. On the wedding night he exclaimed, *'God, what I do for England!'* In fact, he could not perform, and there was a divorce. She was to stay quietly in England and given the title of *'the King's Sister'* and as part of the divorce settlement received seven manors, one of them the recently confiscated manor of Standlake.

Fast forward to the Second World War. A retired headmaster, Captain Sir Henry Chittey, lived in the house, at that time in a very run down condition. When it rained he used to wash the dishes in the scullery, the roof of which was in very bad repair, wearing his tin helmet because water was pouring through. He was an obvious choice to command the Standlake Home Guard.

A Nissen hut headquarters was erected on his land as its base. Exercises consisted of battle between the Home Guard in Northmoor and the one in Standlake. Northmoor had to defend its village against Standlake and each village lined up troops and built barriers at the bridge on the road to Northmoor. The Northmoor men were to attack Standlake and Standlake built a strong defence on the road. But the men of Northmoor decided to go through the fields, invaded from the south, liberated the Standlake headquarters Nissen hut in which all the beer was stacked, and were drinking copious amounts whilst Standlake Home Guard waited for the invasion at the bridge.

We bought the house and six acres of grounds from a failed mink farmer. Mink cages littered the area – and tiny skulls and bones of the departed. He had hung the pelts in a large shed which is now transformed into Uwe's study and dressing room. The walls are thick with nails from which they were suspended. Elderly villagers told us that the smell of dead mink seeped into the High Street. It was strong and revolting. Occasionally mink escaped and ravaged neighbours' poultry.

The Manor House Garden And Paddock

The paddock and garden at the rear of the house facing the back of my flowery courtyard are now packed with bay trees and herbs, hanging flower baskets, pot plants, climbing honeysuckle and brilliantly coloured creepers. One arm of this courtyard leading to the main garden we closed in to make a conservatory and library to connect our two studies. Walls and ceiling are resplendent with vines that produce heavy bunches of grapes which our entrepreneur grandson Sam turned into juice and wine. I stencilled vines all over one wall where the trunk is to encourage the grapes to grow.

We don't know when the garden, *'the football field'*, and the paddock were laid out in their present form. In 1860 we realise from the auction particulars that the Manor House had 233 acres of land attached – but by the time we bought it in 1966 all but a little over six acres had been sold off.

In the 1930s there were several magnificent box trees in the upper garden: but when we took over only the lovely old walnut tree remained. It used to give us masses of nuts in the 70s, but then a bad summer drought marked the end of that bounty. The white and red roses of York and Lancaster climbed up the Cotswold stone walls.

The *'football field'* became far more interesting when Jon, Tess's partner, dug a pond for Uwe. It is visited by all sorts of birds, often a pair of mallards, but mainly pheasants. They are almost domesticated. One winter when only three cocks survived we gave them six hens for Christmas – and if there was snow on the ground they pecked at the back door to make sure Uwe didn't forget to feed them.

The paddock has had no weed-killer or fertiliser on it for decades, and when the girls were young it was inhabited at various times by Shaggy the shetland pony, Tinker the old horse, Hetty and Hannah the goats, and then by a Jacob ram called Joshua.

There have always been birds, too: doves, busy, scuttling bantams, peacocks and peahens. I was once attacked by a peacock as I emerged from the house into the garden putting up a multicoloured parasol. He obviously thought I was competition and wasn't letting me get away with it.

We planted the paddock with expert help from the Kingston Bagpuize Wildlife Gardening Centre to develop it as a habitat for insects, birds and other creatures. Their idea was to spread out a wide diversity of native plants, so there are white and silver birch, wild cherry and crabapple, hornbeam and hawthorn, holly and goat willow, guelder rose, dogwood, rowan, hazel and alder buckthorn. They planted a variety of native herbs and flowers, too – water mint by the old well near the middle of the paddock, pimpernel, woodruff, bugle and hellebore.

The tree trunks left rotting helped provide worms and bugs for the birds, and in the evening there is a white owl and lots of bats. Ground level there are hedgehogs, moles, foxes and squirrels and also some muntjac deer given to raiding the vegetable patch and anything they can munch in the garden.

Gwen Rankin, my long term friend and colleague, writes: '*I remember one happy encounter with Sheila which came out of the blue. My route took me near Oxford, so the opportunity was there to drop in and see her – if she was home that day – and that was a chance not to be missed, to catch up with a valued friend.*

'*I rang the door bell. No response, but remembering how casual the family were about locking doors, I tried the handle – and it opened at once, allowing me to walk in, and shout "Sheila?" No response – and now I began to worry that she might be in need of help. I walked round, calling her name, until I reached the kitchen; and there was evidence of her being at home, as a breakfast tray was on the side, ready to be carried – where?*

'*A quick search upstairs showed me that she had just risen, and left the bedclothes thrown back. Only the garden now remained as a possible place for her to be, so I went back downstairs and opened the kitchen door and stepped out into the garden. And there she was! In nightdress and gown, walking back to the house from the garden shed (where they kept goats). She looked at me, and simply said, "Oh hello Gwen, so sorry not to be there to greet you. I'm in bed with flu." I started to laugh, and said, "I see you are!" She began to explain that one of the goats was in difficulties giving birth and she had to help it out – but that was all now resolved. Her response was pure Sheila, unafraid and welcoming.*

'*We drank tea, caught up with family news, and I went on my way, leaving her back in her warm bed, with a hot drink, and a telephone to reach; I drove home laughing and happy to have been with a unique woman for a few valuable hours.*'

Depression

When Jenny was six weeks old in 1963, Uwe had been depressed. He had always experienced mood swings, and this was an especially bad time for him. We decided to have a holiday, so I asked my parents to look after the older children and we booked a week at the very comfortable hotel on Tresco in the Scilly Isles.

We flew from the mainland of Cornwall in a bi-plane constructed of balsa wood and painted canvas, patched up with what looked like sticking plaster.

There were just the pilot, Uwe and me, and the baby in her carrycot – and a large bunch of flowers tucked in behind the pilot. The plane shuddered into life, running down-hill for the take-off, and we rattled our way across to St Mary's, landing going up-hill, and coming to a safe stop. As we disembarked Uwe asked who the flowers were for. *'Oh, that is for my co-pilot who is in hospital in St Mary's. He crash-landed yesterday.'*

We went by boat to Tresco and settled into the hotel. Little sailing boats bobbed all around in a sparkling sea. It was like a Dufy painting. I suggested that Uwe look after Jenny for a bit while I went across to the big island to the book shop. I came back with a Penguin introductory book on sailing by Peter Heaton. Uwe read it avidly and the next day asked the fisherman if he would give him a lesson. He asked for another lesson but the fisherman said, *'From now on you will teach yourself. Hire a boat and get sailing.'* So that is what he did. Once he had got the hang of it I decided to join him, and we left Jenny asleep under the watchful eye of another friendly guest, the editor of *Nursery World*, who seemed a very suitable guardian. We sailed in sight of the shore, so she could hail me if Jenny woke for a feed.

From then on Uwe was a sailor, with boats on the Solent and in the Mediterranean, and a dinghy in France. His identity underwent a radical transformation. He was a happy man! Depression conquered without pills!

Bages

In 1968 we decided to look for a holiday home in France. Uwe is a great Francophile and wanted the children to absorb French culture. It also had to be a place where he could keep a boat and sail.

So we drove along the coast from Nice south towards the Spanish border, buying local newspapers and checking out the obituaries to get hot news about who had died and find likely properties. We found the ideal place in Languedoc just south of Narbonne, a *'village perché'* (a fortified hilltop village) among the vineyards on a salt water lake that connected with the sea, the *Étang de Bages*, crowned by an old church. There was a placard announcing its presence: '*Village d'Art*'. It had been a base for pirates who raided ships bringing goods from the Eastern Mediterranean. It looked like a quiet fishing village.

Only it wasn't quiet. The fishermen shouted from boat to boat across the water and along the cobbled streets, elderly women dressed in black sat on straight-backed chairs outside many of the houses, watching the world go by and exchanging local news. Everyone coming along the road shouted greetings, and conversations took place from window to window across the narrow alleys and from upstairs windows down into the street. It was a hive of activity and vibrant community life. Cats of all shapes and sizes roamed along the gutters as fishermen cleaned the slippery eels. When water rushed down open gullies at the sides of the road with tiny crabs, oysters and sprats bobbing in the flood stream, cats slithered and sprung to capture them, and then lay replete and glossy in the sun digesting their feast. Children played freely in the open, and as dusk descended there was the heavy clump-clump of *boules*. Festivals such as the *Sardinade,* which were held throughout the region in summer, involved everyone, villagers and visitors, and fire crackled as fresh sardines were cooked on open fires down by the shore to feed them. It seemed that every saint's day was celebrated with a dance in the village square and often with appearances from rock singers. The songs of Johnny Hallyday regularly livened things still further till the early hours of the morning. To all this was added the raucous cries of seagulls fighting over tit-bits and the clacking of marsh birds as the sun rose. The concept of noise pollution did not exist and you had to organise your life around these things.

There were no modern buildings. Islands were dotted between the inlet and the open sea. Sparsely planted vineyards scattered the lowland. The nearest supermarket was outside Narbonne. As we climbed into the village we entered narrow, cobbled lanes with room for just about two people to walk abreast.

Women were gathered at the *lavoir*, the communal washing area, scrubbing linen on flat stones and spreading it on the wide sides to dry in the sun. Hawkers were bringing in local market produce and their latest catch of fish. On Sundays many of the housewives stamped on live eels in the streets to get them to shed their scales – a task nowadays performed by cement mixers in the gardens. There was a bistro and bakery that sold bread and cakes still hot from the oven. We had found Bages!

The house we were looking for clung to the side of the rock, its windows facing the water, and beyond the gardens there was arid scrubland between it and the lagoon, with space to moor boats and a small, rickety jetty.

It was a three storey building. The *grenier* had a towering raftered ceiling and we realised that we could open up the whole wall facing the water, extending it with sturdy sliding glass doors onto a balcony. There was no sanitation and no reliable mains water supply, but that came after a few years, when top quality water flowed from the Rhone and the thirsty land could drink its fill. Then the whole area flourished and vineyards spread everywhere.

In high sun lizards slithered across the floor of the vast upper room, and as dusk approached bats flew in and out, and swallows and swifts swept through. Fortunately the dense clouds of mosquitoes, which had kept the whole region from tourism for so long, were fast disappearing as the land was being drained.

It wasn't easy to negotiate buying a house because often each room was the property of another member of the extended family, and getting agreement between them was a long and arduous task. The house we bought in April 1968 was right on the waterfront and built in about 1900. The stable was at street level, and it would also have been stuffed with wine barrels, fishing gear, and a boat squeezed in, too. People lived on the first floor. At the top the spacious and lofty *grenier* incorporated a tiny room where the stable boy slept.

We learned this from Mademoiselle Denise, an unmarried lady in long skirts and a floppy Victorian flowery bonnet, who was eager to let us know the history of the house, and said the stable boy had been her lover but never came back from the First World War. She had special memories of that little room. A shaft ran from one side of the *grenier* down to the stable at the bottom, and he forked hay down for the animals' feed. A stone circular staircase with black iron balustrades and glass knobs on it twisted its way up from street level to the loft.

The superb dimensions of the *grenier*, splendid exposed beams and red floor tiles presented an opportunity to create a huge living room, on one side a stairway leading to a pine balcony overlooking the main room, and an extra bathroom between the stairs and the back wall, the window of which opened onto sheer rock. Uwe designed it with great flair and did detailed architectural drawings that were followed minutely by the local builder and carpenter, Monsieur Dellong.

The light from the Mediterranean sky reflected in dazzling water thrilled me, and I knew I would want to paint – something I hadn't done since my teens. With the wide expanse of tiled floor I could handle large canvases of wood, silk stretched out and weighted at the corners, or hessian fixed to a big frame, and crawl round them with ample space surrounding. I could spill water or paint

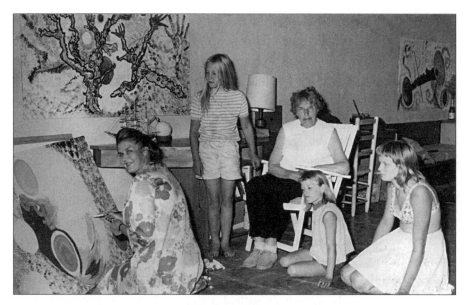

Painting in Bages

and clear it up easily, and leave work in progress overnight without having to
tidy it away. Lavishly decorated wall tiles and china cups and jugs would dry
off in the warm air and then be baked in the oven on the first floor. Uwe was
off sailing, and often the children too, and it was easy to see when they were on
their journey back across the water, so I could estimate their arrival time and
get a meal on to greet them. And when I was tired or inspiration faded I flopped
on a king-sized bed under a massive mosquito-netting tent, a good base, too,
for reading and writing and correcting proofs of articles and books.

I painted birth goddesses, several huge portraits of Uwe in the bath and
eating shellfish with gusto, the village cemetery with its family tombs, vineyards
stretching below, hoofed pan spirits eating grapes, and angels abundant
overhead, and vivid symbolic representations of dramatic world news, triumph
and disasters: earth and moon at the time of the first moon mission, Dubrovnik
under attack, lit by flames, with families sheltering in the cellars, and long lines
of starving people seeking food at distribution centres in Africa. The very first
painting was a pattern of the girls' heads and shoulders, focusing on the special
shape and angle of each, and their inter-relationships. I painted forms that
evolved from the shape of the spiral staircase, and the life that teemed around
and in the house, the rough grey stone walls with lizards and insects, moss and

leaves in their interstices, and a snake that slipped in if we left the back window open. Then there were the birds – the wetlands of Narbonne are a bird paradise – including pink flamingos, great flocks of them feeding in the *Étang*. Uwe's mother stayed with us and I painted her arthritic hands as the knotted branches of old olive trees. And there were sky and lakescapes with dramatic changes in the weather, dawn and sunset, and storms that came up with thunder and lightning crackling across the water, when it seemed the earth shook.

Though the first long drive down through France was stressful with five children in the car – for them as well as us (Celia nibbled at the car upholstery and Uwe was convinced she had eaten a sizable portion of the window frame on her side) – it was wonderful when we arrived. We towed a caravan for the first time so the children loved to sleep in it. When we stopped overnight at a luxury hotel the children slept in the caravan in the car park, and came one by one and on their best behaviour to have a bath in the hotel. I think the staff were rather bewildered by five blonde little girls all dressed alike – or was it one having five baths?

We stopped to buy provisions at little towns and stocked up with picnic foods for the children. This didn't prevent them standing outside the restaurant where we were dining, their noses pressed against the window. Waiters took pity on them and emerged from the kitchen with trays of fruit and other delicacies. I don't think French parents treated their children this way. They would have been sitting at the table until 10 at night.

Life in Bages allowed the girls great freedom, and they could roam and explore all round the village as they wished. They invented a hide-and-seek game they called 'Smith', because it linked to a book they enjoyed reading. All but one girl would hide in the nooks and doorways of the alleys, while another set out to find them. As each was discovered she joined the seeker. The hunt entailed jumping over sleeping cats and dogs and any other hazards. They always came in fresh-faced and shining from their game.

A small 12-foot, gaff-rigged dinghy came with the house, and seemed perfect for the children so that they could have adventures along the coast and into the canal.

We met the other foreigners in the village: Dr Dubost, a radiologist from Toulouse, who bought his house the same day as us, and he and his family became close friends.

The children's boat quickly acquired a name – *Trouble* (as trouble arrived every time they got in it). Our friend Margaret joined us with her daughter Miranda and the girls went on adventures together and there was one occasion when they didn't come home at nightfall.

A Letter To My Father, Summer 1972

My Dear Father,
We are having a gorgeous holiday. The weather is hot and sunny, with plenty of wind for sailing, and the children are all getting on very well together.

I have already done four paintings, one on the balcony wall and two on wood. At the moment Uwe has gone with Polly in Trouble, the little boat with the engine, to try to find Tess and her crew of Miranda, Nell and Jenny, who went out for a day's exploring of deserted islands at 10.30 a.m. this morning and are still not back at 8.30 p.m. No sign of a sail on the horizon, and soon it will be dark! But there is a breeze, unusual in the evenings here, so they should be able to get back. I don't know what we do if they don't turn up. Uwe's engine only takes fuel for an hour or so, so he couldn't get to all the islands to find them. Margaret has gone to Arles for the day. Still, they are good swimmers. I think that perhaps they wanted to go to different islands and so Tess dropped them off in different places and now can't find them to pick them up, or something of that kind. They will get cold, but beyond that I don't suppose any harm will come to them.

2 Days Later:
Well, that letter never got finished, because the girls did not turn up. Margaret got back to find her daughter still not returned and the sun setting. It was clear that a storm was brewing. The sky darkened, the wind roared.

No other boats were around. They had all scuttled to harbour. Hour after hour passed and night fell. There was no chance of them sailing back now. Polly and Uwe tried to reach the nearest islands in a very choppy sea, and came back not having sighted their sail, and with no indication of where they might be. We thought they might have made the mainland at Port la Nautique, the other side of the Étang, so Margaret and Uwe drove there (it is only half an hour or so away by road) and hoped to see the boat by a railway crossing which runs close to the water. It was pitch dark with only a little shrimp of a moon. The wind was blowing hard by now, and there was no sign of them.

We had got together food and drink and sleeping bags and blankets and hot water bottles, but when they returned without the girls we put them away and wondered what to do next. There are no coastguards here, so there is no rescue service on which to call, and one simply depends on friendly fishermen. We had no petrol for the engine of the little boat and Margaret fetched some from Narbonne. We had found a torch, although a very faint one, under Nell's pillow. It was now about one in the morning. Doors were banging with the wind and shutters flapping. Uwe went up to Dr Dubost who has six children of his own and a fast motor boat, but all the lights were out and he didn't want to disturb them. It was decided to go to bed and start the search again as soon as light dawned.

Of course, once we lay down we really started worrying. Had the boat floated away while they swam? Had one of them tried to swim after it and drowned way out in the lagoon? Had one of them stuck in deep mud near one of the islands and sunk? Had someone been hit on the head with the boom as it jibed and been knocked unconscious into the water? Uwe had said they need not wear life jackets all the time if they got in the way and hampered their movements, provided they had them on board. I thought of nasty men encountering a little girl on a lonely island. Were they all together, or had they split up? We had heard them say they wanted to visit different islands. What about Jenny? Had she become exhausted with swimming and exposure? Uwe felt terribly guilty for letting them go.

As soon as the sky got a bit lighter I made coffee and found extra jerseys for them in case they were weak with exposure and dehydration and Margaret and Uwe went off in the motor boat at 5.20 a.m. It takes about 2 hours to reach the island, a speck in the distance, on which it was most likely they had stayed if all was well, except that the wind was too awkward for them to make it back again. As a result I was left in suspense for some six hours (watching the horizon, and seeing if I could glimpse the wreckage of a boat) before they returned to say that they hadn't found the girls, but they had discovered the boat, intact and in good order, with a note tied to the mast saying that Tess, as captain, had decided the journey home was too difficult against the north wind and that they were sleeping on the island, on beds of seaweed in one of the deserted houses. The note said they intended to walk back around the Étang keeping as close to the shore as possible, but omitted to say which way round they were coming. Margaret said it was signed by everyone except Jenny, so we weren't sure that Jenny was all right. Inside the boat was a well kept log of the journey.

Uwe and Margaret chugged back, towing the boat behind them. They were soaked to the skin, and since we didn't know where to find the girls and they had neither of them had any breakfast, we had some bread and cheese, and then the idea was that Uwe and I should drive one way and Margaret in her car in the opposite direction to see if we could find them, with ample supplies of food and water. I could imagine them fainting by the roadside and baked by the sun, which was now very hot. Margaret left, and just as we were walking out of the door Tess came loping in, bright pink, hair wet and matted, and looking worried at what we would say. She made for the shower saying, "The others are on the road between here and Peyriac. Could you pick them up? Their feet are cut about by stones and it hurts them to walk." We rushed off and first encountered Nell and Jenny, grinning broadly and looking as if they had walked 50 yards or so, gaily hitching a lift from us. They had quarrelled with Miranda who was still back near the next village. In fact she was pretty near too, but her flipflops had split and she could hardly walk in them.

They had had a marvellous time. "It was fun", said Jenny, "Only we were worrying about you worrying." They had found a ruined cottage and sheltered behind its stones. The mosquitoes buzzed all night and attacked them. Tess made a plan of campaign, and as soon as they could see a short distance in front of them she started them paddling across the isthmus to a spit of the mainland that projected into the water, and they walked round the bay in the direction of Bages for about 5 kilometres. They had walked a good twelve miles back by following a railway track that runs between a finger of land extended into the lake, wading through shallow water and climbing over rocks, and then gone through fields and along lanes and roads in the direction of Bages.

They treated it as a great adventure and their first thoughts were to write it up in full in their diaries. They had suggested to some boys who were going back from the island that they ring the police in case we rang them, but the police never contacted us. They had not thought of taking our phone number with them and as it is not yet in the book did not get anyone they met to ring us, which would have simplified matters.

We scooped them up, listened to stories of their exploit with relief and admiration, and returned them to civilisation, showers and food.

We have just about caught up with our sleep, but not Uwe, who went down with a migraine, because of being so exhausted and also, I think, so anxious, and he has been sleeping all day solidly. The children have been flopped on their beds for long periods too, but Jenny and Polly have been learning water skiing with Dr

Dubost, and I gather Jenny is getting quite good at it. She has boundless energy, that child. She has been out with him twice already today, although the second time there was a lot of wind and she didn't like having her mouth full of water much of the time.

We have heard from Celia who had Josie staying with her, and was just off on a pacifist demonstration in Stratford and a Quaker youth walk in George Fox's footsteps round the north of England, and then to a meditation session with Hindus or Buddhists or someone, and I think she plans to spend a week or so in London.

Polly and Jenny have been cooking supper and I hear Tess's motor coming in across the lake. She has Miranda as crew and they went to fetch back Trouble, the little rowing boat, which Margaret and Uwe left at the island when they brought back the Bosun which the children had been sailing.

Uwe and I are going up in the Pyrenees and to have a look at Andorra while Margaret looks after the kids the week after next before she leaves. Later this week Margaret, Uwe, Nell, Polly and Miranda are cruising in the big boat, She, down to Spain. Tess likes to be captain of Fertility, so she is staying here.

Both fridges are working well, which is a blessing. The washing machine started as soon as it was plugged in, too. We have bought a liquidiser to make lemon drinks, grate cheese, etc. The house is much easier to run than it was three years ago! Tess jumped on the end of Miranda's bed yelling 'The lady likes Milk Tray' or something the significance of which I don't see, and it crashed to the ground. So we shall have to get the carpenter round.

Love Sheila

Another time Polly and Jenny were arrested by the police in *Trouble* on the canal between the sea and Narbonne. They had no identification and no evidence that they owned the boat. They were locked in cells and given some police magazines to look at. They used their incarceration to put tails on all the pictures of policemen and write '*cochons!*' beneath each. They were allowed to phone me. I got hold of Dr Dubost as quickly as I could and he drove to the police station and explained, as he rescued them, that the English had different educational methods from the French and wanted their children to be adventurous, not '*sage*'.

CHAPTER SIX

LECTURES AND BOOK TOURS

USA

From 1968 onwards, I travelled back and forth to the United States lecturing and publicising my first book *The Experience of Childbirth* and according to the dynamic feminist Norma Swenson, founder of Our Bodies Ourselves, and on the Faculty of the Harvard School of Public Health, had a *'groundbreaking role in changing the discourse in childbirth'*.

Norma invited me to lecture to the Boston Association of Childbirth Education. She flung open the doors of my career in challenging aggressive interventions in childbirth, *'just in case'* obstetrics and ceremonial birth procedures (those carried out by rote whether they are needed or not). It was my first visit to the United States since my time in Chicago in 1950 and I came face to face with a system in which male gynaecologists monopolised women's health care, having completely eliminated competition from midwives, and claimed exclusive access to and control over the organs of female reproduction.

Caring for patients was trivialised and gynaecologists only began to learn how to talk with and listen to them when competing for private patients, and probably did not acquire it at all if they worked with women in clinics. Interaction with patients was often depersonalised. Norma describes some doctors as *'surgical seducers'* who listened to women *'pretending an emotional involvement and interest, and many women responded to this by offering OBS their trust'*, the trust that later meant they accepted whatever advice and judgements were pronounced.

Scopolamine reigned. It had been the standard treatment for pain since the 1950s and was called *'Twilight Sleep'*, because women could wake up and be presented with babies they did not know they had because it removed all memory of birth, almost as if it had happened to someone else.

Dr Guttmacher promoted a three drug mix that should be given to all mothers. *'In favourable cases, under the influence of the drug triad, the patient falls into a deep quiet sleep between pains, but groans and moves about in a restless manner with each pain. The somnolent stage continues into the second stage of labor and frequently for several hours after delivery. When the patient awakes, the obstetrician is rewarded by hearing her ask, "Doctor, when am I going to have my baby?" The quickest way I know to prove that the child is already born is to have her feel her own abdomen. A newly restored waist-line soon convinces even the most sceptical.'*[10]

In fact, women did experience birth, but it was often like a bad dream and they had no control over it. When a woman had been *'scoped'* she screamed and tossed around helpless to do anything about it. Maternity wards sounded like torture chambers. The management solution was to corral patients in high barred cots, thickly padded so that they could not harm themselves, and with canvas fixed over the top to prevent them climbing out.

Introduced by a woman, Bertha Van Hoosen, an obstetrician who reported in the *Wisconsin Medical Journal* that it *'solves the problems of child-bearing'*,[11] the most enthusiastic advocates of Twilight Sleep were feminists, who saw it as the answer to birth pain to which every woman had a right, together with obstetricians who used it as a way of asserting their professional domination of childbirth.

The American College of Obstetricians and Gynecologists (ACOG) was established in 1951. The uterus was treated as an organ that could be whipped out without any problems (and still is today). It was just a useless little bag. By the 1980s more hysterectomies were performed in the United States than any other surgery – with the exception of caesarean sections. Data from the National Centre for Health Statistics shows that more than a third of American women will have a hysterectomy by the time they are 60. Statistics from the 1990s showed that women aged 40–44 years were more likely than any other age group to have a hysterectomy.[12]

Diana Scully's ground-breaking study[13] of the training of *'OBS'* and *'GYNS'* in two Boston hospitals was published a few years after I visited Boston and revealed that obstetricians were trained to prefer politely submissive patients. One explained, *'The main thing is that she understands what I say, listens to what I say, does what I say, and believes what I say.'*

Diana Scully also looked at the medical literature about female psychology and sex. Women have, for example, a pre-menstrual phase in which *'an oppressive, cyclic cloud ... stops them functioning in a logical, male fashion,'* according to the prestigious *American Journal of Obstetrics and Gynaecology,* and one text book stated that a wife *'should make herself available for the fulfilment of her husband's sexual drive'.*

In her interviews with obstetric residents in training she learned that *'medical judgement'* and *'surgical skill'* were the most important elements: *'You know what you are doing, you take it out, and the patient gets better.'* She asked students how they learned about female sexuality. Answers ranged from *Playboy* to the army. Though women expected gynaecologists to be able to counsel them sexually, few in the profession had read any parts of Masters and Johnson's classics.[14] One doctor who was about to give sexual counselling said that he had not actually *read* them but had seen the authors on television.

In their first year residents used forceps for delivery more frequently than later on, since this was the special skill they wanted to learn then and were required to have as part of their training. As one put it: *'I use them a lot to gain the experience of using them. There is almost no time when you can't use them, unless the woman delivers before you get the forceps on.'* They gained status with colleagues as surgeons, not 'baby catchers'. They were not interested in normal birth because they didn't think they learned anything from it and used women as teaching material. They were concerned to gain experience in doing hysterectomies and caesareans and to repair injured organs: *'I need more hysterectomies ... I thought I would never have enough sections, but eventually I said I had enough. ... I have to see an injured bowel and injured bladder.'* So they negotiated with colleagues and developed techniques for talking women into having unnecessary operations. One resident described what he would tell a patient with small fibroids: *'I would explain to her ... that these fibroids may sometime in the future grow bigger, may get symptoms, may cause her trouble; she may need surgery at some point in time, and if she would like to have surgery done now, it can be easy surgery ... She won't have any more children, but she won't have any fibroids, and she won't have any potential for disease.'*

* * *

With the Boston Women's Health Collective Norma and her sister activists challenged the male monopoly of women's health and in the first edition of a remarkable book, *Our Bodies, Ourselves*, urged women to be responsible for their own bodies, demand genuine informed choice, and the opportunity for undisturbed birth in an emotionally supportive setting. I was privileged to be part of that movement.

In a recent communication, Norma kindly said of that time, '*You were a breath of fresh air, and sophistication – almost as if you came from another planet! As I told Uwe, I still remember the dress you wore not only to a public lecture in the church we used but also to an afternoon tea reception for the doctors held in someone's house. It was a black crepe dress, and had large ladder faggoting all down the long sleeves from the shoulders, making a dramatic effect each time you gestured, which you did often and expansively. The doctors who came were drawn to you like some kind of sexual magnet, could not take their eyes off you, and crowded around to have a look and press flesh (your hand, I mean), leaving the rest of us to languish in our usual frumpy respectable Boston "meet the doctors" get-ups, otherwise reserved for church. Nothing of that dramatic impact had ever happened before, and it put me, and BACE, on the map, so to speak.*'

How Not To Push A Baby Out

While I was teaching prenatal classes in Cambridge, Massachusetts, in 1969–70, Uwe was Visiting Professor of Government at Harvard, replacing Henry Kissinger who had gone to work in Nixon's White House.

All the fathers turned up for the classes because this was expected of couples who were doing Lamaze training. In France a woman's obstetric physiotherapist guided her. When psychoprophylaxis crossed the Atlantic the male partner took her place. Elizabeth Byng adapted French psychoprophylaxis and produced a new equally rigid American version.

The male partner managed the breathing training, and supervised it during labour, in a way that struck me as highly intrusive. Men came to classes with stop-watches, to time contractions and regulate breathing with precision – so many breaths at precise '*levels*' in the first stage, and in the second stage commands to the woman to hold her breath for at least 30 seconds. In order to push effectively, the longer she could hold it, the more *successful* she was. At that time birth education classes, and above all the Lamaze method, put strong emphasis on strenuous pushing and prolonged breath-holding.

Women were also taught to contract their abdominal muscles while they pushed. Yet a woman who pulls in her abdominal muscles usually simultaneously tightens her pelvic floor muscles, resisting the descent of the baby's head, and causing herself unnecessary pain. For these muscles are completely released only when the lower abdomen is allowed to bulge out, the opposite of a sucking-in movement. It struck me that women were being trained to do something which was quite unnatural. Our home in England was on the edge of the Cotwolds – sheep country. Walking past fields in which ewes were giving birth at the peak of lambing time, I was fascinated to see how they breathed. They pushed their young out with short, rapid breaths and open mouths. Cats and dogs do the same. They do not go in for all the huffing and puffing and breath-holding that women are taught to do. Nor do they get into the extraordinary positions which are often required of women in labour, lying flat on their backs with their legs in the air. They are in a semi-upright position and, with the pelvis tilted, move around and often shift position during the expulsive stage.

When a woman does what comes naturally she is likely to breathe in the same way as other mammals. It is a breathing pattern like that of sexual excitement and orgasm.

In orgasm breathing is at least three times faster than usual. As a woman reaches a climax her breath is involuntarily held and she gasps, groans, sighs or cries out. When it fades her breathing gets slower again. If it is a multiple orgasm (waves of desire and fulfilment, with intervals between each) her breathing speeds up with each new wave and she holds her breath for a few seconds. She may do this up to five times at the height of orgasm. Her breathing slows down as it passes.

This is how a woman breathes when she acts spontaneously pushing out a baby, too. If she is not told what to do, she usually breathes quickly, holds her breath for a few seconds, breathes out, continues to breathe fast, holds it again for a few seconds, and so on, until the contraction starts to fade. And just like a woman having an orgasm, she wants to hold her breath like this between one and five times at the height of each contraction.

In conferences around the world I demonstrated this on stage, lying on

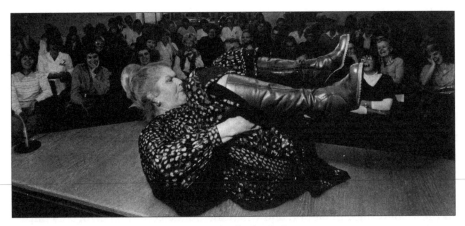

How not to push the baby out

my back on any table that was handy. I remember doing it in Milan lying on a judicial bench in the council chamber under the gaze of portraits of city notables and local saints.

I was always fully dressed with a cape and jewellery of course. I might be wearing long boots, and often a hat. I admit it produced a comic scene. But that was my intention. The performance often brought the house down. I huffed and puffed and strained and blew. I groaned and gasped with gaping jaws. At this point I adopted the role of the encouraging midwife, who admonished me sternly, '*Close your mouth! You can't push with your mouth open!*' So I clamped my jaws together and did it again, drawing a huge breath and hanging on to it, and blew out my cheeks, went red in the face, and my eyes popped. There was a fresh wave of laughter, because midwives had seen it all before, even though they hadn't realised how ludicrous this frantic pushing was.

I saw this enacted in real life in delivery rooms, '*Push! Push! Don't waste your contraction! Take a deep breath and hold it. Now come on, you can do better than that! Push as if you were constipated! Take another breath and hold it for as long as you can!*'

A male physiological model was, and often still is, imposed on women. The characteristic pattern of male orgasm – stiffen, hold, force through, shoot! – (I usually accompanied this with dramatic arm movements!) distorts our spontaneous psycho-sexual behaviour. Instead of the wave-like rhythms of female orgasm, bearing down is treated like a mighty ejaculation. A woman must carry on as long as she can and then sinks back, exhausted.

* * *

There is an endocrinological connection between sexual arousal and the intense sensations of childbirth. Identical hormones pour into the woman's bloodstream. Endorphins, the body's natural opiates, are not only pain-killers. They make us feel good. Pleasurable athletic activity, sex and birth all involve the release of endorphins. In the 70s, Niles Newton explored the action of oxytocin, which she called 'the psychoactive hormone of love and breastfeeding' in sexual arousal and childbirth. A rush of oxytocin pours into her bloodstream when a woman is sexually excited, when she has a passionate urge to bear down in the second stage of labour, and when the milk ejection reflex occurs during lactation. But this 'psychoactive' hormone is easily inhibited.

Women who have had a distressing labour often tell me that sexual excitement and feelings during birth can have no possible connection with each other. Yet the energy that flows through the body in childbirth, the pressure of uterine muscle that is contracting spontaneously, the downward movement of the baby, and the fanning open of soft tissues, can be erotic. A woman who is enjoying her labour swings into the rhythm of contractions as if birth-giving were a powerful dance. She waits for the contraction, and focuses on it, like an orchestra following its conductor. When she pushes it is an expression of sexual energy, of longing and fulfilment, and if she has the loving support to achieve harmony between mind and body, it can be a psychosomatic experience of transmutation and metamorphosis.

Many women never have a chance to experience this because the second stage is managed as a battle to get a baby born, under instructions from their attendants. It is turned into a contest in which a woman struggles to push the baby down through the barriers of flesh, spurred on by everyone present. In hospitals around the world I have seen cheerleading teams urging a mother to greater effort, more sustained and deeper breaths, more energetic strainings.

This not only makes her feel that she is falling short of a standard impossible to attain, but imposes stress on the second stage which sometimes adversely affects the baby. When a woman is exhausted with straining, bursts blood vessels in her face and eyes, and tries to hold her breath for as long as possible, there is a risk of cardio-vascular disturbance that affects the baby's heart rate, oxygen supply, and acid base balance.[15] If a woman holds her breath and strains for a long time her blood pressure drops. This reduces the oxygen available to the baby. Then, when she can push no longer, she gasps for air and her blood pressure shoots up above normal. But long before this stage is reached the flow of oxygenated blood to the fetus may already be reduced. What often happens then is that the dips in the fetal heart rate which persist after the end of the contraction are taken as a signal for her to push still harder and hold her breath longer. This has the effect of cutting down the baby's oxygen supplies further.

For me the power of birth is like the strength of water cascading down the hillside, the power of seas and tides, and of mountains moving. There is no way of ignoring it. You cannot fight it. Techniques cannot enable a woman to control it as she might be in control of a car or a computer. I believe that whoever is helping should aim not to manage, conduct, or coach, but to give her strength and confidence as she allows her body to open and her baby to press through it to life. Midwives can help use this powerful sexual energy to keep birth normal.

Decca Mitford

I spoke at exciting conferences in America in which mothers and midwives got together to explore the possibilities of birth in a setting where women were free to do their own thing, learn about recent research, and plan campaigns in their communities.

I first met Jessica Mitford when I was lecturing at a conference in support of midwives in Oakland, California, and she joined me on the platform. Decca was no feminist and seemed surprised by the feminist fervour of the meeting. She always loved jokes, and indeed, her way of coping with distress and tragedy in her life, of which she had a heavy dose, was to laugh. This wasn't a joke. She opened her talk by turning to me and saying, *'I didn't know that I was going to be at a revivalist meeting.'* Information about birth was not really her metier and she contemplated it with something approaching horror, and midwives, I think, with suspicion.

Decca and her fellow Communist human rights lawyer husband Robert Treuhaft later visited me following the enormous success of her book *The American Way of Death*, which described funeral homes, the mortician industry, and the whole ritualised monopoly of dying and being laid out in the United States. She was researching a book on birth.

We discussed possible titles and I suggested *'The American Way of Birth'* because, in much the same way, it was an exposure of the obstetric system. Kenneth Galbraith, the economist, a close friend of hers, was doubtful about this because it was 'hitchhiking' on the earlier book. I introduced her to 'the empathy belly' designed to involve expectant fathers in pregnancy – a heavily weighted inflatable apron that a man should wear to learn what it was like to be pregnant, and how it slowed a woman down, caused backache, and made it hard to get comfortable at night, or even to sit and walk. I also told her about 'the intra-uterine university' to start early education of the fetus, which involved listening to its heart beats and playing music to which the baby could respond.

Subsequently I sought her advice about publishing and getting an agent, and she put me on to a woman who had been like an adopted daughter to her, Mary Clemmey, who remained my literary agent for some years.

When Decca died of a rapid cancer she faced it with huge courage and planned her funeral in San Francisco with a glass antique hearse pulled by six plumed horses. A marching band, led by a saxophonist friend, followed the cortege, blaring out rousing hymns, including 'When the Saints Come Marching In'. We celebrated her life in an upbeat way in London. Her friends gathered in a theatre to extol her and focus on her colourful personality with a party afterwards.

Palo Alto

At a big International Childbirth Education Association conference in Palo Alto, California, in 1979 I spoke about rites and ceremonies in childbirth. My joy in acting was expressed in my style of lecturing. I didn't want to stand at a lectern and orate. I aimed to use my body to bring to life the different scenarios of birth in various cultures and draw dramatic contrasts. At Palo Alto I acted how women in Jamaica gave birth with strong pelvic movements, chanting with cries to the Lord, and drew on the passionate experience of 'getting the spirit' in revivalist worship up in the hills with dance and song.

Margot Edwards and Mary Waldorf described it this way: 'Sheila acted a scene from a Caribbean revivalist church where women worshipped through song and dance. She rocked and gyrated in rhythm, stunning her audience with a dance that put the West Indian women in touch with the mysteries of their common past and opened them to a shared future.'[16]

I didn't just talk about but demonstrated how medicalised birth trapped the mother by immobilising her and forcing her to lie on her back, often destroyed her capacity to give birth spontaneously by eliminating oxytocin liberated in the blood stream, and turned birth into an ordeal, so that the whole process was reduced to one of pain.

Margot Edwards and Mary Waldorf went on: '*With equal drama, she described a different sort of ceremony, the rites of high-tech birth. The patient, dressed in hospital-issue gown, lies in bed with catheter in one arm and others inserted through her vagina into her uterus and infant so the contractions and fetal heart rate can be recorded on a machine. Communication between women and man is limited since she is immobilised and he is intrigued by blips on the monitor. Already the woman has undergone initiation into the patient role by ritual shaving and cleansing. She undergoes further humiliation in a delivery room filled with surgical equipment and peopled by masked figures.*'

I showed how when an obstetrician isolates with drapes the lower half of a woman's body, it becomes *his* sterile field. But it is clearly neither his nor, because of the juxtaposition of vagina and anus, sterile. It is a convenient fiction, however, by which he asserts his rights and insists that the woman keeps hands off her own body, which becomes out of bounds.

Niles Newton

It was at one of the American conferences that I first met Niles Newton, an amazing woman who did research with her husband Michael, an obstetrician and professor at Chicago University, on the impact of '*happiness*' hormones on feelings, mothering behaviour, lactation and birth. She did a lot of work with mice, demonstrating the effects of disturbance on labour, and discovering, by introducing swabs soaked in cat's pee into the cages of mice when they were having their pups, that they had longer and more difficult labours and were more likely to give birth to dead pups. Environmental disturbance can be dangerous.

She researched the environment for breastfeeding. Studying the effects of distraction and stress, she revealed that it affected the release of milk and the ability to breastfeed. Michael plunged her feet in icy water or asked her complicated maths questions while she was breastfeeding and compared the milk flow then with other days in which she could concentrate. There were two kinds of distraction days: in one Niles had a placebo injection of salt water or artificial oxytocin – she didn't know which. When she had oxytocin and was distracted the quantity of milk she produced was almost equal to days on which she was not disturbed.

In her book *Maternal Emotions*[17] she showed how lactation rites common in hospitals, including washing or wiping the nipples with an alcohol swab, damaged women's chances of breastfeeding. She had deep insight into birth and breastfeeding as part of a woman's sexuality in which, when she was undisturbed, there were oxytocin surges in her bloodstream. There was tremendous resistance to this from many people, as I found, too, whenever I wrote about the sensuality of birth. Niles had studied with the anthropologist Margaret Mead in the 60s and, like me, developed a cross-cultural view of birth and breastfeeding.

One outcome of Niles' research on oxytocin, however, was that keen breastfeeders who were determined to do everything right added an oxytocin nasal spray to their breastfeeding kit, along with a curvy banana-shaped feeding cushion, a pump to extract milk and store supplies in the freezer, bottles and teats, and nipple creams and sprays, even though her research specifically showed that these were counter productive.

South Africa

In the early 70s I was invited to lecture in South Africa and had the opportunity to visit hospitals and indigenous birth practitioners in Johannesburg and Cape Town to learn about birth there. As a midwife bustled me through the labour wards of Cape Town hospital, the largest in the southern hemisphere (the register in the maternity department said *'Admissions 1973: 20,601'*) she remarked *'The Bantu aren't noisy in labour. It's the staff who make the noise.'* It sounded as if life was very stressful for them. I glanced down the list and saw categories for *'ruptured uterus'*, rare in the West, for *'symphysiotomy'* (slicing open the front of the pelvic cage), though this drastic operation had gone down from 87 in 1963 to only four in 1973. Groans were coming from the 25 cubicles in the delivery room, women writhing, mostly alone, with great puddles of blood on the floor. *'For God's sake turn off that drip! The fetal heart is down to*

80.' The patient, sweat pouring off her, was lying flat, her head pushing against the bars at the top of the delivery table as she struggled not to bear down yet. *'Forceps – quickly!'*

All the maternity patients in this hospital were likely to be high risk cases. For most women had to be delivered at home, whether they wished it or not, in the African township outside Johannesberg where the Bantu were herded in row upon row of small concrete and tin-roofed shacks, up to four families living in each.

We went into a dark, unfurnished room where the women were kneeling on the pitted concrete floor. Elisabeth, an impressive matron with a number of small foster-children clustered round her, indicated that I should kneel in front of her. She was in training as a witch doctor, was a trained nurse for seven years before, but now felt it was her vocation to do Zulu tribal healing. Her mentor, Dorcas, an established witchdoctor, knelt shyly in the corner, hiding behind the child on her lap. They told me about herbs which, taken in pregnancy *'make the baby play free inside'*, how to deliver a baby when labour is prolonged by smearing the hands with bone marrow and helping it *'get through the road which is closed'*. *'She must follow the pain, keep quiet and listen.'* The mother holds the baby and kisses it immediately, for *'the child must know who is the mother'*. She confirmed that grandmothers breastfeed when the mother must be absent at work, but said that there was more and more bottle feeding. I had noticed the hoardings for artificial baby milk as we drove through Soweto *'Mom fed me on KLM'* and for SMA, the most expensive milk on the market.

We talked about sex too. When the baby is three months old, the husband says he is going to *'grow up the child with intercourse'*. I asked how the woman felt about it. Elisabeth rolled her eyes and exclaimed, *'The wife feel sweet – oh! Oh! Oh! – Then!'* *'When he feels the wife has felt it he discharges outside until the child is one year.'* Then she went into a trance and started to prophesy.

I also interviewed Vusamazulu Credo Mutwa who knew ancient Zulu practices and lore which were no longer understood by most of the Zulus in Soweto. Although he had written a book, an epic of tribal myth, *Indaba My Children,*[18] and I expected to meet an author living in fairly comfortable surroundings, his home was the same kind of dwelling as those of Elisabeth and Dorcas. Europeans keep their pigs or chickens in similar huts. We squatted on mats. A storm was building up and the sky was black with clouds, I could no longer see the carvings, drums and sacred objects crowding his dwelling. The air was electric and the heavy rumble of thunder came nearer and nearer.

I asked him if male witch doctors had anything to do with childbirth. He told me that in the past a witchdoctor should be present to bless the ground on which the first-born was to be delivered, and to help in cases of need. Maidens smeared cow dung on the floor of the grandmother's dwelling where a woman usually gave birth. 'When the child is born it must look on something beautiful, for this will affect its life.' So coloured beads and special childbirth carvings decorate the room. 'The first minute of life is the most important.' If the woman bleeds too much, the witch doctor orders a red calf to be sacrificed and she drinks some of its blood. After delivery she is always given a special dish of spinach to make her blood strong. A retained placenta is delivered by getting the mother to blow into a bottle. This is an almost worldwide practice for dealing with a delayed third stage.

It was the custom for a male witch doctor to deliver his own child so that it might inherit his spirit. He said hospitals make this impossible – doctors and nurses 'do not realise that the forces that activate the birth are much older than humanity itself. They turn birth into a spiritual nightmare'. He told me Zulu children are taken to see a birth 'to instil in them respect for human life' and 'to regard birth and death as part of life'. Not all women were allowed to bear children, and girls of 16 who have irregular periods use a pessary made of gum, hair and Kaffir beer water. Swazi women considered unfit for childbearing have a tiny stone inserted in the uterus.

When the great migrations took place tribal elders sought forgiveness of the ancestors, animals were killed and their livers used for divining, and the ceremony of 'closing of the gate of the mothers' was performed, using stones from a sacred river.

It became increasingly difficult to hear Credo's soft words as torrents of rain beat on the tin roof, and lightening ripped across the sky, followed by an enveloping roll of thunder.

In the third month of pregnancy the Zulu woman was taught by a folk midwife how to breathe 'to give life and strength to the child'. Each morning she went outside the hut and facing the East, took three deep breaths, followed by a long breath out, to cast out all evil. In labour she focused all her energy on breathing alternately through her mouth and her nose 'to lessen her consciousness of pain'.

In the second stage, Zulu Shangaans and the Bechuanas kneel in labour, whereas the Bushman woman make a space in the bush, like a nest of grass, and tying a rope to the branch of a tree, bears down while holding the rope. Traditionally there was an opening to the sky in the centre of the roof of a Zulu dwelling. *'She must kneel, concentrating all her attention on this space, through the hole where she can see the stars. We say of a woman who is in labour: she is counting the stars with pain.'* I later included what he told me in my book, *Rediscovering Birth.*[19]

The next day I was invited to visit the most luxurious private maternity home in Johannesburg. It was like moving between two different worlds. *'There's the woman, varnishing her nails, a box of chocolates at her side, the radio blaring and the baby hanging at one breast, and she is supposed to be trying to feed it ... They're spoiled little rich girls in here!'* said the obstetrician, (who made his living out of them). This clinic was designed to provide rooming-in for mother and baby, but now according to doctors, was losing money because the patients could not tolerate having their babies with them, and preferred nursing homes where newborns were lined up in central nurseries to be looked after by the staff.

Sister told me: *'Lots of mummies are silly. They handle their babies as if they were little china dolls. They go home with a Sister, and often two Sisters, one for the day and one for the night, and when they leave an African nanny takes over.'* I asked what education was provided for women in caring for and relating to their own babies, and she said, *'Mummies like to cuddle too much. They spoil the babas.'* And indicating the glass doors leading from each mother's bed through to the nursery, *'Of course, we lock the hatches when the daddies come. They are not allowed to touch the babies.'* At night, according to the paediatrician, the mothers were fed several Mogadons, and the babies removed and sent to the central nursery. The women wake up *'with breasts like footballs'.* I said that it was not surprising that parents who were not encouraged to explore and handle their babies failed to develop confidence. *'But,'* protested the obstetrician, *'we can't have women mollycoddling their babies!'* This, I was told by the Association for Childbirth Education, was the most progressive maternity home I would see. I went away shuddering.

In the private maternity home where Grantly Dick-Read introduced what were then his revolutionary ideas of birth without fear, the nuns sat in a circle of beaming faces and fresh white habits, offering tea and cakes. But here babies were not with their mothers at all, but in solid masses of plastic cribs in rows like cemeteries for the war dead. '*Oh, it's rarely that a mother asks for her baby*', Matron said. '*We believe mothers need a rest.*' The nuns glowed as they tended '*their*' babies. Fathers were taboo, and although some were present to watch the delivery, most were sent to the fathers' waiting room downstairs where they smoked and worried together, and – latest development of modern technology – viewed the births on a TV screen. Mothers and mothers-in-law turned up too, and sat with vicarious pleasure or suffering watching their daughters deliver. All the mothers were white. Apartheid might have been beginning to crumble – but only just. '*We have to get permission from Community Development when perhaps an Indian doctor's wife wants to have her baby here, and she has to be kept separate. We have a room downstairs where we can keep her.*'

The Politics Of Birth In South Africa

At the end of the 70s I did a lecture tour and spoke at the PACE conference and visited both private and public hospitals in the Transvaal. The public hospitals were like cattle markets.

Change started to come in Cape Town, which was ahead of the rest of South Africa. Home birth was becoming popular, for example. One childbirth activist wrote, '*Traditionally coloured midwives have always practiced among their own people – they are trained nursing sisters. However, no more training for them has been provided for some time, so their ideas are often archaic. The idea was to phase them out and move the women to hospital. But now there is a group of young white midwives becoming active. It's sad to say, but because they are white they have more clout. I have a large number of American and German couples, with other European countries well represented. I am also seeing a small number of coloured (not black) Indian and Malay couples. It is especially hard for Malay (muslim) fathers to attend, because they are considered "perverted" by their families. I have one such couple at the moment, and while the parents' families are trying to make plans for ceremonial treatment of the baby and the placenta, all the young people are interested in is getting the full Leboyer birth right (complete with sitar music!) This is a real clash of generations.*'

In 1983 I received an invitation from the National Childbirth Association and the University of the Witwaterstrand in Johannesburg. *The Experience of Sex* had just been published there and my publishers were keen for me to appear because it was selling very well. The book was banned at first by the Censorship Board, which allowed publication only after seven photographs had been removed. I declined the invitation telling them '*It would be wrong to condone a society which is based on apartheid*'.

CHAPTER SEVEN

EMOTIONS IN CHILDBIRTH

I have always been passionate about what I believe. Not for me cool, unengaged opinions. Body, mind and spirit, I get involved. How we give birth is an important element in feminism.

In Sylvia Pankhurst's book *The Suffragette*[20] I couldn't find one single reference to babies, pregnancy or childbirth. Yet for the majority of suffragettes babies were as much a part of daily existence as the wind and weather. Most struggled, as they themselves proclaimed, with *'one hand tied behind their backs'* trying to pack in a revolutionary cause between feeding a family their dinner, the cries of a baby for the breast, and cleaning up and running a house. Unpaid domestic labour, the bearing and nurturing of children, runs as a common thread between the lives of the suffragettes and those of us who are mothers today.

Until recently those common patterns have been considered by feminists less central to the struggle than rights to abortion and free child care.

When the childbirth movement started after the Second World War it was anti-feminist, part of a wave of idealisation of motherhood, social pressure for women to return to the home, and psychoanalytic teaching about motherhood as emotional fulfilment. The ideal woman seemed to be the breast-feeding mother-at-home clustered around by cherubs. (You could almost see her halo and the enfolding wings.)

In *Giving Birth: Emotions in Childbirth*, published in 1971, I wrote from a radical perspective: *'Birth is treated as if it were a pathological event rather than a normal life process and this has an effect on all those working professionally with childbearing women as well as on the women themselves. By concentrating* almost exclusively on the training of obstetricians and midwives on the diagnosis and treatment of disease and malfunction and on intervention, our society has succeeded in producing professionals many of whom have never seen a natural birth and who know nothing of the skills of supporting the normal physiological process. It is important for those working in maternity care to understand labour also as women experience it and this is much more subtle than just saying "It's painful" or "It's painless".[21]

'The woman who attends the antenatal clinic or who is in labour is supposed to be a 'good patient'; that is, she is meant to be quiet, placid, polite, appreciative of what is being done to her, quick to respond to instructions, able to comprehend and remember what she is told without requiring the information a second time, clean, neat and self-contained and should not disturb other patients, or the staff, by emotional instability of any kind. The word "patient" itself derives from "passivity"; the patient is someone to whom something is done...

'In achieving the depersonalisation of childbirth and at the same time solving the problem of pain, our society may have lost more than it has gained. We are left with the physical husk; the transcending significance has been drained away. In doing so, we have reached the goal which perhaps is implicit in all highly developed technological cultures, mechanised control of the human body and the complete obliteration of all disturbing sensation.'[22]

I found myself in conflict with feminists who saw birth in very simplistic terms of women's right to labour without pain, and failed to analyse it in terms of institutional power and women's relative powerlessness.

In 1975 *Spare Rib*, the radical campaigning feminist magazine, tackled the subject of childbirth. It followed what amounted to a revolutionary article in the *Sunday Times* of 24 October, 1974, by Louise Panton and Oliver Gillie, who claimed, 'Normal childbirth in hospital has become pathologised'. Birth had not been debated by feminists before this, perhaps because it seemed less to do with women's political and social rights than with female biology.[23]

Spare Rib quoted from the British Medical Association's handout for pregnant women *You and Your Baby*, and exposed its sexism.

The authors went on to quote from the National Childbirth Trust's *Expectant Fathers*: 'A woman is inclined to link the big moments in her life with clothes so when she is going to have a baby her thoughts run on "little garments" ... Your *wife may well be attracted by a pram that either looks like her neighbour's or is the exact opposite (!) depending on whether she is an individualist or the reverse; it will be up to you to see that the brakes work and the handle is the right height for easy pushing. Don't forget that you may want to take your child out yourself sometimes!*

Caring for a baby may have little in common with a manufacturing process but your wife's gratitude will repay you if you simplify feeding, bathing and cleaning routines with intelligent application of a little time and motion study.[24]

The *Spare Rib* article focused on pain as the main issue. It called for the development of medical technology to make birth pain free: *'It is the right of every woman to give birth painlessly'*. At that time feminists were not concerned with the power imbalance between the medical system and women giving birth and unselfconsciously lent their support to the system that I believed was abusing them. Without producing any evidence the authors asserted, *'Undoubtedly, hospitals with all their faults are the safest places in which to give birth. For this reason we think we should press for improvements in hospitals rather than support a move to more home confinements'*. I was appalled at how my sister-feminists could fail to support woman-centred birth.

When the British version of *Our Bodies, Ourselves* came out, it unfortunately described birth in American terms, as if it were always conducted by obstetricians, assisted by nurses – and ignored the role of midwives. I believed that the failure to support midwives was a big mistake and meant that, in effect, feminists were promoting an American model of childbirth in which the male obstetrician was king, to such an extent that the book talked throughout about 'him'.

Revolution started in 1982, with the Royal Free Protest, when 5,000 women came out on to the streets for the right to move around and give birth in any position they wished, to be active birth-givers rather than passive patients. The childbirth organisations, feminists, midwives and mothers joined hands and realised their common cause. Women could no longer be ignored. To reclaim the uterus women have to confront the might of the medical profession, the power of the international drug companies – and all our *own* self-doubts and fears and anxiety. I believe each one of us who dares to be assertive speaks for other women who have no voice.

Birth is a major life transition. It is – must be – also a political issue, in terms of the power of the medical system, how it exercises control over women and whether it enables them to make decisions about their own bodies and their babies.

Researching Induction Experiences

Department of Health statistics published in 1976 revealed that 41 per cent of labours were induced. Many labours were also accelerated, having started spontaneously, and these were often not recorded. In fact, some hospitals set up intravenous drips for all labouring women. It meant that 70–80 per cent of women in these hospitals were attached to an oxytocin drip to stimulate the uterus. It stretches the imagination to believe that this proportion of women had something so wrong with them that they could not be allowed to labour spontaneously.

When I had studied women's experiences of induction in the 70s it was obvious that most women didn't want to be induced unless it was absolutely necessary. A minority sought it for social reasons, but the vast majority had little opportunity to discuss whether they wanted it or not, and it was often done without explanation or consent. The result was that they felt assaulted. Some were lucky to have explanations because these were given to students and midwives over their supine bodies. But for most women who were induced the birth experience was marred by a sense of helplessness. There was wide variation between hospitals, too. Some induced an astonishing 75 per cent of labours, while in others inductions were below 12 per cent, even though the women were the same mix of high and low risk.

Active Management had aimed at medico-surgical control of childbirth and women's spontaneous activity became industrialised. Its inventors explained that it resulted in *'a regular and orderly turnover of work in a planned manner'*. It *'rationalises work flow in delivery suites which usually are "bottle-necks"; continuous fetal monitoring for every woman, with monitors placed centrally at the nursing station so that observers can see the state of the fetus without needing to stand beside the patient's bed, and the management of labor so that it is short … The Active Management of labor necessitates that obstetricians take over, not just a single aspect of delivery, but responsibility for the whole process of parturition. Our control of the situation must be complete.'*[25]

I was influenced by the research by Iain Chalmers and others who analysed 9,907 births in Cardiff between 1968 and 1972, where one obstetric team imposed Active Management and another had a more relaxed approach. There was no difference in the condition of the babies, but more urinary and genital tract infections in the actively managed mothers, and the authors concluded that active management had done nothing to improve perinatal outcomes.[26]

Professor Alec Turnbull, in Oxford, commenting on the way in which maternity units competed with each other to introduce new techniques, pointed out that because the national perinatal mortality rate fell steadily over the period when these manoeuvres were increasing, a cause-and-effect relationship was assumed which engendered a false feeling of security about the value of obstetric intervention. Much of the technology now used in obstetrics was introduced, and became routine clinical practice, without adequate research and with no strong evidence of its advantages. It is difficult for a woman who is told, '*This is done for the benefit of mother and baby*' to query the use of electronic fetal monitoring or an oxytocin drip, for example. Moreover, many hospital rites are taken for granted by members of staff and performed as a matter of course, so that to question them seems almost insulting.

A Birth Revolution Starts

The 1970 British Perinatal Mortality Study had revealed that with induction three times more babies suffered respiratory depression than after spontaneous labour. Of course, labour was induced in some cases *because* the babies were at risk. But a combination of the powerful, rapidly recurring contractions of induced labour and pain-relieving drugs to enable the mother to cope with this kind of labour may have contributed to breathing difficulties in the newborn baby. There was also an association between forceps deliveries, Caesarean sections, babies going into intensive care and rising trends of induction and acceleration.

Yet rates of induction multiplied. Tim Chard, a professor of Reproductive Physiology, commented: '*Spontaneous labour is now an abnormality.*'[27] In 1975 the latest statistics available from the Department of Health were for 1972. There was a 30 per cent rate then, compared with 26 per cent in 1970 and 18 per cent in 1958. By 1974 some hospitals were reporting rates of over 60 per cent. It could be assumed that the average was a good deal higher than 30 per cent. Kick-starting labour, along with time limits on the stages of dilatation and expulsion, came to be a routine element in the obstetric control of childbirth. Induction was just another way of managing labour.

A television programme in 1975 contributed to altering the induction rate in the John Radcliffe Hospital in Oxford overnight: in the three months before the programme, the induction rate had been 61 per cent; in the three months after the programme on induction, the induction rate was 37 per cent. It demonstrates the effect of television publicity.

Professor Alec Turnbull, who had been a strong proponent of induction and the active management of labour, lowered the rate to 9 per cent following the study in Cardiff.[28]

Research on induction is fraught with difficulties. One problem is that as the rate increases more low risk mothers get included in the induction group and perinatal mortality falls in that category. Effects of induction *per se* are no longer being measured. This can give quite an erroneous impression that synthetic oxytocin is less hazardous than it is. Women at greatest risk are those who go into labour pre-term. Pre-term babies weighing less than 2,000 gms accounted for 60 per cent of neo-natal deaths were included in the group of labours who were not induced, giving the impression that it is dangerous to begin labour spontaneously.

At that time there was no research into women's personal experiences of these induced labours. Yet accounts I was receiving suggested that induction profoundly affected the experience of birth, as well as leading to a host of other interventions.

Though I had no funding and there was no question of doing a randomised controlled trial, I decided to explore women's experiences and in 1975 asked those who had attended National Childbirth Trust classes around the UK in the previous year to let me have copies of the birth reports they sent to their antenatal teachers. I did not ask any specific questions about induction or the use of oxytocin to control labour. 614 women whose labours had been induced responded, and 224 women for whom labour had started spontaneously. This is a self-selected sample, and they were not asked to express opinions about induction, which was an advantage to an investigation that was not directed at value judgements but experiences.

There was often no explanation of why labour was being induced. The general pattern seemed to be that they were told they were on a list for induction, and most accepted whatever reason was given or did not expect a reason.

Many felt at a disadvantage during an antenatal examination: '*He didn't give any reason. Being minus my tights and pants I didn't feel I was in the best debating position, and meekly accepted my lot*'.

Some women had been given '*convenience*' reasons. Several had been told by their obstetricians that they were going on holiday. One mother, who was induced with this explanation and gave birth to a three week pre-term baby, said she was *'bullied'* into induction. Others were induced because they lived a long way from the hospital and were told that this would *'save the journey in labour'*. One obstetrician was described as going into the antenatal clinic, having *'a look around for anyone that looks about ready'*, and saying, in the women's hearing, that she wanted to *'clear out'* all her due and nearly due patients. A woman who was attached to a syntocin drip overheard a midwife remarking to that *'These three girls are being induced because there is nothing doing this afternoon'*. Another, three days past the expected date of delivery, said she was *'very shaken'* when she went to the appointments desk to arrange admission for induction at the end of the week, which she was told by the consultant was hospital policy, and the clerk said, *'We are very busy then. Come in* now.*'*

Acceleration of labour once it had started was also occasionally explained as necessary in terms of administrative convenience. One woman said she was told by the obstetrician, *'There are not enough beds for you to hang about.'* For some obstetricians induction was a privilege and they were surprised when it was not accepted. A woman said that her consultant said, *'I guarantee no more than a 10 hour labour. When do you want to have your baby?'* Another informed a woman in early pregnancy the date when her baby would be induced and anticipated a delighted response from her when twins were diagnosed by ultrasound at 16 weeks and he announced the day, at 38 weeks, when he would deliver them. Some consultants offered a *'package deal'* of induction and epidural anaesthesia. Women who declined found themselves in an invidious position: *'I was informed that I would be having the baby in the next 24 hours, so they might as well induce me. I reacted rather definitely and said that I'd rather they didn't break my waters or put me on a drip. I was immediately branded as a "nervous one" who had been "reading too much and watching too many TV programmes"'*.

A woman was told at her antenatal checkup, *'Everything is normal. I see your baby is due on Thursday. If you have not had it by then, come in that day and we will induce you.'* She asked if she could wait until she started labour before being admitted as she wanted to have a natural birth. *'What on earth do you mean by "natural"? All birth is natural'*, the obstetrician said, and told her categorically that she must come in the very next day. Some women describe their anxiety on learning that they were going to be induced: *'The doctor said that I should come in at five and be ready for labour to be induced the following morning. I was completely shattered. I pleaded for just two more days, but he was adamant and told me to "come in tomorrow". No reason. I asked why. He shouted, "Don't believe everything you read in the newspapers!" I was angry.* A woman felt threatened when induction was ruled necessary because she was four days past term. When she said she would like to avoid this the obstetrician threatened her, *'If anything goes wrong, it will be your fault'.* Another spoke of *'strong emotional blackmail'*: *'When I was 34 weeks he told me that labour would be induced. I said that the baby wasn't due, so why? And he said there was uncertainty over the date of my last period. I was very upset and asked more questions. He agreed that I was very fit and said it was because the placenta gets old if the baby is overdue, and if I wanted to go full-time it was at my own risk.'* Another woman was warned that there might be *'placental insufficiency'*, was tested for this, and after it revealed that *'everything was in order'* was still induced, against her clearly expressed wishes. Others were told, *'You have lost weight over the last two weeks'*, *'You have gained too much weight'*, or *'Your weight is static'*, or even *'The baby is above the British national average.'*

Once a woman had already been admitted in labour she became completely dependent. Many said they felt *'taken over'* by the hospital. One woman who queried setting up a syntocin drip was told by the obstetrician that nearly everyone was on a drip anyway, as they didn't like mothers to have a long labour. She said that her previous labour had lasted 12 hours and she felt happy about it. *'He said that 12 hours was far too long, and that they expected labours of six to eight hours.'*

Some women learned that the cervix was not ripe at induction. They tended to have particularly distressing and long-drawn-out labours, which were sometimes *'switched off'* at night. They were given pethidine or sleeping pills and then restarted with an oxytocin drip in the morning. This sometimes went on for several days. Nearly half had an assisted delivery or a Caesarean section. Almost half of those babies went into intensive care, too, and a further quarter had breathing or sucking difficulties.

Some women whose labours were induced had previously had births that started spontaneously, and they compared the induced birth with natural labour.

A minority described this labour as better than last time: *'If I ever have a third child, I would do everything in my power to arrange for an induced birth'*; *'My husband's always been worried about when he should take me into hospital, and it does mean no midnight car rides and wondering what to do with the other* children'; I liked being completely organised'.

But most women said the induced labours were worse: 'There was no rest between contractions'; 'There was only one minute between contractions'; 'Without warning. WHAM! Contraction after contraction, with no break between'; 'If it had been my first I would have been shocked, disturbed and frightened'.

Women were often left for long periods of time with their legs up in lithotomy stirrups. Some became very anxious. Some got cold. Many reported feeling faint. Being stuck in lithotomy stirrups resulted in pressure on the vena cava and postural hypotension.

Rates of induction varied widely between different hospitals. Hospital authorities, while able to provide statistics on induction rates, were often unable to give acceleration rates, because that information was not available even to their staff.

The issue of mounting rates of induction of labour was debated strenuously in the media and in parliament. I worked closely with Lady Micklethwait, Chairperson of the NCT and Audrey Wise, Labour MP for Coventry South West, to raise this issue publicly by getting the topic into the media and challenging the Government to investigate what obstetricians were doing.

My report 'Some Mothers' Experiences of Induced Labour' was presented to members of Parliament in 1975 and Audrey Wise arranged an inter-party meeting to discuss the findings and recommendations with representatives of the National Childbirth Trust. I said that many people thought objection to routine induction was restricted to middle-class articulate women; I referred to more research I was doing on letters written to the *Sun* after it had given publicity to induction early in 1975. These were clearly from women many of whom were in lower socio-economic groups, and of 103 which I had analysed, 76% were negative about induction, 22 per cent positive, and 2 per cent not clear. Furthermore, 60 per cent expressed regret that their partners had not been with them during labour or delivery, or said that they had been lonely during labour; 21 had had severe post-natal depression; a further 20 had experiences that resulted in childbirth phobia and the decision to be sterilised.

Hansard of 8 July 1975 reported an interchange between Audrey Wise and David Owen, the Secretary for Social Services. In an official enquiry initiated in December the year before Dr Owen disclosed that induction as a percentage of all hospital births in England had risen from 13.7 per cent in 1963 to 31.5 per cent in 1972. Audrey asserted: 'Pregnant women are not a production line.

Interference with this process without adequate knowledge is reprehensible.' Other Labour and Conservative MPs also voiced their concerns. Mrs Knight said induction was as high as 50 per cent in some hospitals and added: *'Most women believe that delivering babies is not a nine to five, Monday to Friday business.'* And Mrs Colquhoun stated: *'Women are being asked to have their babies in office hours only.'* Dr Owen agreed: *'There is justifiable concern at the possibility of induction taking place for administrative convenience.'*

The debate about induction started a series of enquiries into what was happening in childbirth and vigorous public debate about the risk of unnecessary obstetric interventions. This provided stimulus for further research and – very important – funding of randomised controlled trials, more Government enquiries, and the publication of papers stating policy for the future: the Winterton[29] and the Changing Childbirth[30] reports, and a new focus on psychological and social consequences of a birth experience that had become dehumanised for many women and completely out of their control.

A Home Death

I was working on a new book, *Education and Counselling for Childbirth*, when my Mother had a brain haemorrhage and asked me to come to her. As I walked into her room, she said, *'You have done birth, Sheila. Now do this.'* She was in bed by a window looking out onto the garden, vivid with flowers and trees, surrounded by bird song.

The book, which would be published in 1977 the following year, was the first one ever written for antenatal teachers. I sat by her with my reference books, knowing that she would be happiest if I got on with things while I stayed close. She opened up her spectacle case, took out her glasses, put them on, but obviously could not see. So she simply, and with a conclusive gesture, carefully folded them, slipped them in the case again, and placed it on her bedside table. That was that! It was a gesture of acceptance.

Mother could no longer swallow, and I knew that she would not want to be kept alive artificially. So apart from making sure that she was well hydrated, and wiping out her mouth with a glycerine swab so that it was moist and comfortable, I concentrated on lapping her in luxury. I gave her bed-baths using her favourite soap with a strong carnation scent, reckoning that the sense of smell may stay strong till the end.

The GP visited and suggested that we move her into hospital so that she could be tube-fed. I consulted Father and we both agreed, 'No. *She would want to be at home. She wouldn't want invasive procedures.*' Later he told me that he wished he had the courage to care for his father that way when he was dying. Instead, he had him admitted to hospital and everything was done to prolong his life by every means possible. Looking back on it, he thought it was wrong, and now he felt guilty.

Three days and nights passed. Suddenly she gave a little cry and stopped breathing. I had just gone off to the bathroom. I think she felt there was a space. It was how she wanted it to be.

Her friend Theresa Hooley wrote:

She died at Candlemas; her bright spirit –
a world's white candle – burns upon its way
to other spheres of service and of merit,
a living light in the Eternal Day.

Lucy, my brother David's American wife, had come to stay, taking over at times when I needed to sleep. She was shocked that Mother was not in hospital. She was very distressed. Afterwards she told me how utterly different it was from how it would have been in the United States: there death was removed from the home wherever possible, the family would not have been expected to deal with dying first-hand, and for her it was all too painfully intimate. People were insulated from it – specialists took over – first hospital, then the morticians. She needed time to come to terms with this and to talk about the cultural differences as she was finding this much too difficult to cope with emotionally.

Mother's death was a practical demonstration of something Dame Cicely Saunders, who founded the hospice movement, once said to me backstage at a conference where we were both speaking, '*You and I are doing the same work*'.

Death is the next great transition that we all go through. We need to prepare for and reclaim it, as we are now reclaiming birth.

CHAPTER EIGHT

CHALLENGING THE SYSTEM

The Place Of Birth　　　　＊

In the early 70s just about everybody assumed that hospital birth must be safer than home because that was where the experts and all their latest equipment was based. I thought about ways of bringing obstetricians, paediatricians and birth activists together to explore ways in which the environment for childbirth shaped what happened and affected both the woman and her baby.

One idea of mine was to arrange regular lunch meetings of doctors, researchers and others at the NCT in London, offering some interesting salads and cheeses, good bread and a glass of wine, at which a practitioner or researcher gave an informal paper and we discussed it in a relaxed, non-partisan atmosphere. The first of these was in 1958 and they were collaborative rather than confrontational, focusing especially on home birth. The result was a star-studded group of obstetricians, neonatologists, general practitioners, psychiatrists and psychotherapists, sociologists, midwives, breastfeeding specialists and mothers.

John Davis, professor of Paediatrics and Child Health at Manchester, and later Cambridge, discussed how a centralised, impersonal and bureaucratic maternity service inhibited spontaneous physical function, and called for the humanisation of hospitals. Michael Moore, a family doctor, spoke about the importance of good antenatal care so that women could choose home birth if they wanted to.

John Ashford, professor of Mathematical Statistics at Exeter, analysed regional neonatal mortality figures at home and in hospital and asked whether they were too high in hospital births – 48 per cent in consultant units and 20 per cent in GP units, according to the latest available figures from 1958. He doubted whether this made birth any safer. Iain Chalmers, an obstetrician and statistician at Cardiff University, presenting an epidemiological view, made a case for experimental studies of home and hospital birth to evaluate different birth places, and suggested that hospital birth could introduce its own risks.

Marjorie Tew, a statistician at Nottingham University, produced evidence to support the case against hospital deliveries. David Baum, the bright, shock-headed young neonatologist at Oxford, described a way of organising neonatal intensive care so that it supported families.

Martin Richards, Social Psychologist at Cambridge and specialist on the consequences of early separation of mothers and babies, showed how, though it was assumed that it must be better, hospital failed to provide a place of safety. Gerard Kloosterman, Professor of Obstetrics at the University of Amsterdam, and Director of its Training School for Midwives, described the Dutch system of home birth and was a powerful advocate for it.

Luke Zander and Michael Lee-Jones, both GPs, and Chloe Fisher, a midwife in Oxford, spoke about the role of the primary health care team in pregnancy and postnatally and showed how GP obstetricians needed to work with a closely integrated group of midwives, nurses and health visitors. Chloe described the opportunities and frustrations of a community midwife. Luke drew on his work in undergraduate and postgraduate education, and Michael looked at the details of administration. Whereas in 1948 over two thirds of GPs were in single-handed practices, by 1971 over 80 per cent were in partnerships or group practices, with a range of paramedical staff attached. Lewis Mehl stressed home birth research in the United States and revealed the disadvantages in the current technological trend in childbirth.

Joel Richman, Head of the School of Sociology at Manchester Polytechnic, and Bill Goldthorpe, Consultant Gynaecologist at Thameside Hospital were working together to study patients' perceptions of illness. In our group they spoke about what can be done to make birth a positive experience for fathers and talked about the 'cultural conspiracy' against fatherhood, described how it started in pregnancy, and made recommendations. They pointed out that fathers present at birth are generally more satisfied and in the United States sue less frequently!

A Freudian psychoanalyst, Peter Lomas, and former GP specialist in postnatal breakdown, focused on elemental features of the helping relationship. He pointed out that behaviour in hospitals is not always as rational and scientific as it seems and that a lot of action is heavily ritualised.

I reported on my first small study of women's experiences of birth at home, and described the research I had done in 1975, asking women who had attended NCT classes how they felt about home and hospital. Perhaps other women wouldn't agree with them, but the chances were that they might put into words something which others found it difficult to say, and a random sample of 2,000 mothers all over the UK by Maureen O'Brien of the Institute for Social Studies in Medicine published later that year bore this out. Women chose home birth largely because they wanted to be protected from interventionist obstetrics, could have one-to-one midwife care from someone they knew, and thought that they could bond more smoothly with their babies in a setting where stress was reduced. At that time women in hospital were often separated from their partners during birth and from their babies afterwards. Women chose hospital birth because they thought it was safest. They were much more likely to describe distressing labours than home birth mothers.

But it was hard to get permission to have a baby at home. I asked, *'Is pregnancy an illness of which a woman must be "cured" by an obstetrician? Or is it part of a developmental process in which a couple grow to be parents and the family welcomes a new member?'* Decisions made about the quality of maternity care should be the concern of society as a whole. These are not exclusively, nor even primarily, medical decisions, but ethical ones. They involve a responsibility we must all share.

We built up a heap of evidence about home birth, looking at it from many different points of view and bringing a wide range of skills. I compiled this material, adding contributions from other specialists. I approached Oxford University Press and asked them if they would be interested in publishing it as a book. *The Place of Birth* came out in 1978, edited jointly by John Davis and me, and sold well.

Professionals And Campaigners Start To Work Together

It was also in 1978 that the National Childbirth Trust approached obstetricians and heads of midwifery, proposing to acknowledge that women had a right to make informed choices about how they were treated in pregnancy and childbirth.

Tony Smith, editor of the *British Medical Journal* interviewed Lady Micklethwait, the NCT President, Professor Richard Beard of St Mary's Medical School, London, an obstetrician who listened to, and learned from, women, and Kathleen Shaw, Divisional Nursing Officer for Midwifery at the West Middlesex. The result was a joint paper, *Expectations of a Pregnant Woman in Relation to Her Treatment.*[31]

Tony Smith asked Philippa Micklethwait what requests a woman was most likely to have. She said that she could if she wished have a person of her choice with her throughout labour, and when her baby was born could hold it as soon as possible, feed when she wished, (unless either mother or baby required urgent attention) and that professional advice would be readily available to her for as long as she needed it when she returns home.

Richard Beard did not consider it simply a matter of explanation, and observed, *'The obstetrician and midwife are considered the guardians of the fetus and a mother with any ideas of her own presents an obstacle to care and put its life at risk.'*

Perhaps this reads as rather low key now, but it was the start of a breakthrough in communication between campaigning organisations and medical professionals.

Learning From Women – 'The Good Birth Guide'

Maternity hospitals were first set up in the eighteenth and nineteenth centuries as charity institutions for impoverished women and unmarried women giving birth in shame and degradation, who often had to give up their babies afterwards. They offered the raw material for obstetric practice and were used to demonstrate obstetrics and gynaecology to medical students.

Hospitals remain bureaucratic and hierarchically organised institutions. They have to be managed so that the different parts of the whole structure work together efficiently. In these circumstances it is easy for a caregiver to abdicate responsibility for focusing on the needs and wishes of those they are supposed to be looking after and the main concern is to oil the wheels of the system.

In the 1970s it was very difficult for a pregnant woman to find out anything about maternity hospitals in her area. If it was her first baby, she might not even know the questions to ask, or if she had recently moved to a different part of the country, have only the vaguest idea of what lay behind those imposing doors.

I believed that we needed information. My idea was to learn about women's experiences of large and small maternity units all over the country, to hear what they appreciated, what they did not like, and how they thought things could be improved, and collect these together so that pregnant women had a basis on which to find out more. I also discovered that midwives and doctors themselves often did not know what was being done in other hospitals.

It struck me that we had books that rated restaurants and hotels, but nothing to help women choose where to give birth. My brother-in-law Hilary Rubinstein had published *The Good Hotel Guide* where people wrote in about hotels in which they had stayed. Unlike the Michelin guides it didn't rely on experts, but was based on descriptions by guests. Why not find out about women's experiences of hospitals across the UK in the same way? A woman can't know what she wants until she knows what is *possible*. She may not be aware that she can give birth squatting, for example, or in a birth pool, or that there is a midwife-led unit where she can have one-to-one midwife care, or a home birth.

So I conducted a breakthrough study of around 300 maternity hospitals in Britain, using accounts of care antenatally, during labour and postpartum from 1,500 women in response to my questions to those who attended NCT classes. I did programmes on radio and TV, and wrote articles in magazines and newspapers asking women to tell me about their experiences. I wrote to each hospital asking for statistics of induction, acceleration of labour, forceps deliveries, Caesarean sections and episiotomies, and about any changes that had taken place over the last few years. I asked about the care they aimed to provide and their policies.[32]

As a general rule I only included hospitals about which I had received information from at least 24 women, except in the case of GP units, for which I used 12 accounts.

Some hospitals sent sheets of grateful letters from satisfied parents. Though I realised they would be unlikely to send letters from those who were less satisfied, wherever possible I incorporated positive comments. Some stood out as offering women choice and giving sensitive care. These earned a star. Some even got two stars!

My colleagues in the NCT didn't want to be involved because they thought any criticism of hospitals would jeopardise the relations with staff that they were so carefully cultivating. One admonished me, *'The Matron invites us to sherry parties now. Criticism would put an end to that. We believe in tact and persuasion.'*

In 1962 Professor Norman Morris, a professor of obstetrics and gynaecology, was one of the founding members of the International Society for Psychosomatic Obstetrics, and its president for nearly 20 years. He teamed up with progressive obstetricians from France, Italy and other continental European countries as well as from further afield – including my friend Murray Enkin in Canada. There was a launch conference in July that year in Paris, at which I spoke. Norman respected women and told them, *'I can't guarantee you the labour you want, but I'll do my best for you with the labour you have.'* Norman was a friend of mine and I admired him.

I asked him to tell me the episiotomy rate at Charing Cross Hospital, where he was the professor of the Medical School. There was a long pause. No records were kept. He didn't have a clue and was appalled about this. I said that I considered routine episiotomy our western way of female genital mutilation. Immediately he instructed that records must be kept.

I asked some senior obstetricians and midwifery managers about their statistics. Replies varied from curt refusal to give any information at all to very generous four or five pages of A4. One consultant said that since these were matters of a technical nature he did not wish them to be the subject of public comment, so was unwilling to let me know anything. I was often told that these requests had never before been made by their patients. This happened with gentle birth, rooming-in of mother and baby, including at night, and the father being allowed to cuddle, change and bath the baby. The replies usually went on to state that if such requests should be forthcoming in future staff would be glad to make arrangements. It seemed a bit like a shop. The assistant says, *'We don't have any demand for that, madam,'* but if enough people ask, and go on asking politely, the management realises that there *is* a demand after all and sees what it can do about it.

Women often didn't ask for what they wanted, and felt intimidated by the organisation of a hospital, however kind and helpful individual members of staff were. Or perhaps they asked, but whoever happened to be on duty, who might be a junior or student midwife or an auxiliary, dealt with it to make least fuss.

Human Relations

The most important thing was the quality of personal relationships. Staff were *'friendly'*, *'treated women like equals'*, *'as an adult'* or *'an intelligent human being'*, or on the contrary came over as *'cold'*, *'impersonal'*, *'distant'*, *'brusque'*, *'patronising'*, *'condescending'*, *'rigid'* and *'bossy'*. Women said they were treated *'like dim-witted or naughty children'*: *'They were so busy and preoccupied I felt I should have almost apologised for being there'*, *'I felt I should be saying, "I am so sorry I am having a baby. It won't happen again."'*

Women felt they must be on their guard against being seen to be *'knowledgeable'* or *'demanding'*: *'The most delicately worded questions were interpreted as sinister threats'*. A midwife exclaimed, *'You've been reading books!'* or asked sarcastically *'Who put those ideas in your head?'* There were striking exceptions to this in a few hospitals. A woman who was in pain asked for pethidine and *'Sister said, "Do you really want it? I don't think you have much longer to go"'.* And the mother delivered happily shortly after. Another asked for an epidural, though she had said beforehand that she hoped to be able to manage without one. In this case the anaesthetist suggested that she was doing so well that she probably did not really need it and stayed with her, helping her with her breathing and relaxation during every contraction. She looked back on what was obviously an ordeal at the time as a very positive experience. But it is clear that drugs for pain relief were often used in place of emotional support, and that some caregivers were adept at undermining confidence: *'She said, "You don't know how painful it is going to be. You haven't any idea".'* The midwife said, *'"I've never seen relaxation work yet."'I was greeted with, "So you are another of those huffers and puffers".'*

Continuity Of Care

Contributors to the research set high value on continuity of care and being able to get to know well those people who looked after them through pregnancy, labour and the postpartum period. Those with GP/midwife care saw fewer professionals than those who had consultant care.

But even where care was given by a large number of professionals, women appreciated being greeted by name and welcomed by members of staff introducing themselves. This acknowledgement of individuality, being treated as more than just one more bulging abdomen, was important. Antenatal clinics provided for most of these women their introduction to the worst aspects of fragmented care. Clinics were described as *'badly organised'* and even *'a shambles'*. Women told of long waits, sometimes exceeding two hours, being moved from queue to queue, and coming away from the clinic frightened, depressed and humiliated. Even in units where care in labour was personal and intimate, in the antenatal clinic work tended to be task-centred, not woman-centred, and 'the *only continuity was that of written notes'*. There were several accounts of notes being lost.

Women wanted to be remembered in the antenatal clinic and to meet the same people in labour whom they had already encountered in the clinic, and liked the midwife who delivered the baby visiting the postpartum ward to see how the mother and baby were getting on. During labour shift changes sometimes caused confusion and distress and a woman had to work at establishing a link with a different midwife and to redefine her wishes with members of staff whom she may never have met before, often when contractions were coming thick and fast in the late first stage.

In some hospitals women were left alone for long periods and described members of staff popping into the room to ask rhetorical questions such as *'Everything OK?'* and passing on before they could answer. They also described people *'wandering in and out'* sometime when the mother was in the shower, on a bedpan, or physically exposed in the second stage. They said they did not know who most of these people were, but it included *'tea ladies'* and other ancillary hospital personnel. *'I felt like an animal with so many people present during a vaginal examination'* one woman said, and another, *'There was a succession of nurses and midwives, none of whom I had ever seen before or saw again after the birth'*. One woman even laboured with a window cleaner clinging like a limpet to the delivery room windows, apparently fascinated by the view of her perineum.

Satisfying personal contact was most likely to be remarked on by women who had GP unit deliveries and continuing care from a community midwife through pregnancy, labour and the immediate postpartum period. This was sometimes stated as the reason they chose GP/midwife care in the first place.

Information

Women stressed the importance of being able to get accurate and unrestricted information. Nearly every account contained references to the ease or difficulty with which information was obtained about, for example, the progress of labour, alternative courses of action, the side effects of treatment and such things as the measurement of blood pressure and the outcome of a scan. Where women had free access to information they said things like, *'All my questions were answered fully'*, *'They explained everything they were doing and asked if I consented'* or *'The midwife consulted us over every issue'*. There were other women, however, who felt taken over as if they had been sucked into a complicated machine. This process of feeling treated like an object acted on by doctors and nurses started for many women in the antenatal clinic. Care in the labour ward and delivery suite was sometimes more intimate and personal than in the antenatal clinic at the same hospital.

A woman's satisfaction with the information which she was given and being asked to share in all decision-making was only indirectly related to the degree of obstetric intervention. Though in high-tech hospitals women said they felt manipulated even in some very straightforward labours, in some complicated labours other women felt free to make informed choices between alternatives, and said they were consulted and their views respected. One woman who had a forceps delivery, for example, said, *'The doctors explained what they were doing in such a gentle, respectful way that it was as if they were suggesting what they would do.'*

Autonomy

Support for personal autonomy was important in every account. *'It was a team effort, with me as Captain'* one woman stressed. *'It was my labour and they were there to help if needed'*, another said. Their autonomy was supported where the system was flexible and the woman's needs and wishes recognised, and caregivers made it clear to mothers that they had freedom of choice and could ask for what they wanted and staff co-operated to adapt to the wishes of the individual. In those hospitals a woman felt that it was she who was having the baby, not the staff. One woman said that after lifting her baby out of her body, she turned to the doctor as she was cuddling her daughter and asked if the baby was all right, *'He replied that he hadn't seen her yet and then we all realised that he had just stood in the background and let us get on with it.'*

Yet in many hospitals the mother's freedom to decide what she wanted and to act spontaneously depended on whoever happened to be on duty and it was impossible to know in advance if she would find allies or whether it would be an uphill battle.

Clockwatching

Time was also a central issue, time given for discussion with the mother, and time for her to feel that she could work with her body instead of battling against it to get the baby born.

When women praised the birth environment they often said it was *'a relaxed atmosphere'*. *'I never felt rushed'*, *'I could ask him anything, however trivial, and would always get a patient answer.'* One woman wrote, *'When I asked about the size of the baby in relation to the pelvis the doctor disappeared and returned with a bright blue rubber pelvis and a doll and delivered the child several times, this during a particularly busy afternoon.'*

Some women discovered that an intravenous oxytocin drip was set up as part of the admission procedure, often without asking permission or explanation other than a comment such as, *'We'll just help you along. You don't want a long labour, do you?'* It was common practice to do an amniotomy (the artificial rupture of the membranes), fix an electrode on the fetal head and set up a drip to stimulate the uterus shortly following admission. These women felt taken over by a baby-producing institution. They said things like, *'I felt like a tin of beans on a conveyor belt.'*

In the second stage some had time to find their own rhythms without being commanded or coaxed to push, but many said they were *'rushed'*, *'harried'* and urged to push harder and longer. *'I was hectored by a jolly midwife who seemed to have done her training on the lacrosse fields of some girls' public school'.* Women were sometimes told it was the rule that they could be in the second stage no longer than one hour, and then it must be forceps. Occasionally this was restricted to 45 minutes. They described the anxiety, desperation or sheer panic this caused.

Time was also of primary importance following birth and most women referred to time with their partner and baby. They valued having unlimited and undisturbed time together and where it was restricted to a statutory *'ten minutes bonding time'*, after which the partner was told to leave and the baby often *'whisked away'*, said they felt *'frustrated'*, *'cheated'*, *'sad'*, *'lonely'* and even *'disoriented'*.

Technology

Whereas some women felt trapped and immobilised by electrodes and catheters, a small number felt more secure when the fetal heart was monitored continuously and many used the monitor to help them prepare for contractions, watching the print-out to see when they should start using breathing and other techniques learnt at antenatal classes.

But most described how it made them anxious, distracted them from concentrating on relaxation and breathing, or restricted movement. They often said that the staff took no notice of the print-out and there were frequent descriptions of monitors not working properly or breaking down completely: *'Various members of staff came in and kicked it. They said to ignore it. It was always doing that.'; 'It was on the blink and emitting a piercing whine.'; 'They left us alone with the monitor for an hour. I couldn't see the point of it, since no-one even looked at it.'; 'It wasn't recording anything properly. It seemed futile to have the electrode on the baby's head and to have to lie still when it wasn't registering anything.'; 'A doctor came in and pointed out that the belt was monitoring my heart rate, not the baby's.'*

Technology often prevented a woman's spontaneous behaviour. It was difficult or impossible to move or get into a comfortable position. *'I sat up to see the head and was told off for disturbing the drip.'* Some women said they were instructed to lie on their backs so that the monitor could more accurately register the fetal heart, so they had to adopt a position which tended to put pressure on the inferior vena cava and reduce the flow of oxygenated blood to the fetus. Women often acknowledged the skills of obstetricians in dealing with the abnormal, but in many high tech units felt the constant threat of intervention in normal labours.

Ritual Interventions

I learned that shaving of pubic hair, a practice that started in hospitals created for the indigent poor to eradicate pubic lice, together with the routine enema, were still seen as part of 'clean midwifery'. Women were often told that the shave was done to have a bald area for episiotomy and suturing the perineum. A few years later midwifery research showed that shaving did not reduce infection, but increased bruising and caused multiple abrasions around the hair follicles. Though the enema had become an almost sacrosanct element in the management of birth, research was to show that it, too, was of no benefit, and if a woman had an enema she was more likely to pass liquid faeces as she gave birth.

In the 70s Active Management was the norm, membranes were routinely ruptured on admission, and other interventions, dictated by the clock, took place from then on.[33] In some hospitals it was possible, provided she made it clear that this mattered to her, for a woman to try to deliver without an episiotomy, but most women were cut in the end because staff had no idea of how to help them give birth so that they didn't need one, and they were urged to push harder even though they didn't want to.

Continuous fetal monitoring, with monitors located centrally at the nursing station without having to stand at the patient's bed, and management of labour to last not more than six hours from six centimetres dilatation in women having second and later babies and 11 hours in those having first babies, were more or less routine. Membranes were ruptured artificially early in labour, often when the woman was admitted, when she might be only two to three centimetres dilated. Then an electrode was attached to the fetal scalp so that continuous monitoring could take place. Unruptured membranes were thought of as getting in the way of the progress of labour. But early amniotomy exposes the baby and the uterus to invading pathogens. Infection is directly related to the length of time between amniotomy and birth.

Iain Chalmers wrote, *'Thousands of existing questions have not yet been investigated in systematic reviews, and thousands of systematic reviews have shown that the existing evidence does not answer important questions about the effects of many treatments. This challenge will not go away – indeed, resolving one uncertainty almost always results in the recognition of additional uncertainties...*

'The consequences for patients of acquiescing in therapeutic ignorance can be disastrous, yet, perversely, current attitudes to, and restrictions on, therapeutic research are powerful disincentives to people who wish to confront uncertainties about the effects of treatments. It is up to clinicians, patients, and the public in general to decide whether they wish to continue tolerating this bizarre state of affairs.'[34]

Fathers

I campaigned for acknowledgement of a father's role in childbirth. In those days a male partner was allowed in the birth room only in the role of *voyeur,* and back in the 60s, the first man to be with his partner in a big American teaching hospital had to handcuff himself to the delivery table before he was allowed to stay.

Fathers couldn't be turned out at home, and the midwife often depended on a man to learn the geography of the house and where she could find things she needed.

In hospital men often had to wear gowns, masks, caps and overshoes. As an anthropologist I could see that protective garments play a ritual role denoting status in the hospital hierarchy, and the lower down in it an individual is, the more protective clothing he has to wear. This produced a barrier between the woman and her partner. For one thing, they couldn't kiss each other. A mask used for 15 minutes is no longer sterile anyway. It has only a ritual function. One hospital that undertook bacterial counts when overshoes were used found that there was no statistically significant difference, so discarded them. Caps rarely covered the hair, so they had a ritual function, too.

The father was treated as an optional extra. Most women wanted their partners or some other companion with them. Hospitals usually allowed a single labour partner, but sometimes only for the second stage to witness the delivery, because first-stage wards opened onto each other and were inadequately screened. In many when a woman was admitted in early labour, or having labour induced, the partner was sent away because *'It'll be hours yet'*, or was told to eat or have a smoke because *'Nothing's happening'*. He was only there on sufferance.

If he was present he might be told to watch the monitor print-out to tell the woman a contraction was coming. His eyes were focused on the machines. Occasionally a midwife tried to form a feminine bond with the mother by saying, *'We women understand each other. Men can't know'*, or something of this kind. In a disturbing number of hospitals the man was asked to wait outside during minor nursing and obstetric procedures. This included admission procedures, amniotomy, the insertion of an IV, when she was using a bed pan, and vaginal examinations. Staff often forgot to invite him in again. Sometimes drugs for pain relief or an oxytocin drip to accelerate labour were given without him being told. He then came back to find there was no room beside her because a machine had taken his place, or that she was drowsy with pethidine and he could no longer help her handle contractions with techniques they had practiced together. He was barred from attending a forceps delivery or Caesarean section, just when she was most likely to need him.

Drugs For Pain Relief

Freedom of choice with knowledge of alternatives was especially important when it came to drugs. In some hospitals women were persuaded to have pethidine or an epidural and nurses stood over them asking, at the height of each contraction, *'Don't you want something to take away the pain?'* or words to that effect. When staff gave warm approval to a woman's determination to cope without drugs and supported her in her decision, the way was opened for an almost conspiratorial collaboration which boosted morale and made it much more likely that she did not, in fact, need analgesics or anaesthesia. This mutual aim formed a strong bond between a woman and her caregivers; *'I said I didn't want pethidine. I wanted a natural birth and the midwife was delighted'*. They worked together with a sense of common purpose and it gave spice to the relationship.

Writers referred often to ways in which midwives offered pain relief through strong emotional support and in the words they used rather than through drugs. Non-pharmacological relief of pain was provided by touch and holding, eye contact, massage, changes in position, moving around, and unswerving praise. A good midwife gives of *herself,* not only of techniques.

Women were also told that they had a *'long way to go'* in labour when, in fact, they were almost fully dilated, and in some cases given a high dose of pethidine, and when they asked what was being injected, were told, *'Never you mind. We know what we are doing',* or words to that effect. It was possible to ask for a mini dose of the drug, but difficult when a junior midwife felt that she couldn't give a lower dose than one that was normally prescribed, and sometimes a woman had to choose between not having pethidine and having a dose of 150mg. That is enough to cause extreme drowsiness, nausea and vomiting, confusion, amnesia, visual disturbances and hallucinations. It makes the baby less likely to breathe spontaneously at birth, especially if given close to delivery, may make it sleepy in the days following birth, be slow at sucking, and interferes with the interaction between mother and father.

In some hospitals epidurals were *'pushed'.* Women offered a package deal of an epidural and induction were told that even if they didn't have pain relief at that point, they were bound to need it later, so they might as well have the epidural *now* while the anaesthetist was around. They were not told about possible side-effects and were surprised when their blood pressure suddenly plummeted, they felt weak and faint, and their bladders had to be emptied with a catheter. They also didn't realise that an epidural increased the risk of a forceps delivery.

Spreadeagled And Harpooned

While I was researching material for *The Good Birth Guide* I also did a small study into opportunities to move around in labour. This was based on detailed birth reports from 48 women. I found that many birth attendants assumed that women would be in bed. They were expected to lie down or sit propped up. Pillows kept slipping, and any foam wedge was often not high enough to give good back support. Women in labour were often in acute pain when lying or sitting, but were given no help to kneel or get on all fours, and there were often not enough big cushions on which to crouch forward and rest between contractions. Beds were too high to get on and off, and there was no stool. Beds were too hard, too. This was commented on especially by women who were immobilised with an intravenous drip and/or a fetal monitor. Midwives and doctors palpating the uterus and doing vaginal examinations expected the woman to lie flat on her back. This increased the pain.

They took it for granted that she must deliver on the delivery table or bed. All but five hospitals assumed that a woman would deliver on her back. These five offered the choice of lying on her left side. After a vaginal examination many women found it too exhausting to turn into a more comfortable position, so remained supine. Even those who had enough pillows in the first stage often felt they had insufficient in the second stage. When they were moved to a delivery table some were not permitted to take their pillows with them, and were left with only one or two. The delivery table was too narrow and they felt suspended in space. They worried that they would fall off, and when the lower end of the table was removed, that they would push the baby out with no-one ready to catch it. They were particularly anxious if the birth attendant turned away or was talking to anyone else and not concentrating on them. In some hospitals a midwife got the mother to lie with her feet on her hips, in a simulated lithotomy position. But if the midwife twisted away she was lying with one foot supported and the other suspended in air. Women were often told to put their hands on their thighs and pull their heads and shoulders up when they pushed. Many found this very tiring. Though most described the baby being placed on their tummies, some wanted to watch and help lift their babies out, but could not because they were lying too far back. When they asked if they could be more upright caregivers refused to allow them to change position.

In the early 70s the John Radcliffe hospital in Oxford was the first to use a foam support, shaped like the back of an easy chair but with the bottom part, behind the lower spine, bulging outward. 'The Kitzinger Cushion' was designed by an architect/interior decorator friend of mine, Martin Sylvester. This hospital also introduced polystyrene-granule filled bean-bags for women who wanted other positions and to lean or crouch forward. Meanwhile discussion had started about the dangers of the supine position because of reduced blood flow to the fetus, and an obstetric chair was invented in Sweden that enabled a woman to sit up.

Change was in the air, but women needed courage to ask for what they wanted.

Caesareans

With the explosion of technology Caesarean rates were rising. The lowest rates were in the Netherlands and some of the Nordic countries where around 10 in every 100 women had Caesareans; in the United States and Canada Caesarean rates were much higher and in some countries (Brazil and Mexico) 30 to 40 percent of all women are given Caesareans. In British hospitals Caesareans were often performed because labour was exceeding the time limits. Women were told that they would not be allowed to labour beyond 12 hours, for example, and many felt the whole thing was a race against time, with the threat of intervention hanging over them.

Following a Caesarean, babies routinely went straight to the nursery. Some remained there for no other reason than that everyone was busy, postnatal wards were understaffed, and ward routines took precedence over responding to mothers' and babies' needs. Communication between postnatal wards and the special care baby unit was very poor. A mother felt trapped on a ward far from the unit where her baby was cared for and reluctant to interrupt busy nurses with requests to see her baby. When she did get there she might find the baby had been fed, though she had wanted to breastfeed.

Staff encouraged breastfeeding, and sometimes were enthusiastic about it. Unfortunately, advice and assistance did not always match up to enthusiasm, and the biggest problem was conflicting advice which led to confusion, and at times despair, and resulted in the mother losing confidence and giving up breastfeeding.

The night after delivery was an ordeal for many women because of rules that the baby must be in the nursery. I believe that a mother and baby belong together. This can be arranged safely if clip-on cribs are provided. I would like to see the day when all hospitals have large double beds in which mother and father can be together with the baby in a crib attached to the side. Hospitals, even those which say they offer 'family-centred care' are usually highly unsuitable places in which a family can be born.

Bonding

Towards the end of the 70s, as a result of research in the United States by paediatricians Marshall Klaus and John Kennell – both colleagues and friends of mine – the word '*attachment*' used by John Bowlby to describe the close relationship between mother and baby was changed to '*bonding*'.[35]

I was happy about this new emphasis on falling in love with your baby. Yet I had trouble with the word '*bonding*' because it was commonly seen as a magic glue that makes the mother and baby stick together. Hospitals started to advertise and promote bonding. In some of them caregivers turned into bonding sleuths who watched new mothers to see if they responded to their babies in the correct way. If they didn't, they might be reported to the social services. I went back to the hospital administrators to ask them about their policies. In many of the letters from managers there were statements such as, '*Time for bonding is allowed in the delivery room*', '*Staff understand bonding*' and '*Bonding is encouraged*'.

I wondered if this was another imposition on women. It often happens that after a birth in a hospital setting a woman needs time to find herself. That is a normal phase in the moments after birth in an alien environment. I believe she should be able to follow her own feelings.

Breastfeeding

In the 70s it became generally agreed that women should be encouraged to breastfeed their babies for the first months of life and that feeding whenever the baby wanted it was better than a strict schedule. This was largely the result of the Oppe Report of 1974.[36] Yet in many hospitals babies were still being given additional fluids, especially at night, with the intention of letting the mothers sleep, sometimes even if they were awake and listening for their babies. In some paediatricians insisted on babies being given water before they went to the breast to rule out oesophageal atresia (obstruction in the upper digestive tract). There was no evidence that observing a feed with water was safer than observing one when the baby was getting colostrum.

Some mothers felt bludgeoned into trying to breastfeed. One said she was handed her baby for a feed and the nurse said, '*Poor little baby, your mother doesn't want to feed you herself. You're only getting a bottle*.' On the other hand, some nurses who were concerned a woman did not have enough milk were pleased when the baby was given a bottle and said things like, '*It'll be all right now*.'

In many hospitals women said that nurses and midwives did not know how to help. Different ones tried different ways and women were subjected to conflicting advice. One nurse came up and positioned the mother with the baby's head in the crook of her arm. Another came and moved it so that she could control it with her hand. Another came and suggested that the baby's legs would be best tucked under her arm. A fourth placed the baby on a pillow. So women had to keep a look-out to see who was approaching and quickly switch the baby round to the '*correct*' position. This made an athletic exercise of even the simplest feed. This was later corroborated by Jo Garcia in the Community Health Councils Surveys on Maternity Care.[37] She pointed out that rules about feeding were too numerous to be described. One was that a mother must feed her baby in the nursery at night, so as not to disturb other patients who were sleeping. Women had to sit on hard, straight-backed chairs set in a row, lights glaring, sometimes with pop music playing non-stop. Occasionally there was even a queue for the chairs.

Another rule was that women had to fill in the baby's sucking time on a chart. This occurred where the hospital had moved on from schedules to '*demand*' feeding, but staff had such little confidence that it could work that it was necessary to record the length of each feed or nibble. Women often made these times up, partly because they found it difficult to be sure when a baby was sucking and swallowing or simply enjoying sucking without swallowing, and partly because the more experienced mothers realised that according to hospital rules the babies were supposed to feed for three minutes on the first day; five, seven and 10 on the second, third and fourth days, and not more than 10 minutes each side after that.

The worst problem for most women was the constant stream of staff requiring information or wanting to do something to them, which made their stay exhausting. Some sent detailed diaries of events during the 24 hours. It was a kind of torture.

Day And Night

Care at night was dramatically reduced and created problems for breastfeeding mothers who wanted to feed their babies as soon as they woke. A completely different system was often introduced when the nightshift came on, which was made up of agency nurses, often unaware of the unit's ethos concerning breastfeeding. In some hospitals people were walking around, chattering, and waking mothers, while babies were left to cry. Women left these hospitals exhausted.

They were not supposed to labour at night in some hospitals. Labour had to be at the right time, which was in office hours. In one hospital a woman in an antenatal ward with rapidly escalating contractions was told, 'Go back to sleep and stop imagining things'. The night staff must have realised she was in labour because when they handed over to the day shift they passed on this information, and a midwife examined her and found her in the second stage.

In some hospitals, too, if a woman was admitted during the night she was sedated, her partner was directed to go home, and she was put in a darkened room and told to sleep. For some women this meant that they were deprived of their partners' support, and of help from staff, when they most needed it, and either passed hours in anxiety and pain until the hospital started up again, or had a sudden dash to the delivery room in the early hours of the morning, while being ordered to stop pushing. Occasionally their partners missed the birth.

Certain methods of managing labour, notably the use of an oxytocin drip or regional anaesthesic, often depended on the time of day, too. A woman labouring at night was unlikely to have drugs to stimulate her uterus, or have an epidural. On the other hand, if she went into labour in the daytime, laboured through the night, and was still in the first stage when activities started in the morning and doctors' rounds took place, she would automatically be put on an oxytocin drip. Active management related to social divisions of time, rather than the progress of that particular labour.

At night, too, a woman was less likely to be allowed out of bed and to move around. Her spontaneous urge to rock her pelvis, stand up, or go on all fours, might have produced more effective contractions, but an oxytocin drip was used in place of simpler methods of stimulating labour.

There was wholesale distribution of sleeping pills at night time. One mother said that they were 'handed out like candy' and staff lacked sympathy and understanding for women who said that they wanted to be alert to respond to their babies, or were concerned about contamination of breast milk with sedatives.

Rigid routines meant that all mothers were woken at 5.30 or 6.00 a.m. to feed their babies, regardless of the fact that some had been feeding during the night and had just dropped off to sleep again.

Cosmetic Changes

Putting up curtains and hanging pictures improved the look of wards, but creating a positive environment is a matter of *people*. On the other hand, women don't like having to give birth in boxes. I was appalled when I was taken to see the labour and delivery rooms in a large American hospital. We went down to the basement. There, with all the plumbing, birth took place underground without daylight.

Women appreciate being able to see living, growing things through the window. Many hospitals have been built in which labour and delivery rooms have no windows. There were detailed descriptions of ceilings. When women are in bed the view may be restricted to a wall and a clock. Ceilings were often cracked and stained. One woman encountered a blood-stained ceiling over the delivery table, but luckily had already been warned about it by a friend who had a baby there two years previously!

Many women had lights shining directly in their eyes. It is difficult to surrender to a natural psycho-sexual process with your whole body and mind in such surroundings, and labour has been turned into a clinical event.

The Good Birth Guide was originally published in 1979, the first time anyone had asked patients what they thought about the care they received and published the results. It was a daring venture and bound to attract criticism – even outrage. But my book stimulated a range of enquiries and what amounted to a fresh approach to birth. I can be proud of that.

CHAPTER NINE

THE EIGHTIES:
INSTITUTIONS OR INITIATIVES

The University

One of my few experiences of a *'proper job'*, working in an institution, was in 1981 when I enthusiastically joined a university as a lecturer and Team Chairperson to create materials for community education. Perhaps I'd better not identify the university I worked for given what I am about to say about the experience. I expected social idealism expressed in practice, a shared spirit of adventure, and a stimulating environment. Working there was a shock because they seemed to me cut off from other vigorous organisations that were shaping the way women thought about pregnancy, birth and motherhood.

Our team was supposed to revise an existing course. This tied our hands, and it was difficult working with the original authors, who had set ideas about how their material could be updated.

My main concerns about writing fresh courses on birth and parenthood were that we should draw widely on all the help we could get from professionals and parents, and that materials should be made readily accessible to a much wider public than in the past. They should attract those who would not normally think of doing a university course, be written in an easy, flowing, warm style, starting from readers' own experiences and the challenges facing them in their everyday lives.

Film was an essential part of the course material and the BBC gave me speed training in the basic skills of video-making.

When Esther Rantzen came to film it was a high spot. She arrived wearing a capacious leopardskin coat, heavily made-up for TV, and with her new baby. She and I went out to a pub for lunch and the baby got hungry. Already the men in the pub were eyeing and talking about her. She just pushed back her fur coat, pulled out a breast, and fed the baby, who nestled under the pelt like a baby cub sucking from its mother. It was a superb demonstration of the ease of breastfeeding and how to incorporate it into a busy life.

I had a lively and excellent secretary, Helen, and became very fond of her. She was pregnant, resigned when I did, had her baby, and died of cancer of the cervix when her daughter was just over a year old. Her mother had disapproved of her choice of partner, especially when she became pregnant. In her last letter to me Helen wrote: '*My mum still won't talk to me. I was shopping last week and saw her and she totally ignored me. She didn't even look at the baby. Never mind. I rang her to try and make peace and asked her if she'd like to come and meet the baby. She told me she didn't want any "intruders" in her family. Oh well – at least I tried.*'

I was informed that all work in the department should be done with doors open so that there was easy access. Nobody worked in isolation. In fact, everything took place by committee, and I was very bad at working this way. It was very slow. I felt sucked into a machine which ground up everything I wrote and spilled it out as slobber, and confronted ingrained smugness which was resistant to ideas coming from outside the building. Committee language was churned out, drafted and redrafted, then redrafted again. Decisions were delayed until everyone agreed, sometimes out of sheer exhaustion. The custom was to write everything and then look to external organisations to rubberstamp the material.

Topics were put into second draft stage by a small group on which I was not represented. They were written in a pseudo-academic, patronising style, mixed with jerky, short and disconnected statements. Many vital educational points were thrown out or ignored, without any reason being given although some of my phrases were included in this general indigestible pudding. Finally, discussion on the course team was terminated by the Project Co-ordinator concluding that the whole course should be 'put on ice' and that I must get on with writing yet another set of first drafts for the second course – more work to be fed into the sausage machine.

I was keen to draw in professional health and birth activist organisations and star journalists for advice right at the beginning. Dee Remington, who had been

Assistant Editor of *Woman's Own*, and Davina Lloyd, Features Editor of *Woman*, advised us on how to reach a target audience. I showed them the material that had been handed over to me. They commented that the writing style talked down to readers, at the same time as going over their heads, using complicated language and terms but failing to explain them. There was no glossary. It did not discuss emotions, dilemmas and challenges in any depth. They pointed out that *'ease of reading is related to the cadence of sentences and phrases, not just the words used.'* Under the title of each topic there should be a *'come on'*, to draw the readers into the subject. Starting off each with a statement about the learning objectives *'is like an eighteenth-century novel in which the author tells the plot before you start. It makes it very dull.'* Activities should be fun to do and be realistic. It's no good telling the reader to spend an hour talking something through with her partner. She won't. At the end of the running copy salient points should be picked out with bullets. I thought this was all spot on, but my colleagues did not welcome the suggestions.

It was exciting to get a breath of fresh air from outside when an American researcher, Marjorie Walker, joined the team. Marjorie wrote to me saying that she had a doctorate in the education of young children and wanted to develop TV programmes. She had done research with Kathy Sylva, professor of Educational Psychology at Oxford – who suggested she contact me. (I knew Kathy because she had come to me when she was pregnant). Marjorie had no work permit for the UK so offered to work voluntarily for six months. I grabbed the opportunity, found a new ally, and she took over after I resigned in 1983.

One reason why I found my role difficult was that I was used to working independently, while drawing on advice on an international scale from a wide circle of friends in the birth movement, and health professionals.

I was writing a book for Dorling Kindersley called *Woman's Experience of Sex* and had a very good photographer, Nancy Durrell McKenna, who also worked with the United Nations and was commissioned by charities such as Save the Children Fund and Oxfam. She submitted a photograph, from a South African Family Planning Clinic, of a mother holding a mirror so that her daughter could see how her genitals looked, and discuss the difference between a child's and an adult woman's. Though addressed to the Course Team Secretary, someone opened this package, was deeply shocked, and reported me to the Director of Continuing Education. I was accused of passing on sexually explicit and obscene photographs and this led to my resignation.

I never worked for a mainstream institution again, remember my stint at that university as an ordeal, and was pleased to get away. I decided that if I was to create change I probably could not do so through any authoritarian organisation.

The Royal Free Protest

April 1982. Three days before. The phone rings and I am selecting clothes to wear – my choice a Stetson and a flowing cape – at the Birthrights rally outside the Royal Free hospital in three days' time. '*The Chief Constable here. You won't be able to have your meeting by the hospital – too many people are coming. You will have to march to Parliament Hill Fields. I have arranged for mounted police to escort you.*' I ask how he knows this and how many he reckons will come. '*Coaches have been ordered and will be arriving from all over the country. There'll be around five thousand.*'

Five thousand people out on the streets protesting at an obstetrician's decision that in future, in his hospital, all women must give birth on their backs on the delivery table, '*until, and unless, it can be proved safe to do otherwise*'. Many of Janet Balaskas's clients had their babies in this hospital and some had been prevented from giving birth actively.

The day came, and I watched the crowds swell. There turned out to be about 6,000 of them: mothers and babies, couples, single women, women medical students, midwives and students, doctors, feminist activists, home birth supporters – a great tide flowing around the hospital. We walked, (you can't march with toddlers in pushchairs and it is difficult with a newborn tucked into a carrier against your body), to Parliament Hill Fields, together with Anna Ford, the TV presenter, Michel Odent, who introduced waterbirth to the UK, Janet Balaskas, founder of the Active Birth Movement, who fired us with her organising and publicity skills.

The band struck up, and we were away!

5,000 JOIN NATURAL CHILDBIRTH RALLY
by Annabel Ferriman, Health Services Correspondent, *The Independent*

'*More than 5,000 mothers, fathers and young children marched across Hampstead Heath in north-west London, to demand choice in childbirth and the right for mothers to give birth by natural methods.*

The demonstration was sparked off by a ban on natural childbirth at the Royal Free Hospital, Hampstead, and the hospital's refusal to allow women to give birth in whatever position they want: squatting, standing up, or on all fours.

The hospital's contention, and the belief of many obstetricians, is that the use of high-technology equipment during labour, such as fetal heart monitors attached to the baby's scalp, improves the safety of childbirth.

The organizers of the rally claim that such equipment forces women to take a passive role in labour, makes it necessary for them to stay still and consequently slows up labour, making it less safe and less satisfying.

Banners with slogans such as 'Squatters Rights', 'Stand and Deliver' and 'Don't Take it Lying Down' were carried by the marchers, who came from all over the country.

Dr Michel Odent, the French obstetrician whose non-interventionist methods were recently shown on television, told the rally that the day represented the end of an era, a period when human beings had been dominated by technology.

'Today we are awaiting hopefully another human being who might have a different mental picture of the Earth, who will use technology in the service of life', Dr Odent said.

Technology itself was not to be feared, but only the glorification of technology. He hoped new methods of monitoring a child's heartbeat during labour would be developed which would be non-invasive and would make present obstetrics practice obsolete.

Mrs Sheila Kitzinger, a natural childbirth campaigner, who organised the rally, called for the establishment of alternative birth centres in the National Health Service, which would be staffed and run by midwives.

Anna Ford, the former Independent Television newsreader, told the rally about the birth of her first baby at the West London Hospital, Hammersmith. She had been allowed to give birth in the squatting position. Other women should not be denied that right she said.'

This Royal Free protest, was called to demonstrate against an edict by Ian Craft, Professor of Obstetrics at the Royal Free Hospital, that all women must push and deliver lying down, 'until, and unless, it is proved safe to be in other positions'. The spark that lit the beacon came from the Senior Lecturer in Obstetrics, Yehudi Gordon, who was encouraging women to get into any position that was comfortable for them and keep active. Midwives were developing alternative positions for birth and suggesting that women move around right through labour.

Mounted police accompanied us on the march, and those who were dads were eager to tell us about the births of their children and what their partners had been allowed, or not allowed, to do, so there was animated discussion throughout the march.

Following the protest the Professor resigned, left obstetrics and went into embryo research. He said it was nothing to do with the public protest.

Janet Balaskas

The joining together of mothers and midwives in the protest marked the rise of the Active Birth Movement.

Janet Balaskas had studied with me to become an NCT teacher and I realised that she was a special discovery. Like me, she did not toe the line and simply repeat Grantly Dick-Read's method of relaxation. This brought her into major conflict not only with the medical system but with the NCT, which threw her out, and there was a split between those who advocated active birth and others who stuck to the standard Dick-Read methods.

The NCT dreaded further polarisation between professional caregivers and pregnant women making what they saw as excessive demands. But soon NCT teachers started to examine research results and to incorporate pelvic movement, upright postures and spontaneous dance-like activity in their classes, which changed from '*think positive, flop and breathe deeply*' to what was virtually '*listen to your body and keep active*'. There was a new synthesis.

Radical midwifery was born. The Association of Radical Midwives, founded in 1976, chose the word '*radical*' not to suggest violent revolution, but because of its literal meaning of '*going back to the roots*'. This ginger group was concerned to improve the education of midwives and pushed for extension of the three-year direct entry training (so that midwives did not first have to be nurses) to centres all over Britain. They claimed that midwifery was quite distinct from nursing. The leaflets they produced were illustrated with lively cartoons by Polly, my daughter number four.

Childbirth Is Shaped By Culture

A common picture of childbirth in primitive life is like that of anthropoid apes. It is wide of the mark. It is *always* shaped by culture.

In traditional cultures around the world divination and incantation is widely used. Hawaiian midwives, for instance, use magic spells to take the pain from the woman and an incantation gives it to an animal. In one birth I attended the pain was conveyed to a very lazy brother-in-law.

In Jamaica a woman who is having a difficult labour can be helped by the midwife if a sweaty undershirt belonging to the father of the child is put near her and she takes some good sniffs. Then the baby is born speedily. Most births are without an acknowledged father, so the sweaty undershirt indicates that there must be a man around. This gives the mother a sense of security because it indicates the man is going to take paternal responsibility.

In Polynesia there is an incantation that midwives chant over a woman in labour, '*Now the living child, long cherished by the mother beneath her heart fills the gateway of life. There is room to pass safely through. The child slips downward, becomes visible, bursts forth.*'

Just as there is ritual in traditional societies, there is ritual in modern hospitals.

In a high tech culture women must go to hospital. Visits are allowed under restricted circumstances. The woman is separated from her partner and he (or she) is in a dependent situation, not allowed to affect the treatment of her or the baby, and often heavily patronised. In fact, a father usually has a humorous role and is supposed to be in a state of confusion and hopelessness.

In our technological birth culture obstetric incantation is when the doctor says, '*Don't bother your head. Leave this to us, woman.*' Or '*Keep your hands away from my sterile field.*'

The mother tends to be treated as if she were a sardine can and professionals open it to get at the contents. Technical terms are kept from her, and things said over her supine body which she is not supposed to understand. She may not be allowed access to her case records.

It would be incomprehensible in a traditional society for the baby not to be given to the mother. In a technological culture a woman is not so much a mother as a sick person. She is not responsible for her baby, and the coming together of her and the outcome of pregnancy is regulated by the hospital. In

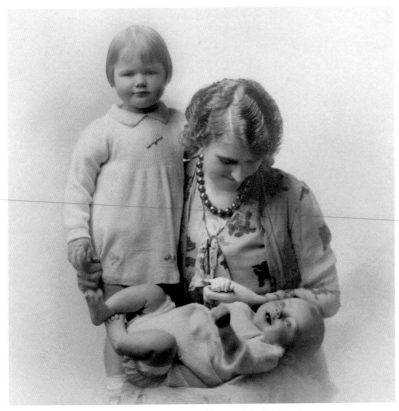

With my beautiful mother and baby brother

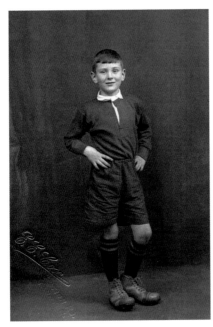

My brother David

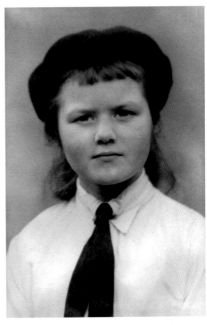

Teachers found me difficult

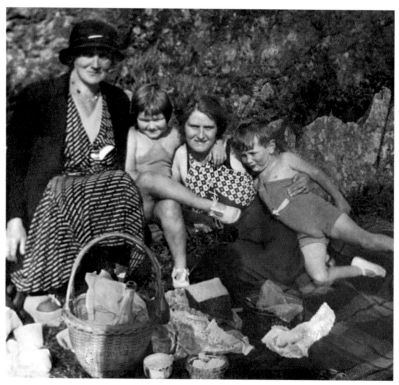

Father's photograph of a family picnic

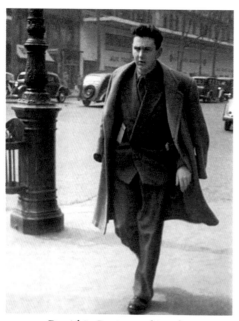

*David in Paris, working for
the World Student Federalists*

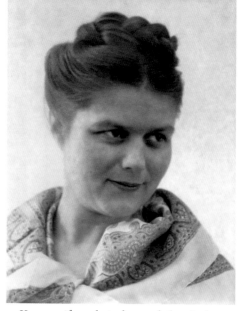

Young wife – photo by my father-in-law

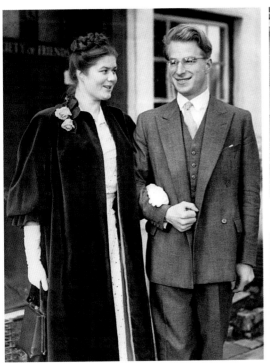

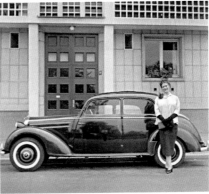

Pregnant diplomatic wife, 1956

*We married each other in the Quaker Meeting
House, Oxford, 4 October 1952*

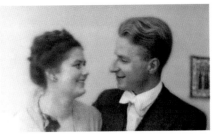

Strasbourg in the early 1950s

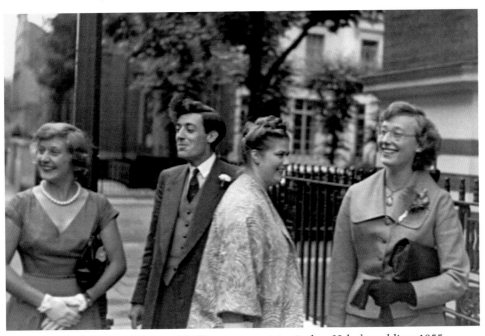

With Shirley and Bernard Williams at my sister-in-law Helge's wedding, 1955

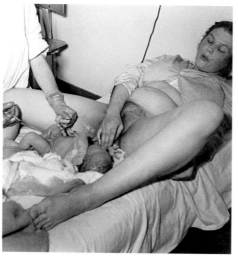
Celia's home birth in Strasbourg, 1956

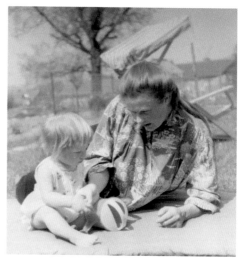
Enjoying parenthood, 1957

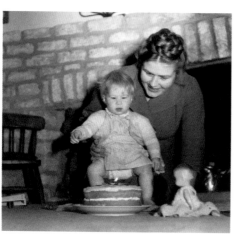
Celia's first birthday cake

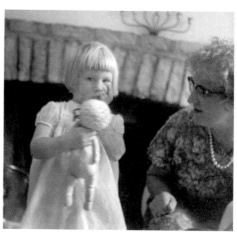
Celia with my mother Clare

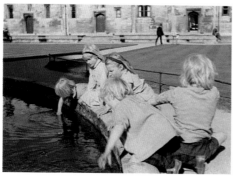
Tom Quad, Oxford:
Jenny, Nell, Celia, Polly, Tess

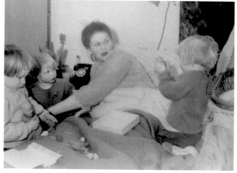
Playing with Mr Potato Head
just after Polly was born, 1961

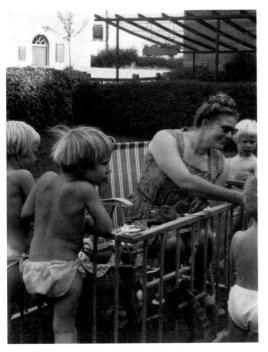

My retreat – the playpen

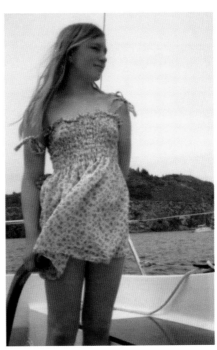

Polly at the helm off France

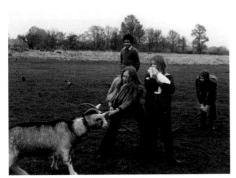

Polly, Jenny, Nell and Richard Ifill in the paddock with some of our pets

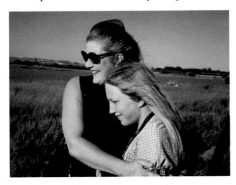

With Polly near Bages in the 1970s

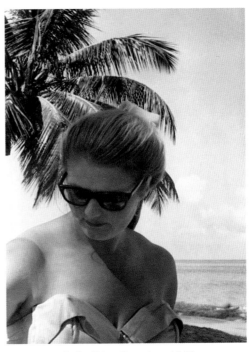

Ocho Rios, Jamaica, 1965

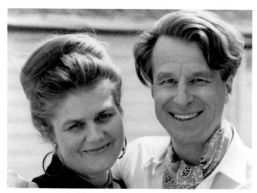

*Us together three days before Uwe had an eye
removed because of a melanoma, 1970*

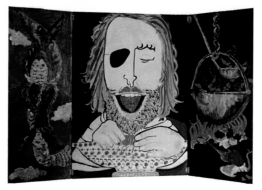

The Lord in judgement (triptych)

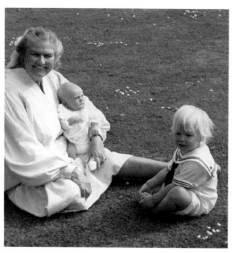

Happy with Laura and Sam

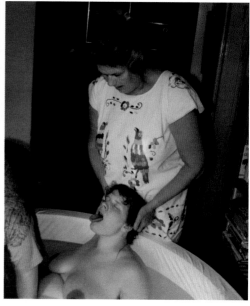

Sam's waterbirth

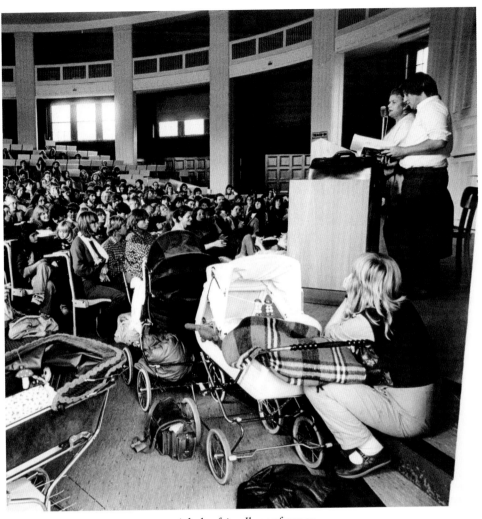

A baby-friendly conference

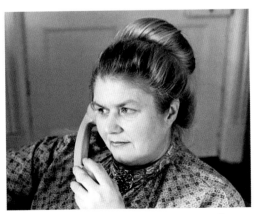

*My family remember me always on the phone,
always listening to women*

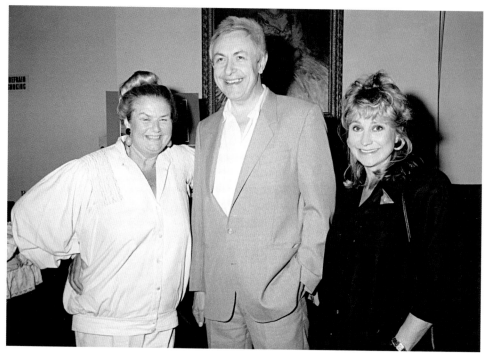

Launching Freedom and Choice in Childbirth *with Michel Odent and Felicity Kendal, 1987*

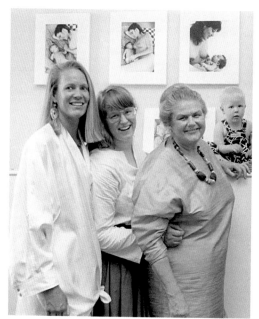

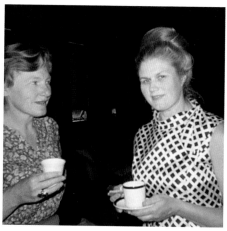

An NCT coffee break

*Nancy Durrell McKenna (left) contributed
her photos to half a dozen of my books*

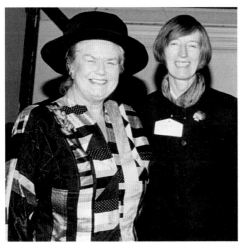

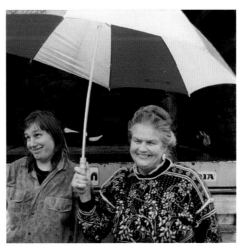

With Wendy Savage　　　　*With Polly collecting for Lentils for Dubrovnik*

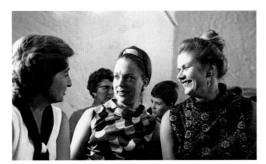

With Joan Gibson and Ruth Forbes

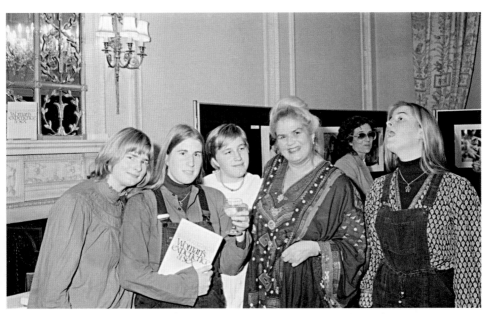

Launching Woman's Experience of Sex *with Nell, Celia, Polly and Jenny, 1983*

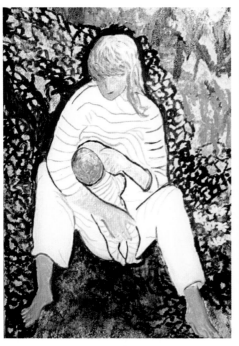

Tess breastfeeding Sam

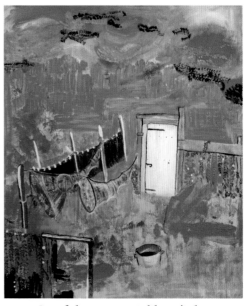

*Our fisherman neighbour's door
to nowhere*

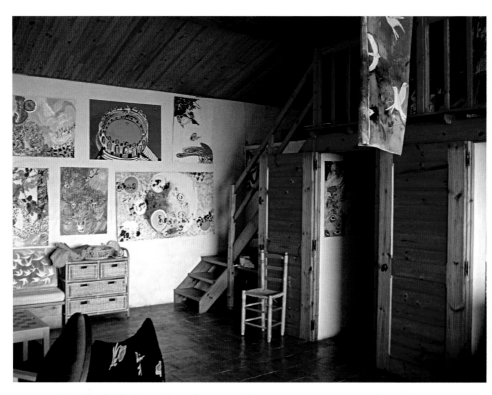

Wonderful light and studio space for my painting in southern France

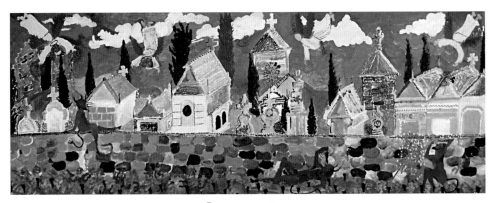

Bages cemetery

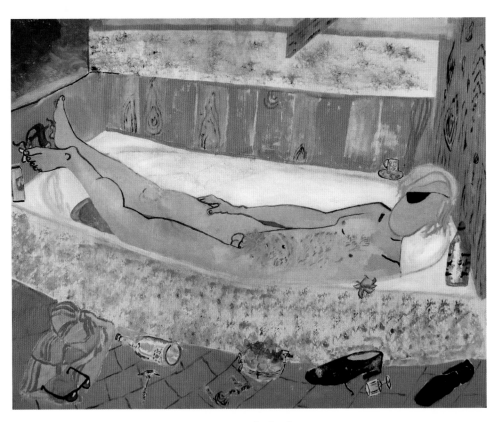

Uwe in the bath

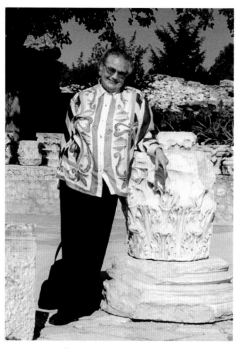

January in Morocco

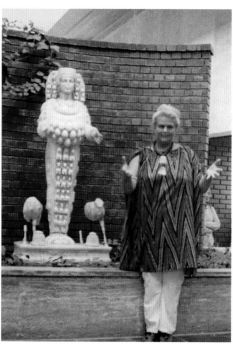

Great is Artemis of the Ephesians

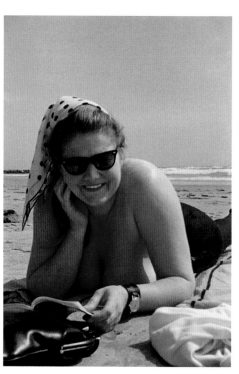

Gruissan Plage, 1968

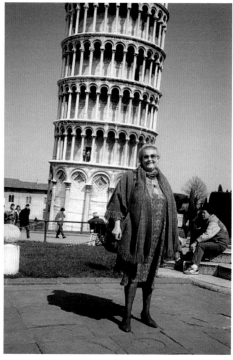

We love Italy

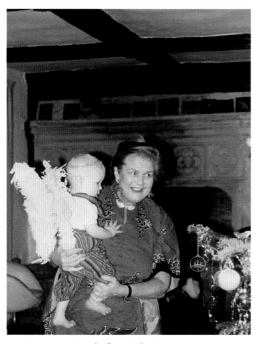

Sam's first Christmas

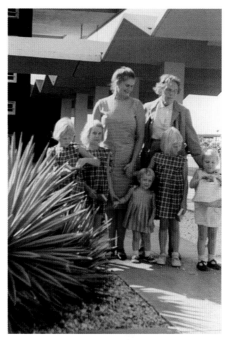

*Kingston Airport: Seeing off
Polly and Mutti*

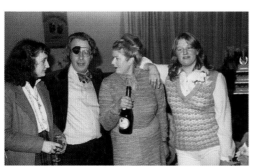

With Miranda at Tess's wedding

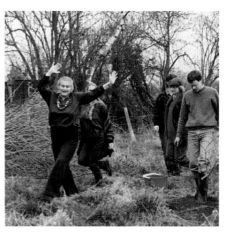

*Inventing our family rituals:
burying Sam's placenta*

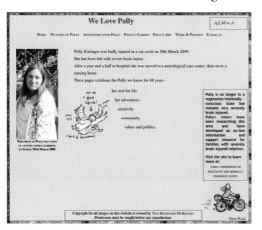

We Love Polly website, welovepolly.org

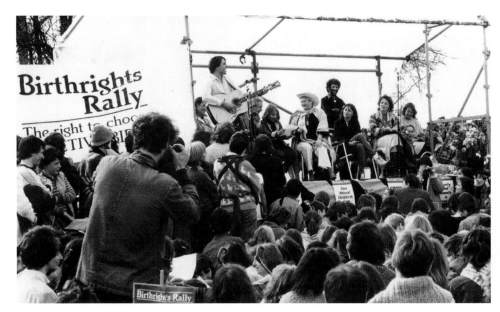

The Birthrights Rally – protesting at an obstetrician's decision that in the Royal Free Hospital all women must give birth on their backs, 1982

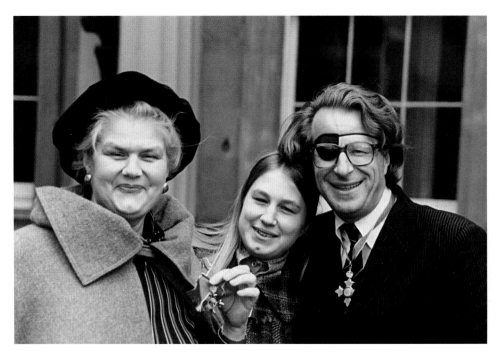

Buckingham Palace, 1982

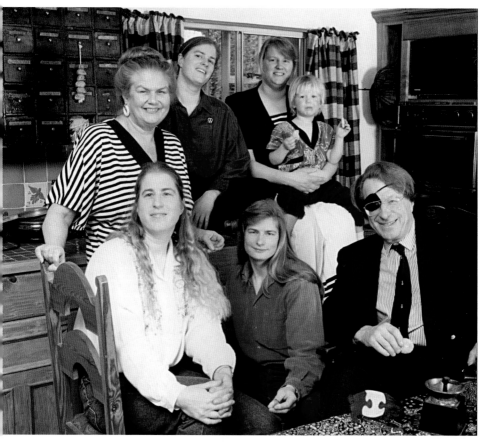

Family kitchen with Sam

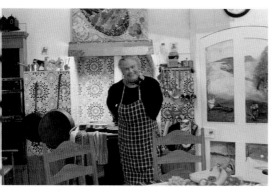

My kitchen: a riot of colour

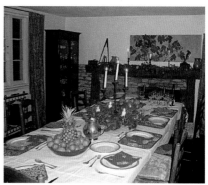

Set for a special occasion

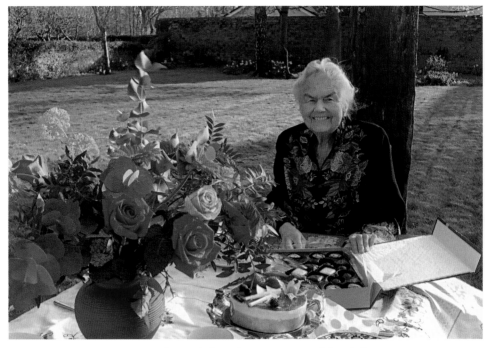

Roses, cake and chocolates on my 85ᵗʰ birthday

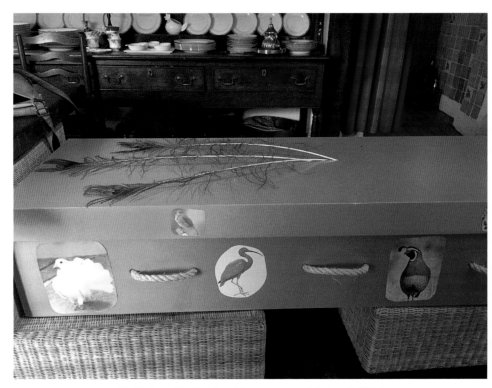

Sheila's coffin in the dining room, 12 April 2015

the United States, and throughout the world where American obstetrics have spread their influence responsibility is taken from both the father and the mother. They become virtually non-persons. The ideal patient is passive and trusting – one who doesn't interfere with hospital routine and is recorded on the case sheet as '*resting peacefully*'.

Yes, there are women who wish to know very little and who don't want to make decisions or even be aware of their labour or delivery. I believe they should have the right to that kind of birth if this is what they want. But birth as a pathological disturbance has now become the norm.

Many women feel the need in and after birth to propitiate those around them. Bowlby suggests that men envy women's possibilities of creative achievement in and through their bodies.[38] Hatred is projected onto women by society at large. How else can we explain '*routine*' episiotomies and '*routine*' use of forceps? By cutting the vagina a culture seeks to gain control over women's sexuality.

There is evidence that continuity of care and care-giving helps make birth a satisfying experience for mothers. A continuous relationship also contributes to a midwife's satisfaction with her work. Though shift work and being a member of a large team means that she can plan ahead, know what she will be doing this time next week, next month – even, perhaps next year – it fragments the midwifery experience, and all too often means that she feels trapped in a hierarchical and bureaucratic institution that regulates and controls her life, where she is just a cog in a machine. Because it denies her autonomy, and makes it difficult to give one-to-one care, it leaves her dissatisfied and frustrated.

Many women struggle to find a way through post-traumatic stress after birth. They suffer nightmares, flashbacks and panic attacks, and describe the birth as a kind of rape, played out over and over in their heads like a video tape that cannot be switched off. It is still not recognised that midwives, too, may suffer from post-traumatic stress. Birth can be emotionally mutilating, for them as well as mothers.

The essence of midwifery is a close relationship with women and their families as they pass through a major life transition. It is an exciting and awesome journey in which challenges are met, personalities revealed, and values explored. Midwives who have worked for many years in a hospital shift system may grasp the opportunity of switching to case-load practice because they are able to offer personal care. At first doubtful about it, and perhaps low in self-confidence, a new world opens up for them, and they use their midwifery skills with a fresh focus.

Being a midwife is not just what a caregiver *does*. It is who this person *is*. A midwife stands at the crossing-point of generations, embodying fundamental values in societies across the globe.

Writing About Sex

'*Why did you have five children? Was it just so that you had material for your books?*' Celia shouted at me when she was 12.

When *Woman's Experience of Sex* was published in 1983 she said this: '*I am always accusing Sheila of being heterosexist. Looking back, I really appreciate the fact that she never wanted us to be the same as everyone else. Above all, she expected us to battle to change the world as she had done, and she always said that we should endeavour to put back more than we took out of life.*

'*It wasn't difficult to tell her that I had become a lesbian. She found that out from the headmaster of the school I was asked to leave. Although I wasn't technically "guilty of the offence", the experience of my mother sweeping in to see him in her flowing cape, and insisting that I be heard and believed, left me with a lasting sense of solidarity. It was clear that, although she would always say, "Fight your own battles", secretly she was on our side, forever willing us to win.*'

Many mothers make it plain that what they would tell their daughters about sex bears little relation to their own experience. Pregnant women in antenatal classes often confess to a difficult relationship with their mothers. With busy lives of their own, they may have no time to be interested in their daughter's impending motherhood. They don't want to get involved.

Since the birth control pill came on the market women find it hard to say '*No*'. Sex is still used as a way of getting your man – and keeping him. Our sexual experiences are not just something to do with the genitals, but feelings about our bodies and the relationship between these and other people's bodies, and about ourselves as women and who we are.

A woman may decide that she doesn't want intercourse. She may want to be celibate. That is a perfectly viable option. Look at all the women who went into convents in the past. Some were trying to escape men – and live their own lives.

Women often apologise for themselves. If things are not good it is their fault. Before I wrote the book I talked to women who had been sexually abused, women who had been beaten, those who had been raped, and almost invariably they asked, '*Was it my fault?*'

The sex book came about because I was fed up with sex being identified as an object and a vagina. A woman's warm, tender, passionate, urgent, ecstatic feelings were much more than that. So I decided to research a book about female sexuality, and to include same-sex relationships and women's feelings about pregnancy, birth and motherhood.

One of the first things I learned was that many women were dissatisfied with their relationships with men. They were submitting to sex, enduring it in much the same way that we often think Victorian women did.

The so-called sexual revolution of the 60s did not liberate women. Sex was a common currency so that women's bodies were more bound to the sexual act than ever before. A great many women thought they were liberated but were in fact caught up in a rat-race to prove that they were sexually successful, and enjoyed the best and most frequent orgasms.

I felt sure that sex was not just something to do with the genitals, or any one particular organ – clitoris, back of the neck, big toe, or anything else. A woman's whole body can become an erogenous zone when she is aroused, sexual energy rushing through every pore of her body – her fingers, her toes, her head – everywhere.

We had built up the idea of orgasm as the heavens opening and angelic choirs playing, so a woman can be quite surprised if it turns out to be quite a little thing for her. Orgasms can be different on different occasions. It depends on your mood and relationship. A purely mechanical orgasm can be unsatisfying. We have become conditioned to think of it as being '*triggered*' because the language of sex is a *male* language. I was also learning a lot from my lesbian daughters.

When I asked women what they would tell, or had told, their daughters, almost invariably it would be a romantic story, even though their own experiences had been grim. One woman said that her husband used her like a rubber doll for his pleasure. Yet she was still claiming that sex was beautiful and uplifting and something to be kept for the right man. In the 80s mothers often taught girls to wait for their prince to come. Young girls expected sex to be a gift conferred upon them, instead of accepting that their sexuality was within themselves to discover. Lesbian experience was still perceived as deviant.

Many women use fantasies to escape from the reality of their relationships. If the way a man makes love is crude – get it up, get it in, pull it out, roll over and go to sleep – all a woman may be left with are the cobwebs of fantasies.

Sexual energy is not only expressed in foreplay and intercourse. As a writer, I must admit that sometimes I feel so alive when I am writing – when things are going right and I am carried away by ideas – that it feels like sexual energy rushing through me.

You can feel sexual energy very strongly with a baby, when breastfeeding is going well, for example. I remember talking to a much older woman whose husband had died some years ago, and she said that when the first grandchild was born and put into her arms, she felt a rush of feeling as strong as anything she had ever acknowledged as sexual. She felt *'This is what these arms are for'*.

I was apprehensive about writing the book because I knew I was not an expert. I was not a sex therapist or doctor, and here I was daring to write for other women. But as I listened and learned from them, I realised that I was acting as a channel for their thoughts.

Before we can accept the validity of our own experiences, we have to disabuse ourselves of the idea that there are experts who know more about us than we do ourselves. Our society told us to rely on 'professional' advice, to go to our doctors and do what they say. The women's movement, drawing on the ideas of Illich and others, was questioning this in the 70s and 80s. We were beginning to draw on our *own* experience. Quite a lot can be done in small groups of women sharing experiences. This was already happening with those who had been through traumatic experiences, such as rape, or who were in consciousness-raising groups. But many women still felt isolated.

In order to share we needed the words to communicate. It was the same with birth. When I first started writing about childbirth, there were few words to describe all the sensations, the firework display of labour, and so I invented them. I had to give other women the opportunity of saying, 'Yes, I *felt like that too...'* The more we could forge new words we could reclaim these experiences as our own. That was how my book *Woman's Experience of Sex* came to be written.

Kitzinger Women

I work closely with my daughters, and we share the same ideals. The 80s saw the Kitzinger women campaigning vigorously for social and political change. Polly and Jenny worked closely together organising '*Women's Strength*' demonstrations flying massed balloons painted with messages like '*Lesbians are Flying High*', '*Lesbians are Everywhere*', and '*Dykes Against the Bomb*'.

Polly wrote to me when I was on holiday in France: '*The Women's Strength Festival was very successful – we had hundreds of purple helium-filled balloons and marched through Carfax on Saturday morning with lots of musical instruments. It POURED down with rain, however, as soon as we'd left the city centre and 150 sodden and dripping lesbians turned up at the Poly for evening entertainments.*' There was a lively social programme, too: '*I had a great party the weekend before. 25 women turned up and we ate and played croquet and things. I hadn't intended there to be 25 women but once I'd invited my special friends, I then had to invite their households and their lovers – and their most recent ex-lovers (just to be impartial) and all their lovers' households too – and then I had to make sure I'd invited women with cars!*'

Jenny worked with Women Against Violence Against Women and was part of a collective which set up one of the earliest refuges for incest survivors. She moved to Scotland to work with the Glasgow University Media Group on communication strategies in the AIDS crisis, and later researched issues such as genetic research and medical ethics. She became a specialist in focus group methods and then went to Cardiff University leading research into science, health and risk.

Celia campaigned for a Lesbian and Gay Section of the British Psychological Society. As a visiting speaker finished his lecture at the annual conference a group of women jumped on stage wearing T-shirts announcing that they were '*visible lesbians*' and challenged the organisation to establish a lesbian and gay section. They won their case! Celia's book *The Social Construction of Lesbianism* was published in 1987. It broke new ground in psychology, presenting lesbianism as a political statement rather than either a pathological condition or, on the other hand, an affirmation of '*gay*' lifestyle. Journalists began to interview me asking about Celia and my disclosure that I had another two lesbian daughters. This continued to perturb journalists for many years. As late as 1997, the front page of the *Telegraph* ran a strap line reading: 'She's the expert, so how did her children turn out?' – with an article speculating about why three of my daughters were lesbian. Was it a reaction to my work in childbirth? Wasn't it a terrible shock for me? I said that I had learned a great deal which challenged my own liberal humanist ideology and led to deeper understanding of the oppression of women.

Lots of people saw my work as *'maternal'*, simply to do with *'natural'* birth and over the top. I was a *'guru'* extolling a weird religion. In the past other radical movements have been marginalised, too. Higher education for women was considered 'unnatural' in the nineteenth century and the abolition of slavery in the eighteenth. When slaves ran away they were described as mentally ill, suffering from a disease called *'drapetomania'*.

Mutilating Sexual Surgery

When I became Co-Chairperson with Baroness Caroline Cox of The Foundation for Women's Health Research and Development (FORWAD) in 1983, it was not with the idea of attacking a tradition that is a rite of passage in the culture of many African societies, including Somalia, Egypt, Ghana, Nigeria, the Sudan, Mali and Ethiopia. For me there was an imperative to challenge genital mutilation in western culture too, and assert the rights of women everywhere to control what is done to our bodies.

Western campaigners against female circumcision often talk about clitoridectomy and infibulation (removal of the labia minora and labia majora) as if genital mutilation were practices of an alien culture. In fact, routine episiotomy in childbirth is our western way of female genital mutilation, and cosmetic operations to reshape the vagina and labia, sought by women who are convinced that their genitals are ugly, are on the increase. In the United States *'designer laser vaginoplasty'* and laser vaginal *'rejuvenation'* are one of the fastest growing forms of plastic surgery.

In Victorian times, in Britain, and the United States, excision of the clitoris was performed to stop women masturbating and in the belief that it cured, among other things, mental illness, insomnia, infertility and *'nymphomania'*. Isaac Baker Brown, an eminent surgeon, published his book *On the Curability of Certain Forms of Insanity, Epilepsy, Catalepsy and Hysteria in the Female* in 1886. Earlier, his paper in the *British Medical Journal* of 1867 describes how to cut out the clitoris using two hooked forceps and a hot iron.

The Swedish Save the Children Fund wanted to make it possible for women in large areas of North and East Africa to choose not to submit their daughters to female circumcision. It is done on little girls, not only Muslim, but often Christian families too, usually between four or five and 11 years old.

In may seem that female *'circumcision'* is a minor operation. But it is not a matter of lopping off a piece of skin, but usually excising the whole of the clitoris, and in much of the Sudan, the Somali Republic, the Gambia and Mali, cutting away the labia as well, and stitching the wound so that only a tiny hole remains, through which urine and blood can be passed. Though in cities anaesthesia may be used, in country areas the operation is usually done without anaesthetic. It is believed that it makes the girl *'clean'* and that if she does not have it she will be dirty, smell objectionable, be too highly sexed, and may not be able to bear children. Infection is common and she may not be able to pass urine for days or weeks after the surgery. She may haemorrhage and become anaemic. Abscesses and urinary tract and pelvic infections lead to infertility. Every now and then a child dies. After a man has tried to open up his bride using a knife, razor or acid, she is often rushed to hospital bleeding heavily and in terrible pain.

The practice persists in Britain, and some Harley Street surgeons specialise in it. Other families send their daughters back to Africa to have it performed, largely because it represents a guarantee of virginity before marriage and is considered proof of chastity. In 1985 the Prohibition of Female Circumcision Act became law in England and Wales, making it illegal to cut off the genitals, the clitoris, labia minora or majora of any child or woman.

Even in those early days of protest I believed that we must put the emphasis on education, not condemnation, and make the education entertaining and fun. I thought that it was also important to understand the social and economic conditions in which this practice flourishes. Some of the African women performing clitoridectomy and infibulation are midwives who are no longer able to assist at births because women are going to hospital or nurses trained according to the western medical model have taken over their jobs. So they supplement their meagre income by doing genital surgery.

When people feel they are under attack and degraded they may cling to traditional practices in order to stress their cultural identity. Somali immigrants in the UK are shocked by the promiscuity they witness here and one way they seek to maintain standards with their young is to have their girls *'circumcised'*.

* * *

The first thing I proposed was to change the name of our organisation from FORWAD to FORWARD so that we presented a dynamic image. It was important to use the media. An impressive film was made by Louise Pantin for BBC TV, and two others on *African Women and Health* for Thames Television. Radio included discussions and talks on Radio London, BBC African Service, Network Africa and Gambia Radio. Articles appeared in the press, notably the *New Statesman*, the *Economist*, the *African Times*, the *New African*, *Third Way* and *Connexions*.

FORWARD contributed to the report from the Women's Action Group on Excision and Infibulation to the United Nations Commission on Human Rights, and its advice was sought throughout the various stages of the Bill on Female Circumcision that came into force in the UK in 1985.

FORWARD was represented at major conferences, including the UN End of Decade Women's Conference in Nairobi, the mass lobby of Parliament on World Poverty, the Gambian Women's conference on Women in Development and the Scottish Catholic International Fund Conference. We were also represented at many other smaller conferences and workshops run by women's development groups, educational institutions, African aid organisations and other bodies.

FORWARD published *Sister Links and Your Health,* the magazine of its African Mother and Child Campaign. In Ghana *Sister Links* was established as a voluntary organisation to distribute that magazine. Information packs went out to many other African countries. Health education material about vaginal health was prepared for rural women in the Gambia and sent in the form of taped cassettes with radio cassette recorders on which they could be played.

The African Mother and Child Health Campaign held workshops on health and beauty which attracted women who would not have wanted to come to workshops that were simply about their vaginas. A make-up demonstration among a group of friends in a woman's home was used as a basis to discuss aspects of reproductive health and issues relating to female '*circumcision*'.

Our offices also became a drop-in advice centre and women came seeking help with personal and socio-economic problems and to find refuge from domestic violence. FORWARD worked with other helping agencies and links were developed with Elders in African communities in Britain.

Educational materials were developed for health trainers – some specifically for non-literate groups. A very successful play was written about clitoridectomy and infibulation and shown in African communities. In all this Efua Graham, later Dorkenoo, worked tirelessly and effectively to spread the message and inspired the voluntary workers. She died in October 2014, just a week after launching The Girl Generation, a global, Africa-led campaign against FGM.

The Crying Baby

In 1985 I started to study what it is like to have a crying baby and to learn from mothers about their experiences. They told me the advice they were given, different things they did to try to stop the crying, and those that worked and didn't work.

The research began with a questionnaire in *Parents & Children* magazine in Australia and *Parents* magazine in the UK, to which 1,310 women responded. I followed this up with interviews with a large number. One subject we discussed was the advice they received from their doctors. Many seemed to know very little about crying babies and treated the matter lightly. They tried to reassure the mother and told her to put the baby out of earshot and leave it to cry. Women often lived in housing where it was impossible to do this so that the screaming was not bothering somebody.

Even when they could put the baby out of hearing, most women believed a crying baby had needs which must be met, and couldn't tolerate the crying, even in the distance, for more than 10 minutes or so. They said they couldn't concentrate on anything else and longed to comfort the baby. I don't think we need be ashamed of these feelings which run counter to so much professional advice. Right through human history these emotions have had biological survival value and have meant that mothers have picked up their babies when they were unhappy, kept them close – and protected them from danger.

Doctors also suggested giving up breastfeeding or introducing bottle-feeds as well. Yet my research showed that just as many bottle-fed babies cried for long periods as those who were breastfed. And many only started prolonged crying bouts after they were put onto artificial milk and other foods. They almost certainly had an intolerance to cow's milk. Though a baby who is simply hungry will quieten down when artificial feeds are added, these babies cried more.

Doctors often reached for the prescription pad, too, perhaps because they couldn't think of anything else to do when they saw a woman obviously at the end of her tether, and also because patients expect a prescription. The result might be tranquillisers for the mother and/or colic medicine for the baby.

I was alarmed to discover that a quarter of all babies had had sedatives by the time they were 18 months old, some for four months or longer. Many had a succession of different drugs – not only sedatives, but also pain-relievers, antihistamines (which also have a sedative effect) and anti-spasmodics.

The drug used most frequently was dicyclomine in the form of Merbentyl syrup and other colic drops. In 1984, 74 million doses of these medicines were sold in the UK alone. But in February 1985 a letter went out in the UK from the Committee on Safety of Medicines and the manufacturers warned doctors that a number of babies had stopped breathing for a while, had convulsions, or went into a coma, and some had died, after being given this drug. Since then Merbentyl had a label on the bottle saying that it is not suitable for babies under six months.

This was a shock to mothers who relied on regular dosing with this medicine to keep a baby placid. One mother described it as her 'liquid gold'.

Babies might have been having much more than the recommended doses if they were fed on demand, since the manufacturers assumed that it was given before every feed on the basis of four or five scheduled feeds a day. But if a woman was demand-feeding and gave the baby the drug every time, this maximum dose could easily be exceeded. There were other difficulties too. It was supposed to be given 15 minutes before a feed and with demand-feeding it might be difficult to know when a baby was going to wake. And mothers said they hated trying to keep a crying baby waiting for quarter of an hour before a feed was allowed.

Dicyclomine could sometimes make the baby even more uncomfortable, with a dry mouth, constipation, retention of urine and skin rashes. Some mothers also described how this drug had been over-prescribed by the doctor, with the result that a baby did not wake for feeds, had to be coaxed to suck, and fell asleep before a feed was finished. The effects of dicyclomine were often increased by combination with other drugs, such as tranquilisers or antihistamines. Sometimes this drug mixture made the baby more jumpy and irritable.

Some babies got a succession of drugs or a mixture that interacted with each other. Vallergan, for example, is a powerful sedative also used in psychiatry and as pre-medication for surgery. The manufacturers warn that it can potentiate symptoms of other drugs. A mother whose baby was on Merbentyl and Vallergan at the same time told me she stopped giving the drugs because *'I couldn't bear to see him so dopey'*.

Occasionally drugs made a baby so sleepy that the mother could not make eye contact with it, mothering became very unrewarding and the baby did not put on any weight. Some of these babies were admitted to hospital for failure to thrive.

Drugs were often prescribed when what the mother really needed was emotional support with a new and frightening task – and help with building up her self-confidence. A 20-year-old first-time mother was prescribed six different medications by her GP including Infacol, Merbentyl, Piptal, and Phenobarbitone, and gave the baby gripe water and whisky as well! The problem, she told me, was that her baby cried for about one hour every day. She needed help for her loneliness, anxiety and depression – and resulting panic when the baby cried – but she never got that. Instead her baby was drugged to the eye-balls.

Yet, if drugs don't work, what does? Since babies cry for many reasons, there is obviously no single remedy. Some babies need more stimulation and by the time they are about six weeks old start crying because they are bored stiff. It is only when they start doing things for themselves and exploring the world around them that crying becomes less. Mothers often said that these babies became happier when life was made more exciting – when they were surrounded by other children, for example, could listen to music and had lots of handling.

But babies can be overstimulated, too, especially those who are premature. These babies only stopped crying when they began to feel more secure. This does not necessarily mean that they needed peace and quiet. What was needed was to recreate something of the conditions a baby experienced inside the mother's body – playing a cassette tape of the sound of the heart and circulation – and cradling the baby close to her body like a kangaroo in the pouch.

Some babies needed a lot of holding and touching. Many women suggested to me that this might have been because they had a difficult birth and as a result had frightening dreams, so that they needed to be soothed again and again. Jumpy babies – who startle and cry in their sleep, often waking themselves up – can find a definitive routine comforting, which may mean parents need to keep to timetables. Some mothers became so tense themselves when the baby was constantly crying that they needed to be alone for a while. Only then could they unwind and the baby settle down: *'What helped me most'* one woman said, *'was to leave the baby in a safe place and go for a walk around our farm and talk to the animals where I am unable to hear or see the baby.'*

Some breastfed babies were not getting a good mouthful when they were at the breast. As a result they seemed to be feeding, but were in fact only getting the fore-milk, and none of the richer hind-milk. Their tummies were never comfortably full and they whined and fussed. When a baby is well latched on to the nipple a good deal of the areola, the brown circle around the nipple, is drawn into the mouth as well as the nipple itself. You can always see when a baby is latched on because sucking produces some movement in the upper cheeks and the ears wiggle!

A baby might cry irritably if a mother was under stress herself – because of family difficulties or problems in her relationship with her partner, for example. Sometimes it was only when these things were sorted out or when she developed a strategy for coping with stress that the baby calmed down.

However much helpful advice she was given, I concluded that the mother was the expert on her baby. Nobody else could know her baby as well as she did. Though drugs sometimes gave a breather so that she had a chance to calm down herself and think straight again, they were not really the answer. A baby's cry always means something and it is those who love the baby most who can learn to interpret what she is trying to tell you. The cry is part of a pre-verbal language which, like all languages, has to be studied before you understand its meaning. It can be the most difficult language of all to learn!

A book grew out of this research: *The Crying Baby*, which was published by Viking in 1989, and with additional material in a new edition, *Understanding Your Crying Baby* published by Carroll & Brown in 2005.

Being Born

Much of my work has centred on finding vivid words in which to communicate and share women's experiences. In *Being Born*[39] I tried to extend the use of language and imagery to share with a small child the amazing process of pregnancy and birth. In the 80s this hadn't been achieved.

I decided that I wanted to write a book for children, and record the unfolding of a journey that each of us has taken, but of which we have only momentary glimpses, or which we cannot remember at all. It is not the story of what happens when a baby brother or sister is born, but about what a child might see, hear, feel and do deep inside the mother's body, and about the baby's experience of birth.

This is different from an approach that explains a mother's pregnancy in terms of the biology and mechanics, and the names of organs so that labels can be put in correctly. Distinct, too, from the teaching of *'human reproduction'* in a detached, dispassionate way as a matter of hormones, anatomy, cellular development and viability, which is often how TV programmes for schools are done.

Children are often treated as completely ignorant of intense experiences they live through. These include sexual feelings, loss and grief when someone close to them dies, and outrage at social injustice. Yet experiences in childhood can be very powerful, even when children do not have the language to express this other than in difficult behaviour or withdrawal, and we should learn how to give them loving understanding and share with them accurate information. They do not live in a world of their own. They live in *our* world.

Language for most things that take place in women's bodies – menstruating, being pregnant, giving birth, even making love – is heavily medical. We just don't have words to say what we feel and know for ourselves.

I wanted to write for three and four year olds and talk to them just as I talked to my own children about pregnancy and birth, drawing on their experiences of their own bodies and their feelings to understand what was happening inside the mother's body, and how it might be for the developing baby. Only in this way could I do justice to amazing photographs taken inside the uterus and draw on the child's wonder at the miracle that was unfolding. So it was all written to the child as 'you'.

Lennart Nilson's photographs were an inspiration for me to write that book. They were perfectly tuned to describing fetal development in a language children could understand, in immediate and warmly descriptive terms that help them imagine how it might be inside their mother's bodies.

Some children's books about birth were comic. Fine! Others were sternly educational. Not so good. There is no need to talk down to small children or make pregnancy and birth jokey. I believe that we should aim to be honest and use vivid descriptive language, linked with visual images with which they can identify. What must it feel like to be curled up in your mother's body? To feel contractions clasping you in labour? To be pressed down through bone and muscles and out into the world? To be held in your mother's arms and see her for the first time?

I wanted my book to use language which creatively and vividly, attracted young children to the book with terminology and simile that was right for their age, and read like a good story book: '*You didn't look much like a baby yet – more like a sprouting bean ... and then, like a tiny sea-horse, you grew little ridges down your back that would form your backbone.*' '*When you had been growing for about five months your mother felt you move. At first your kicks were faint, like butterflies inside her, or little fish swimming, or soap-bubbles that float and pop.*' '*Your mother could feel you go bump-bump-bump. If she didn't guess what had happened she would have been surprised and wondered what you were doing.*' '*Your fingers reached out and felt water. Your fingers touched wet, shiny skin. Your face felt the touch and your fingers felt it too. Then they slipped away again, into the water. Your fingers were the first things you played with. They moved like the fronds of a sea anemone in a rock pool. Then one day your fingers found your mouth and brushed your lips. You liked the feeling and you began to suck your hand.*' '*It was warm in the uterus, like being in a warm bath in a darkened room. Fresh, warm water kept flowing in to keep you comfortable. Your skin had a white creamy coating that kept it from wrinkling in the water.*' '*When you had been six months inside your mother's body you could hear her voice. Often when she spoke you moved, almost as if you could talk to her with your whole body. She spoke and you listened. Then you moved. She spoke again and you stayed still. Then, when she had finished speaking, you would move again. Loud bangs made you jump. Sometimes you went to sleep for a long time. Then, when your mother went to bed and was about to go to sleep, you woke up and bounced around.*' '*When you felt the thick, springy uterus pressing against your foot you pressed your foot down and then lifted it. You took your first step. The stepping movements you made helped you turn upside down in the uterus, ready to be born. They helped you press your way out of the uterus when it was time for you to be born. You had been growing for eight months and now you were beginning to get plump. The fat would keep you warm after you were born. Your fingernails were like tiny shells.*'

Being Born was published in 1986 and earned a *Times Educational Supplement* Award. I think I succeeded in what I was trying to do. A Swedish journalist told how she read the book with a group of four to six year olds and was immediately asked to read it again. She had five children gathered around the book. *'Their individual comments inspired by my readings aloud and their looking at the pictures gave rise to one comment after the other, alternating between delighted screams and laughter whenever they recognised the similarities between the pictures and their own world.'*

For the record, the purpose of this book was definitely not anti-abortion. I support every woman's right to make this decision for herself. This is her body, her baby – her life.

Home Birth

For many women who wanted birth at home in the 80s the whole pregnancy was turned into a struggle involving negotiation with doctors and midwives about their right to give birth in the place of their choice. It still is. Every week two or three women contact me who are battling with the medical system. Most are suffering extreme stress from the uncertainty, and dread that their blood pressure may go up (which it may as a consequence of this stress). In relationships with caregivers they say they are made to feel like someone concerned only with her own emotional satisfaction, and who doesn't care whether her baby lives or dies.

One thing it was important for a woman who wanted a home birth to realise was that GPs themselves were also under strong pressure from hospital obstetricians and from their colleagues to *'play safe'* and turn down requests for home births.

Some of them were very frightened of the whole idea. It was not only that they had had no experience of it. Many had never seen a completely natural birth without any intervention during their training. They distrusted their own skills and did not really understand the skills of the midwife. They felt that if they could not intervene in a way similar to that of a hospital obstetrician, and did not have immediate access to high tech procedures – continuous electronic fetal monitoring, for example – they would be giving less than adequate care and might be guilty of negligence.

This is why it was important to share with GPs all the knowledge that was building up about the safety of planned home birth, and to work to increase their self-confidence in doing home births. One aspect of this was helping to link together home birth GPs so that they did not feel isolated and could exchange information and skills with each other.

It struck me that a way of reducing some of the obstacles for women, and at the same time helping those GPs who were willing do home births, was to contact the Family Practitioner Committee asking that it approach all GPs on the obstetric list to find out which were prepared to do home births.

In 1986 I wrote to the Oxfordshire FPC saying this. I said I realised that no GP could be expected to approve of home birth for all women, and that he or she would have to come to a decision with each woman. It agreed to draw up a list.

This worked well. GPs who were happy to help with home births had come out of the closet.

Germaine Greer's 'Sex and Destiny: The Politics of Human Fertility' Is Published

Whenever any woman whose name is linked with feminism produces a new book announcing a development of her ideas, it is greeted as evidence that the women's movement is crumbling. Articles are published selecting, with glee, phrases which cast doubt on, or seem to be an open denunciation of, what is taken by many to be a received feminist gospel.

Recantations and heresy are bread and wine to anyone trying to review a new book and the reviewer often comments that this is '*mature*' feminism or feminism '*grown up*'. This woman is, after all, just as men have always known women were – finding deep contentment in babies, hearth and home, and longing for the protective arms of a strong man.

Feminism *has* no leaders in the conventional sense. It has spokeswomen but no elected leaders, not even by popular acclaim. That structure of power and submission, authority and passivity, is an integral part of organisations dominated by men. On different issues women speak out, and what comes over as ovarian (no, not '*seminal*') philosophy at one time tends to be subsumed by fresh thinking. There is no creed to which women are required to give assent.

Some find it difficult to cope with this. There are those who long for a firm statement on belief and who reject each one of their sisters who will not vow allegiance to what they consider to be the truth. Yet flexibility is an important part of our strength. The imposition of any creed, however noble it looks, propels us from one schism to another – schisms which are the product of fear: that insidious poison in the relationships between women and their capacity for effective action.

'*Ideological correctness*' is the Marxist term, but this kind of conformity is of course much older than Marxism. It fired the crucifixion of Jesus and the Crusades, the Spanish Inquisition and the burning of witches in Salem, and it is inflaming rival concepts of Islam today.

I was brought up as a Unitarian, the daughter and granddaughter of a female line which believed passionately in free thought, the searching spirit and the death of creeds. This was no limp '*live-and-let-live*' philosophy to avoid fuss and unpleasantness. These women would have said, with Voltaire, '*I disapprove of what you say, but I will defend to the death your right to say it.*' They were anti-authoritarian, anti-establishment, against social injustice and inequality and exploitation. It is a heritage of strong and courageous women who refused to claim that they must always be in the right or understand each aspect of the truth.

With these strongly held convictions, I opened Germaine Greer's book, *Sex and Destiny: The Politics of Human Fertility*, and discovered that she was extolling babies, the family and the oldest kind of contraception in the world – withdrawal.

She presented a very romanticised view of women's lives, but then she always was a romantic! She used to think that fun and spontaneity were tremendously important. When she wrote *The Female Eunuch* 14 years earlier, she advised women to refuse to do things when other people expected or required them to and do them only when they themselves wanted. If you don't like cooking or housework, she said, don't do it! Do away with timetables and routines! She didn't say what a hungry three-year-old was supposed to do when there was no food and mother had gone off to be spontaneous and express herself. And she seemed unaware of the physiological pull a breastfeeding mother feels when her baby cries. She ignored all the gut feelings of being a mother and the emotional umbilical cord through which flows pain and longing that is a good deal more powerful than detached intellectual awareness.

At that time she was toying with the idea of having a baby in a rural Italian setting. She thought that a farmhouse in Calabria might be the answer. She would go there with some women friends to give birth to their children: '*Their fathers and other people would also visit the house as often as they could, to rest and enjoy the children and even work a bit. Perhaps some of us would live there for quite long periods, as long as we wanted to. The house and garden would be worked by a local family who lived in the house ... The child need not even know that I was his womb-mother and I could have relationships with the other children as well. If my child expressed a wish to try London or New York or go to formal school somewhere, that could also be tried without committal.*'

There were two elements in that particular recipe which I found disturbing: one was the last two words – there was *no committal* to another human being; the other was that all this could never be done unless you hired or cajoled other people who *would* take responsibility – the peasant family on whom everything else depended. She must, I think, have realised this herself.

The attraction to feudal solidarity has now become a paean of praise to the extended family, which she calls '*The Family*' to distinguish it from its pale shadow, the nuclear unit of a couple with their 2.5 children. Life with mothers and father-in-law, uncles and aunts and nieces and nephews and cousins-once-removed may be, she admits, difficult. But '*The Family*' has always offered women territory which was indisputably their own, and however disenfranchised they have been in the outside world, in the domestic sphere they have exercised political power. In breaking up '*The Family*', women have been robbed of their own territory. '*The Family*', she says, '*offers the paradigm for female collectivity; it shows us women co-operating to dignify their lives, to lighten each other's labour and growing in real life and sisterhood – a word we use constantly – without any idea of what it is.*' She may be right, but she writes all the time as a '*visitor*' commenting on how other women live. We never hear what these women themselves have to say about their lives.

She also claims that the extended family provides a much better environment for children. '*In our society there is profound hostility to children and those of us who decide against childbirth do not do so because we are concerned about the population explosion or because we feel we cannot afford children, but because we do not like them.*'

Anyone who has had a baby soon comes to realise this. Babies are rarely welcome at adult social gatherings and in Britain, unlike Italy and France, some restaurant owners detest them. *The Good Food Guide* often suggests that parents should leave '*under-14s and dogs at home*'. (I once wrote to the editor, suggesting that there ought to be a special list of restaurants which put themselves out to welcome children.)

Anyone who has tried to carry on a normal working and social life accompanied by their children will know how anti-child our society is. There are many places where you cannot take pushchairs, prams, or even babes in arms, and the effort is so great that many women give up and are imprisoned as if in their own barred play-pens, looking out at the world but unable to take any part in it.

In most of the Third World and in peasant societies, each child is welcomed as a protection against poverty in old age and to strengthen the bonds and enrich the life of the extended family. The child does not belong merely to its own parents but to a whole group of relatives and neighbours.

Our Western society locks families up in concrete or brick containers, piled high in tower blocks, and tarmacs over the green spaces and woods. It crowds two adults and two children into as limited a space as possible and tells them to love each other and behave nicely, and if they are so profligate as to have more than the correct number of offspring and lumber themselves with grannies and other elderly relatives and ill or handicapped children – who should have been '*screened out*' in pregnancy – well, they should have known better!

Children need mud, grass, water and space to explore. Children need the wilderness. We have tidied it all away. It is a thing country children have always had and in Third World societies they still have it around the shacks and pre-fabs that scar the cities like great sores. Even if '*home*' is a two-room hovel with a corrugated tin roof, a worn out motor-car body or packing case by the harbour, at least outside there is a natural adventure playground. The women, babies in shawls attached to their bodies like limpets, meet at the pump or well as they draw water, scrub clothes on stones by the stream, at the market where they sell and haggle, and on the ramshackle bus rattling its way stuffed with grown-ups, children, hens, ducks – and perhaps a goat or two.

It is not, perhaps, the life we'd choose. But, Germaine asks, '*What is our civilisation that we should so blithely propagate its discontents? How can we teach due care for children when we do not care for our own? Why should we erect the model of recreational sex in the public places of the world? Who are we to invade the marriage bed of veiled women? Do we dare to drive off the matriarch and exterminate the peasantry? Why should we labour to increase life expectancy when we have no time or use for the old? Why should we care more about curbing* the increase in the numbers of the poor than they do themselves? Who are we to decide the fate of the earth?'

I've seen stickers on cars in the United States which announce 'Pollution – Your *Baby!*' Perhaps it's all very well for us to lecture each other about the world population, but to foist our solutions and our philosophies on the rest of the world is another matter. Multi-national companies are making large profits producing pills, injections and intra-uterine devices with which, even while we are becoming more and more aware of their danger to our *own* health, we are flooding the developing countries.

Enthusiasm for controlling the breeding of the unfit and the unfortunate is, of course, not new. In 1915 Margaret Sanger, the American pioneer of birth control, chose several down-and-outs and sent them into the most crowded streets of New York, displaying the warning: '*I am a burden to myself and the state. Should I be allowed to propagate? I have no opportunity to educate or feed my children. They may become criminals. Would the prisons and asylums be filled if my kind had no children? Are you willing to have me bring my children into the world? I must drink alcohol to sustain life. Shall I transfer the craving to others?*'

In England Marie Stopes wrote an article in the *Daily Mail* called '*Mrs Jones does her worst*': '*Are these puny-faced, gaunt, blotchy, ill-balanced, feeble, ungainly, withered children the young of the imperial race? Why has Mrs Jones had nine children, when six died, and one was defective? … Isn't it for the leisured, the wise, to go and tell her what to do? … Mrs Jones is destroying the race!*' When Marie Stopes's own son wanted to marry a woman who wore glasses, she wrote to a friend: '*She has an inherited disease of the eyes which not only makes her wear hideous glasses so that it is horrid to look at her, but the awful curse will carry on and I have a horror of our line being so contaminated and little children with the misery of glasses … Mary and Harry are quite callous about the wrong to their children, the wrong to my family and the eugenic crime.*'

Germaine pointed out that, even though we had stopped talking to each other like that, much of what was being said to parents in the Third World countries was on the same level and denied our own responsibility for '*the sudden exponential increase in the global human population as a result of an ecological disaster which happened about five hundred years ago, namely the explosion of Europe.*' Europeans founded their empires, finding stable populations living in circumscribed communities with reproductive strategies some of which had been effective for hundreds of years. '*After the initial shocks, and systematic annihilation by guns, disease and poison, especially alcohol,'* survivors began to expand in a population explosion which spread like a virus. '*When we see the hopelessness of the slums ... we see the latest stages of an epidemic disease ... It was the scourge of colonialism that cheapened human life, that made human dignity a nonsense, that showed the people in the hot lands that their destiny was not theirs to command. They may wish to escape the pangs of childbirth, for they will not wish to be fewer. There is all the difference in the world between family limitation undertaken for positive reasons and family limitation accepted out of despair. If the second becomes the rule, the world will not be worth living in, however few people are in it.'*

Germaine also discovered the joy of withdrawal – *coitus interruptus*. What had those of us who have been messing about with chemicals and bits of rubber been missing all these years? Far from being a sub-standard, risky and thoroughly awkward method of birth control, Germaine claimed that it held delights which most of us have forgotten as we have stumbled on, experimenting with yet more complicated and costly methods with dangerous side-effects.

The trouble with *coitus interruptus* is that there is no money to be made out of it. No international pharmaceutical company is going to market it as a great new technique or arrange jamborees for doctors to discuss its benefits. Yet withdrawal is probably used more than any other method in the world and is associated with some of the lowest birth rates on record. It is how whole populations have been ready to respond to poverty, famine and other economic pressures long before the days of contraceptive clinics and the invention of rubber, and explains why in Europe birth rates went down dramatically the instant that couples decided they wanted to delay having children, or already had enough.

It is generally assumed by doctors that it is both ineffective and harmful. One nineteenth-century writer claimed that it resulted in '*general nervous prostration, mental decay, loss of memory, intense cardiac palpitations, mania and conditions which lead to suicide.'* More recent writers warn about marriage breakdown, anxiety and neurosis and suggest that men have heart attacks because of it!

Whether or not a woman finds sexual intercourse satisfying has little or nothing to do with when or where a man ejaculates and everything to do with what he does *before* and *after* ejaculating. It is very hard for men to understand this because they think that the be-all and end-all of sex is penetration and ejaculation. And all the other delights of love-making are to them merely *hors d'oeuvres* to the main meal, or after-dinner mints! Women enjoy other kinds of touches and closeness, other caresses.

Coitus interruptus is certainly not incompatible with skilled and considerate love-making. And because it demands care and self-control it may even draw out the best in a man. When women have talked to me about memories of adolescent sex, it is this aspect of it which they speak of with nostalgia. The quick screw in the marital bed is a far cry from this earlier long drawn out love-making that was spiced with danger.

In peasant Italy the idea of '*serving*' the woman entails prolonged intercourse with frequent withdrawal, and men pride themselves on their ability to keep going '*all night*'. A man has no intention of getting married and having children until he can afford a house, so couples may be engaged for 12 years or more. The practice of *coitus interruptus* is part of the courtship. The woman who thinks it is about time they got married uses all her wiles to break down the man's control so that, once pregnant, she goes to the altar, as Germaine says, '*dressed in white as a testimony of the chastity of her relationship with the only man with whom she has ever been intimate.*'

Conception in this context is not seen as a disgrace, but as a blessing on the union and evidence of its rightness. After the birth of the first child, coitus interruptus will be used again until the couple want a second child, and so on. A good lover is one who can reserve and control ejaculation and who is considerate; a bad one is a man who just grabs a condom and uses the woman for his pleasure.

In colder climates the practice of '*bundling*' has allowed for the same extended love-making. The betrothed couple were tucked up in bed together, made snug and warm, with a large bolster between them to preserve the girl's chastity. A man needs considerable flair in sexual technique to make love to a woman on the other side of a bolster! And it created a pattern of prolonged love-making and consideration for the woman's feelings which lasted well after the eventual removal of the bolster and the right to lie in their own marriage bed.

Germaine's fireworks about sex and fertility are more than just a dazzling display. They spark off questions which, though uncomfortable, demand to be answered. They challenge the assumptions of those of us who live in the privileged and economically powerful parts of the world and which come from ignorance of values of women in Asia, the Middle East and Africa. We need to think in a new idiom, taking into account and trying to understand the bonds of commitment that tie human beings together over most of the world.

Until now feminism has been a movement mainly for Western women. If it is also to be an expression of the hopes and longings of women in the Third World it is bound to change and may end up looking very different from Western-style feminism. Let's hope that Germaine's particular brand of shock-treatment helps us to understand this and adapt.

My Teaching

I have been accused of viewing birth through rose-tinted glasses and failing to acknowledge the agony and pain that most women experience. The argument is that women should have the right, without any special medical reason, to anaesthesia and be knocked out and wake up after it is all over.

On TV and radio I have always stressed that there is no recipe for childbirth. Choices have to be made and they must be based on knowledge, not ignorance, or on wishful thinking.

In an interview in 1986 I said: *'Birth is absolutely rotten for many women. It's sometimes made rotten because of the environment in which they give birth. The kind of professional help they have sometimes involves intervention which makes them feel trapped and disempowered. I had four home births and they were terrific. There are lots of other women who won't have ecstatic experiences. I fully acknowledge that. But that's why it's so important for women to be educated about what is possible: to learn how to talk to their doctors, how to say what they want and stick to it and learn how to negotiate the kind of birth which is right for them.'*

Woman's Hour

From the 70s on I made quite a few appearances on *Woman's Hour*, first with Sue MacGregor and later with Jenni Murray – both superb presenters – with whom I enjoyed discussing birth.

In an interview in 1986 Jenni Murray drew on the *Woman's Hour* archives to discuss the work I started in the 1960s she said: *'Thousands of women in Britain have had greater control over the way they give birth thanks to Sheila Kitzinger. At a time in the 1960s when childbirth was almost exclusively in the hands of the,* usually male, medical establishment she wrote her first book "The Experience of Childbirth" to "give women a voice". She introduced to them the idea of fathers being present, if the couple wished it, at the birth; the birthing stool, moving around during labour and squatting for delivery, and the birthing pool. Her advice has sometimes been misunderstood as a demand for "natural childbirth" for everybody, causing women dangerously to refuse medical interference in their labours, or to expect an ecstatic experience when, for some, it could be anything but.'

In one of the earlier programmes I had explained how I became enthused about childbirth: 'It was my training as a social anthropologist that led me to my work with pregnancy and childbirth. When I first became pregnant myself, I discovered that we really didn't know much about how women felt and behaved in different countries. All the anthropological work had been done almost exclusively by men, and they hadn't asked questions about birth; there was a big literature on what was done to the placenta, because they had stood outside the birth huts of primitive tribes and had seen that happening, but they didn't really know what went on inside. So I became very interested in what it felt like to be a woman giving birth in different societies, which of course included our own.'

I said, 'We have now discovered – and there's plenty of evidence to support this – that it is much safer for a woman to have at least the upper part of her body well raised, even to be standing, for much of the labour. The uterus contracts better, the woman feels less pain, and the baby is better oxygenated. First of all this was looked at in terms of the first stage of labour, and then also in terms of the second stage. No woman in her right mind would choose to lie down on her back with her legs in the air to push a baby out, because she has to push uphill. Most women, if allowed to do what they want to do, and what comes naturally, will adopt a modified squatting position, crouch or kneel forward, or even get on all fours. Hospitals are now beginning to see that they achieve more effective second stages if they encourage women to adopt any position which is comfortable for them. I think this is marvellous – it means we have to do away with the old-fashioned delivery room beds, and put mattresses on the floor and provide lots of pillows, and something more like the medieval birthing stool – a very low, horseshoe shaped kind of milking stool – which women right through history used to sit on to have babies.

'All this, of course, challenges the current preference in hospitals generally for mechanised, monitored birth. But what is the point of rupturing the membranes, inserting an electrode and putting a clip on to a baby's scalp, and having a woman *lying down and monitoring every heartbeat, if you are thereby producing a dip in the fetal heartbeat? There is also plenty of evidence to suggest that having a woman immobile, and rupturing the membranes artificially, thus taking away the protective bubble of water in which the baby is lying, actually produce the conditions which we then go on to monitor.*

'*Sometimes I hear a doctor say that the one thing that matters is a live and healthy baby. For most families it isn't the only thing that matters. The way one feels about that baby, and the bonds that link you with it, are important too, and there's really no point in producing a perfect, well-oxygenated, healthy little animal unless the relationship between the baby and its parents is a going concern. That's why I think we have to look at the whole culture of childbirth in our society and see what we can do to make it a celebration, a joyous occasion.*'

My own approach to giving birth I described as '*psycho-sexual*', a term I used because I believe birth is essentially a sexual activity. '*By this I mean not only that sex starts the baby off, but that the rhythms of birth are essentially sexual, if we allow them to be. I suspect that most of our hospitals don't let women do this, but treat birth as a medical crisis. If a woman is really listening to her body, however, and in tune with it, the rhythms come in waves – both the rhythms of contractions right through the first stage, and the bearing down urges in the second stage. Often there is a team of people standing over the mother and saying, "Come on, mother, take a deep breath and push. Come on, push ... push ... push ... Come on, you can do better than that ... Hold your breath ... and push ...push ..." There she is with her eyes popping out of her head, little blood vessels breaking in her cheeks and eyes, straining and groaning. In fact it's an awful waste of energy, and she's not helping the baby get born. Moreover her prolonged breath-holding may well be cutting down the oxygen reaching the baby. She looks quite obviously in distress, which can reduce the amount of oxygenated blood flowing through the placenta to the baby. Studies have shown that if a mother holds her breath for longer than six seconds there is a risk that she may cut down the oxygen reaching the baby, and yet people in hospitals still coax, cajole and command women to push.*'

Nigella Lawson

Shortly after Nigella Lawson gave birth to her last child she and I did a *Woman's Hour* discussion together. It was a meeting of minds. Nigella had had a home birth. She was still fresh from the experience, scented with breast milk, luminous, dewy eyed, touched with the extra beauty and gentleness of new motherhood. She spoke about the importance for her of giving birth in her own space, having those she loved around her, being free to move and make the sounds she wanted. It was clear that she was not just a *'celebrity'*. She was a highly committed woman with a strong mind and determination to do what she believed was right, and birth was for her an outpouring of love.

Journalists And Me

I usually enjoy working with journalists, though many assume I'm a midwife. Others cling to the *'earth mother'* stereotype, and I must often try to dissuade them from using the term *'guru'*. They tend to write about natural childbirth without defining it, and imply that this is what I teach. It is a bit like *'natural'* eating, clothing, or for that matter, parenting and education. The way we give birth is an expression of culture. It can be spontaneous and instinctual, but it is still patterned by the society in which we live.

Sometimes a journalist's questions are formal and routine. Do you believe…? Where do you like to go for your holidays? And so on. Sometimes they are zany: What animal would you like to be? I think I prefer the zany ones. Anyway, *Good Housekeeping* asked me that one and I said:

'I rather fancy feathers – lovely to stroke and to ruffle, and pretty to preen. For grand occasions I'd like splendid plumage touched with gold, emerald, crimson, ivory and black. I'd never have to think what to wear – only have to spread wide my peacock tail or flamingo wings. I could adapt to changes in the weather, too, without needing to wear heavy clothing – just a shake or two and I'd be wrapped in a soft, air-pocketed feather duvet, which rainwater would just slide off, leaving me glossy, bright and dry.

'Then I could spread and lift my wings and take flight over cities, mountains and the sea. It would be a terrific improvement on transatlantic flights – I'd no longer be locked in a metal tube and forced to inhale other people's cigarette smoke.

'I'm not sure that I want to lay eggs, though, since the sensations of human birthing are so exciting. Give me a new combination of bird and mammalian physiology and I'll take off, flapping my wings into the sunset.'

It is those women journalists who claim to be *'post feminist'* and who see birth entirely in terms of shopping around, with every option of more or less equal value, who criticise me for apparently dictating how women should have their babies.

Polly Toynbee writing in the *Guardian*, came over very strong on this one. She wrote: '*Natural childbirth, a child of the sixties, was and is largely a nutty fad from a noisy group of lentil-eating earth goddesses.*

'*How extraordinary that those who call themselves feminists fight for women's right to suffer and, in the process, inflict so much unnecessary suffering on women. The right to safe local anaesthetics, properly administered by experienced obstetric anaesthetists, should come first. Of course, the right to refuse it is important too. But the earth mothers have lied and lied again about the risks of anaesthesia and as a result they have denied women a genuine right to choose. For if you are led to believe there is a serious risk to yourself or your child, you would probably opt to suffer the pain, however severe.*'[40]

In my letter back I said: '*Polly Toynbee claims that I, and other "earth goddesses have lied and lied again about the risks of anaesthesia". I want to put it on record that I have not lied, and that I object strongly to her unsubstantiated accusation.*

'*Some women have had traumatic experiences with so-called "natural" birth. (Actually, it's not a term I use. As a social anthropologist I see birth as always patterned by culture). Often this kind of "natural" labour has been under slap-dash supervision, with no real understanding of how to support physiological processes in childbirth, and sometimes with staff who have attitudes towards the labouring woman which can only be described as punitive. My own research reveals that there are other women who have also had traumatic experiences with epidurals. I am working to make birth better for all women, whether they decide they want an epidural or prefer to avoid all obstetric intervention.*

'*Instead of polemics and angry denunciations, we need to explore exactly how care, including different methods of pain relief, can be made more effective, and enable women to make informed choices between alternatives.*'

Rowan Pelling did a witty piece on witchcraft and midwives and, thinking I was both, wrote: '*I made a programme on childbirth earlier in the year and I can state as an unscientific fact that one in three midwives is a practising witch. I knew within one second of meeting Sheila Kitzinger, Britain's reigning birth guru, that she could turn you into a frog by one clench of her pelvic floor muscles.*' It is rather difficult to live up to this image but I continue doing my pelvic floor kisses, and one day may qualify as a witch.

Baby Mix-Up

In 1986 a mix-up in an Irish hospital left two women with each other's babies, and the blood tests that followed to sort it out seemed to justify the nagging doubts of many mothers – particularly those who gave birth in large hospitals where babies were routinely taken away to the nursery.

'Can I be sure that this really my own baby?' they often asked themselves as they removed the name tag when they got home and tucked it away as a memento.

When birth takes place at home it is impossible for babies to be switched by mistake. But when the birth was conducted in a busy 'production line' maternity hospital, and babies were whisked away to lie in rows in plastic boxes in the nursery, returned to their mothers only for feeding, it quite possibly happened more than we know. And maybe in some instances where nobody realised, such mix-ups were never detected.

In the United States all newborns were foot-printed immediately to avoid such confusion and some people pressed for foot-printing to be introduced in the UK, too.

In the past queens always had to prove a baby was really theirs and Queens of England gave birth surrounded by members of the court and in the presence of the Lord Chamberlain. Marie de Medici, one of the Queens of France, delivered in the presence of 200 people. Today, one of the reasons some mothers insist that their partner is present is to be absolutely certain there are no mix-ups.

Another fascinating issue raised by the confusion over the babies is the importance and power of mother/baby bonding.

How can a relationship build up between a mother and *somebody else's* baby in such a short space of time so that when the mistake was discovered the mother at first refused to accept that the child was not hers?

It is well known that adoptive mothers often feel immediate, intense love for babies placed with them. Most women, whether natural or adoptive mothers, are swept into motherhood on a wave of joy.

There is a definite sequence of events as mother and baby get to know each other and, significantly, it is the same between a mother and an adopted baby. It is the beginning of pre-verbal communication, starting with the woman touching the baby so gently and tentatively, usually with her fingertips only, as if the child is too fragile to approach in any other way.

She explores the tiny fingers and shell-like ears. All the time she quite spontaneously speaks to the baby in a high-pitched voice, repeating many phrases – a language that a baby can understand and often finds riveting!

Much was made of one father's insistence that the baby they were given had his mother's nose and his uncle's forehead. But it's much more likely that the instant, immensely strong bonding that can take place between a woman and a new-born child, even when it's not hers, convinced them both that this was their baby.

They each needed uninterrupted time alone with their babies without anyone hovering over them to see whether or not they were bonding. You can't demand too much of your own feelings – testing to discover if you have the right maternal emotions is like pulling up hyacinth bulbs to see if the roots are growing.

CHAPTER TEN

AROUND THE WORLD

Throughout the 70s, 80s and 90s I lectured around the world and built a web of contacts with individuals and organisations in Austria, Switzerland, the Netherlands, Malta, Malawi, Nigeria, Zambia, South Africa, New Zealand, Australia, Kenya, Mexico, Colombia, Canada, Germany, Poland, Belgium, Greece, Finland, Iceland, Norway, Denmark, Sweden, Italy, Romania, France, Spain, Portugal, Abu Dhabi, India and islands in the Pacific. It demanded a lot of energy and quick change focus of attention. Wherever I was, I asked the organisers to arrange for me to be with women in childbirth, so that I could learn about their birth culture. I had some horrific glimpses into birth management as I was conducted by senior members of staff through proudly exhibited labour and delivery rooms. And I've also often been able to learn about and observe traditional practices.

Dublin

Invited by the Association for Improvements in Maternity Services and the Dublin Childbirth Trust, in 1981 I lectured for the first time there and appeared on TV in the evening on *The Late Late Show* with Gay Byrne, who treated me as a dangerous and dotty radical, and a *'flash-Harry'* obstetrician who cited inaccurate statistics from the Netherlands in an attempt to prove that the Irish rate of home births resulted in death and disaster.

Attendance at the seminar was so good – around 400 women and a sprinkling of men – that we had to move to a larger hall in order to seat everyone.

The Master of the Rotunda, Dr Henry, said that for both the mother and baby, all births should take place in hospital. He produced statistics from the Rotunda and compared these with those of the other three largest hospitals, and, in answer to questions said there were no records of epidurals administered, that it was impossible to relate epidurals to forceps deliveries or episiotomy and there was no evidence of any association with postnatal well-being following these two interventions. Nor were there any records of the percentage of mothers breastfeeding on discharge from hospital. He expected that since the members of the audience were asking about these things, they would start to collect such '*unimportant*' statistics.

Birth activists in Ireland were facing a major challenge. They drew attention to practice at St James' Hospital, for public patients only, where still in the 80s it was policy to forbid fathers to attend the birth. A member of staff explained why: '*Because fathers are a nuisance. They get in the way and the proper place for them is on the far side of the delivery room wall.*'

At the Coombe, the Master, Dr Duignan, was keen to give information. He said that enemas were given routinely on admission, and the perineal area shaved. It was also hospital policy to rupture membranes on admission. This enabled staff to see whether there was meconium staining. The standard dose of drugs was 150mg of Pethilorfan, but women could decline it. Approximately 17 per cent of women had continuous electronic fetal monitoring. Patients were moved to the delivery room for birth, where they had to climb onto the table. Fathers were present if they wished. The cord was always cut immediately. Mother and baby were allowed some time together in the post-labour room, but then were routinely separated for several hours. 33 per cent of mothers breastfed, but were handed glucose to give their babies, too. All babies were taken to the nursery at night unless the mother was in a single room. (Public wards were six bedded but in practice often more crowded than this.)

Italy

When I visited hospitals I was escorted through wide expanses of marble halls from the first stage to the delivery wards. Women were wheeled through these cavernous, echoing spaces, on open display. It must have been rather like being conveyed across a London Victorian railway station from platform to platform.

They laboured alone in small cells in virtual solitary confinement. Every now and then a midwife came to check on them and write something in the notes. Staff talked about the patients in front of them as if they could neither hear, see or speak. They were forced to labour flat on their backs on a hard, narrow bed with one pillow at the head.

I remember one woman who was moaning and tossing in pain from side to side. '*The cervix is not dilating. There is no progress*' I was told. I asked if I might stay with her and if I could get her out of bed. The senior midwife looked surprised, but gave her consent.

Once we were alone I smiled and told the mother, '*I have had five babies. I will help you.*' I reached out and lifted her up, and then off the bed. Holding her lightly, I started to rock and circle my pelvis. As each contraction ebbed away I gave a long breath out and was still. When I sensed another was coming I breathed out as it began, and danced and breathed my way through the contraction. We did it together. This went on for half an hour or so. A midwife came in to do a pelvic exam. She was fully dilated. We laughed, and the mother and I hugged each other.

I spoke at conferences in many different parts of Italy in the 80s: Bologna, Rome, Genoa, Milan, Turin and Sicily – helping to form new birth action groups, and to support midwifery and the feminist health movement.

Professor Miraglia at the University of Milan asked me to speak about the midwife's role in birth. I described how in the 60s and 70s there were exciting developments in the UK, with the creation of the Association of Radical Midwives, stimulating three year direct entry training across the country, and the Midwives Information and Resource Centre, and finished by saying, '*Birth is an intense personal experience. Yet it is more than that. The way we give birth is also a political issue. When women are herded into large hospitals like cattle, when their own choices are disregarded, or they do not even realise that there are any choices between alternatives, when the natural rhythms of birth are ignored, when they lie on delivery tables like fish on a slab about to be filleted, and are subjected to the crude assault of routine episiotomy, our Western form of genital mutilation, and when, after birth their babies are taken away from them to be put in plastic boxes while their arms are empty, all women are degraded.*'

Each year in Britain there were now two Research and the Midwife conferences. So research was one major theme contributing to the rediscovery of midwifery. It was a midwife who did research on shaving of the perineum and the use of enemas in labour and discovered that neither practice contributed towards a sterile perineum, shaving caused abrasions through which infection could enter, an enema did not speed up labour, and both routines caused extreme discomfort.

A midwife, too, who conducted a randomised controlled trial of episiotomy which revealed that episiotomy has no advantages over a second degree laceration, and there is less perineal trauma when episiotomy is restricted to cases in which otherwise a tear into the rectum appears inevitable.

It was a midwife who analysed the benefits and risks of the managed third stage of labour and discovered that each intervention, even simple early clamping of the cord, made other interventions necessary and introduced risks. A midwife, too, critically examined the relationship between midwives and women in a modern high-tech maternity hospital and showed that women ask questions of the midwives who are with them longest – usually student and junior midwives – who do not know the answers and who say as little as possible, to be on the safe side. Midwives are often inhibited about giving information, especially when other staff are present, and have subtle techniques to block conversation with their patients.

In Rome I did workshops on posture and movement in childbirth, the rhythmic second stage, and the vitality of the pelvic floor, and lectured on birth pain from an anthropological perspective.

But it wasn't only what I said that got the message across. Meetings were often in ancient, very dignified offices of the city's Mayor and Corporation, a court room or university senate room, with dark panelled walls, massive antique furniture, and oil portraits of ancestors. To demonstrate how ludicrous (and potentially dangerous) directed pushing was I lay flat on my back with my legs in the air on a heavy oak table, huffing and puffing, gasping, desperately holding my breath, hyperventilating, and screaming every now and then. I looked up and between my stretched, wide apart legs could see these worthies staring down at me as I was writhing and straining – with apparent profound disapproval.

In Rome in 1983 I spoke at the Palazzo Valetini, in the conference on 'Non-Violent Birth' organised by the government Social Services Department and helped create an out-of hospital Birth House run and staffed by midwives, and this gained good publicity and was reported in *La Repubblica*.

Australia: Midwives And Convicts

My visits to Australia opened the door for me to learn about the unique history of midwifery there. In 1778 the first convict ships arrived in New South Wales. Most of the female convicts were '*fingersmiths*' – petty thieves and pickpockets, and the logbook of the Lady Juliana recorded that a baby was born at sea to Mrs Anne Whittle. The boat had stopped on the African coast so that the women could '*service*' the crew. Mrs Barnsley, a madam, another of the convict passengers, became one of the first midwives in New South Wales, assisting at home births, and often working under very difficult conditions, especially in the disastrous times when crops failed. Rum was used for pain relief and rags for childbirth linen, and often even these were in short supply. It was the custom to have 10 days lying in, with sometimes an extra day for each previous birth. The birth announcement consisted of placing a cushion on the doorstep with a pink or blue ribbon attached. Everything depended on successful breastfeeding. Sarsparilla was used as a galactalogue and if necessary older women served as wet nurses.

Most women had home births, but in 1841 the first maternity institution was established – the Female Factory, aptly named because the policy was to get women producing a baby every year in order to build up the population. It didn't matter who the father was. '*Lower order*' Irish were sent there and the child was adopted or put into service when five years old. The Female Factory was later renamed the Benevolent Asylum.

There are records of public meetings about baby deaths and the falling birth rate in 1891 and a Royal Commission of Enquiry was set up. The result was that maternity hospitals were established in Sydney and midwives started to be trained: St Margaret's and Crown Street, where I was now lecturing, and the Home of Hope for '*friendless and fallen women*' turned into South Sydney's Women's Hospital.

Working with midwives for change was sometimes tough going. After I came back from Sydney where I lectured in 1983, I learned from Jan Cornfoot, who had organised the speaking tour, that I had left some midwives distressed and angry at the analogy I had made between birth in which women were disempowered and rape. I explained that I could not avoid speaking about this because it was some of the most significant research I had done. Whenever American obstetrics changed care in developing countries, and above all in the

USSR and Eastern Europe, terrible things have been done to women. I also suggested that on my next lecture tour I speak about waterbirth on which I had been working over the last two years.

Jan Cornfoot was the great communicator in Australia. This was before Amazon, Google and the World Wide Web. She edited a popular parenting magazine, had her own successful mail order book company, and ran speaking tours and conferences. She and other bold spirits opened up a vast continent. She organised speaking for me in Perth, Adelaide, Hobart, Melbourne, Brisbane and Sydney. There were public lectures and workshops and seminars in hospitals on *The Rebirth of Midwifery, Birth and the Transition to Motherhood, Massage and Touch, The Second Stage, Postnatal Counselling,* and *Traditional Rites and Symbols* – just some of the subjects on which I lectured and demonstrated.

I met people like Georgina Walker, who worked with rural families in New South Wales. There women often had to travel up to 600 kilometres to give birth in large hospitals. The dirt roads were often impassable during the 'wet', and because of kangaroos and other wild animals, and so they were compelled to leave their homes and journey into the city to wait for the start of labour in huge hospitals. They were utterly isolated, and nobody visited them. These were the conditions in which Parents Centres were striving to promote distant education active childbirth classes with birth videos and phone discussions.

I visited Australia again in 1992. By that time midwives and mothers had joined together in activism. When the Facility of Health Sciences at Newcastle University with Hunter Valley Homebirth organised a conference to explore issues around birth. Nicky Leap, a midwife from England, and who was very experienced in setting up support groups for women, spoke directly midwife to midwife. The conference included input from the Aboriginal Medical Services on *Women's Business: Dream Babies; Belly Dancing,* a discussion of feelings after birth and workshops for fathers.

Japan

Invited to lecture several times in Japan in the 80s, I was also able to do research on Japanese birth traditions and observe practices in large modern hospitals, and midwives' birth houses.

Arrangements for my lectures ranged from addressing midwives in one hospital to facing the Mayor and corporation and their wives in another. In that one the Mayoress broke down in tears when confronted with the memory of her terrible births, and in another my interpreter had to stop because she was overwhelmed by hers. It seemed that the open expression of birth trauma and criticism of routine hospital methods was very suppressed, and when women were at last free to talk it was like an explosion.

Traditionally there is a link between having a good harvest and giving birth, and Suitengu is both God of the harvest and God of easy birth. His shrine is a place of pilgrimage for women seeking a good birth. A bell on a rope hangs in front of it, and if a woman places the end of the rope on her pregnancy belt, or 'obi' – the 'fukutai' – birth will be easy.

Dogs are said to give birth easily. On the Day of the Dog women and their families seek blessing at the shrine. The priest blesses the woman's obi and offers a charm for easy birth – 'itsumoji'. This rite is still accepted as a normal event in pregnancy, at the same time that Japanese hospitals work to a model of medicalised birth, like other hospitals all over the world.

At Ai-iku hospital in Tokyo I learned that 20–30 per cent of pregnant women were assessed as high risk. If pregnancy, birth and postpartum were normal health insurance did not cover the cost, and a woman had to book and pay a deposit for a hospital room at 34–35 weeks.

Waiting times in the antenatal clinic were usually anything up to 4 hours, largely because midwives had little function in the clinic. 95 per cent of women attended childbirth classes, but only 5 per cent of couples went together.

On admission, all women received a partial shave and an enema, and were only allowed fluids when in active labour. Yet, in contrast to hospitals in the rest of the world, drugs for pain relief were rarely used, and the epidural rate was only about 5% at that time. External electronic monitoring took place routinely. In the first stage catheterisation was mandatory and women had to be in the supine position. They were moved from the first stage to the delivery room when fully dilated. Pelvic examinations took place frequently in the second stage, along with routine electronic monitoring.

In spite of protocols dictating intervention, up to 90 per cent of women were delivered by midwives, though a doctor always had to be present. The episiotomy rate was as high as 80–90 per cent for first time mothers, 30–40 per cent for multigravidae. Only about 15 per cent of fathers attended the birth. Another woman companion was never allowed. After birth women were required to lie flat on the hard, narrow delivery table for two hours.

This juxtaposition of traditional practices in pregnancy, when women felt they had control, with a rigid hospital system and technological intervention in childbirth, in a virtually industrialised setting, where women had little say about what happened to them or their babies, was typical of Japan.

Some independent midwives were establishing their own consulting rooms and birth houses, resisting the medicalisation of birth and incorporating the best of traditional midwifery practice. I visited some of these birth centres, too, and saw how, for instance, the midwife laid tatami mats on the floor so that the labouring woman could move freely in her own space, and provided a doubled-over futon to support her in a semi-upright position to give birth.

There were a handful of traditional midwives – 'sanbas' – in their 60s and older – practising too, from whom some younger midwives were learning.

Midwives were joining together with mothers to challenge the medical system and create a culture of woman-centred birth.

Israel

I visited Israel twice, first in 1979 and then in 1986, when I was keynote speaker at the Fifth Birthday Conference of the Israeli Childbirth Education Centre to which I was already an advisor.

A four hour workshop on relaxation and massage in pregnancy was attended by 100 nurses and midwives together with pregnant women and their partners.

It turned out to be confrontational because I hadn't understood how Israeli midwives were thinking and how dogmatic and authoritarian some of them were. The *Jerusalem Post* reported that there was strong opposition from many midwives and that I was '*known for provoking the ire of health-care workers and doctors who, I said, "sell hospital birth without helping women to see the pros and cons of the different alternatives facing them or to be able to plan ahead, knowing that things may not turn out as they hope".*' My suggestion that a pregnant woman might make a birth plan was described as '*one of the more revolutionary recommendations*'. The article continued, '*Furthermore, Kitzinger noted in all seriousness, hospital staff should be "guests" in the delivery room, entering only after knocking on the door, and after receiving the consent of the woman in labour.*' A '*veteran midwife*' who was '*insulted by Kitzinger's comments on the technological take-over in delivery rooms and the lack of flexibility among doctors and midwives'* said that staff *'never force a woman to accept care that she doesn't want.'*

Midwives at this conference argued that fetal monitoring, intravenous drips, and even enemas had reduced fetal mortality. I said that well-controlled randomised studies on obstetric interventions had rarely been conducted, and that wherever research *had* been done the case for routine intervention had not been supported. I proposed regular meetings of the members of the medical establishment and the Israeli Childbirth Trust to exchange ideas and discuss the outcomes of evidence-based research. One midwife was reported in the press as protesting, *'Hospitals cannot allow someone off the street to start giving advice to pregnant women.'*

I discovered that the Israeli Childbirth Centre was in much the same position as the National Childbirth Trust had been 10 years before – trying to legitimise itself in the eyes of the medical establishment and the Ministry of Health.

The Tel Aviv conference happened to take place just as a court case had started against Wendy Savage, an obstetrician who was accused of malpractice in seven births, in which two babies died. Wendy Savage's colleagues, consultants who belonged to the same lodge of the Freemasons, suspended her from practice and fed loaded and heavily biased information to the media. Mothers and midwives who supported Wendy, together with some other obstetricians, organised a march which hit the headlines. Wendy believed that women had the right to make an informed choice and have the kind of birth they wanted in the place they wanted. If they did not agree to a Caesarean section she did not force them to have one and tried to deliver the baby safely vaginally. So I returned from Israel to help organise a massive march, together with the National Childbirth Trust, and the Association for Improvements in the Maternity Services. Choice in childbirth had become an issue of human rights.

Wendy Savage

Wendy Savage is a strongly committed feminist, an obstetrician, and a close friend. She was working as a doctor in Africa when the Abortion Act was passed and returned to England in 1969 to take up a post as Consultant in Obstetrics and Gynaecology at the Royal Free Hospital, the first woman ever to be appointed in London. She had seen the disastrous effects of illegal abortion and believed that women, not doctors, should make the decision about abortion.

Wendy became President of the Medical Women's Federation. She had a hard struggle in her career. Much later, writing in the *British Medical Journal*, her advice to women was: *'Make up your mind what you want to do and know what you are capable of doing and don't allow people to tell you that you can't do it because you are a woman. I have never forgotten being told by the senior obstetric consultant at the London in his Harley Street rooms when I sought his advice about progressing my career in O&G (obstetrics and gynaecology) having had four children in eight years, lived in four countries and three continents and worked throughout that "there was no place for married women in O&G". It gave me great pleasure when seven years later, having been to another country in a fourth continent, I was appointed as the first woman consultant at the London and met him at the Xmas party.'*

Some obstetricians treat each pregnant woman as an ambulant pelvis and every woman in labour as if she were a contracting uterus. Many assume that they know what is best for her better than she can know herself. The Medical Defence Union booklet *Consent to Treatment*[41] stated, *'the Union does not consider that a maternity patient need give her written consent to any operative or manipulative procedures that are normally associated with childbirth. When she enters hospital for her confinement it can be assumed that she assents to any necessary procedure, including the administration of a local, general or other anaesthetic.'* In a book for pregnant women, Gordon Bourne, an obstetrician, wrote, *'You will learn to adapt to the difficulties and to accept the changes that occur. You will learn to co-operate with your professional advisers.'*[42]

In Tower Hamlets, where there were many Asian women who wanted to be cared for only by a woman doctor, Wendy was in the vanguard of doctors determined to improve the quality of maternity services and to listen to women. She went to GPs' offices so that women did not have to make the long trip to the hospital for prenatal care, something no other obstetrician in the area did. She supported the Domino Scheme, a system in which the midwife went to the hospital with the mother-to-be, delivered her baby, and then went home with the family afterwards. She helped many women deliver at home.

We first met when she was accused by colleagues at the London Hospital in 1985 of having failed to perform caesareans on five women who asked not to have surgery unless absolutely necessary, and agreed to a trial of labour. She was considered dangerously non-interventionist and suspended from practice following an enquiry in the blaze of publicity. She said it was part of a 'struggle about who controls childbirth'. Her suspension was a direct attack on the concept of community obstetric care, and I wrote about this in professional journals. The committee that campaigned for Wendy's reinstatement included mothers, representatives of various birth organisations, some GPs, health visitors, medical students, Asian women, and midwives. Never before had such groups worked together for a cause in which they all believed so strongly. To support her, we had a splendid march – her patients and a crowd of birth activists – wearing badges that announced 'Wendy's Best. Investigate the Rest' that achieved good media cover. The enquiry resulted in her being re-instated.

But when she returned to work relations with obstetric colleagues continued to be difficult – so strained that she could not continue working there. It didn't finish. Ten stressful years after this she learned of an anonymous complaint about her actions in a further five cases. At that point she became Honorary Professor at Middlesex University and updated her book *A Savage Enquiry* as *Birth and Power*, with additional chapters from contributing authors, including another extraordinary friend of mine, Dr Marsden Wagner, former Director of Women's and Children's Health in Europe for the World Health Organisation.

Wendy also spear-headed a campaign for keeping the Elizabeth Garrett Anderson Hospital, the first run by and staffed by women obstetricians, in London exclusive to the care of women and staffed entirely by women. She and I met with Frank Dobson, the Labour Secretary of State for Health, to plead for re-establishing a 'woman-for-woman service'. We were unsuccessful, though Wendy set up a pressure group, Women for EGA, on which I served together with other pioneers, including midwife Caroline Flint, who ran an independent birth centre, and the feminist barrister, Helena Kennedy. Wendy doesn't give up easily!

Visual Aids

Every time I attended a large birth conference in the 80s drug firms were exhibiting teaching aids and other equipment. There was invariably a bizarre, often floppy, fetus – either that or a semi-rigid medical specimen sold by other medical equipment firms, paired with a plastic pelvis and drawings that represented birth as a dangerous passage necessitating a narrow scrape between

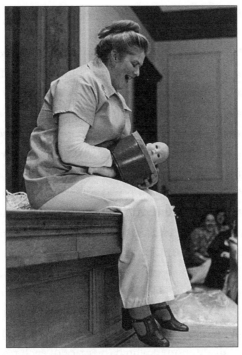

How to breathe a baby out

bones and cartilage – a rigid, immobilised structure. When the fetus was a rag doll it could be twisted into various positions but was nothing like a baby. It looked as if it had been whacked to death.

I decided to construct a pelvis out of a box into which I could place a flexible baby doll that was attractive, and mocked up a foam-rubber vagina through which it could gradually emerge. I sat on a table, legs wide apart in an upright position, as I acted breathing the baby out, stroking the head, and pressing it passionately, little by little, into the world.

Instead of displaying an instrumental technique and delivery by a gynaecologist, I was *being the mother* and breathing my baby out with intense excitement. I acted this with audiences around the world.

This teaching aid came into its own in Canada when we were demonstrating outside the College of Obstetrics and Gynecology in Toronto and marching for midwifery. The police told us that we must keep moving. It was fine by me! I danced ahead of the main procession, birthing my baby through the foam pelvis, making the sounds of pushing, and acted the baby out in waves of excitement. We were doing as the police had instructed us, and I hope they enjoyed it too!

Turkey And Birth Symbols

Carpet-sellers and silversmiths lingered outside their honeycombed shops and bazaars waiting to entice, plead, even order us in to view their wares: *'Come only to see! It is free'. 'Touch this carpet. Feel it! I can give you a better price than any other in the town.' 'My grandfather is selling all. For you I can give a special price because you are the first in the morning.' 'I am a sad man, for my two sisters died in a bus crash as it returned from Caesarea and now my family has no-one to weave. These kilims only remain from my sisters.'*

Once persuaded inside, each shop was a temple of carpets, as ablaze with colour and intricate design as stained glass windows. The patterns were mixed, contrasted and mingled, with enchanting names like the *Gate of Paradise, One Thousand and One Nights, The Tree of Life,* and *The Coming of Spring.* Tea or coffee, sweet, black, rich – a devil's brew – was brought and we were given a magnificent display of combined sales patter, poetry and cultural history. It took a good deal of determination to harden our hearts and announce that we were not going to buy today. Perhaps later, perhaps we'd come again. Even then there was protracted discussion in which the price of each rug was progressively lowered if only we would buy.

Turkey was one of the few countries where I went not to lecture, but on holiday. We retreated to the oasis of our hotel which sat on a projection of white rock with iridescent lapis lazuli water nearly all round it. On one side beneath us was a crisp modern marina with swanky yachts. Opposite, two hours boat ride away, the soaring mountains of the island of Samos seemed to float in the distance. We basked in sun-dappled water, woke to the chatter of birds and a violet shaded dawn sprinkled with feathery clouds, and at night the sun dipped like a huge glazed apricot beneath a rim of sea which ran molten gold and the sky became a glowing, fiery furnace.

This was Kusadasi in the 1980s, then still a small harbour town on the Aegean coast of Turkey, 90 minutes drive south of Izmir, the Smyrna of classical Greece, which was the greatest port of Asia Minor. Though Kusadasi was a perfect place in which to swim and sun and laze, I had come on a treasure hunt. I wanted to search out fertility symbols. The ones I was looking for were not phallic. They were symbols of birth, representing the energy and creative power of women.

Freud introduced us to phallic symbols and since then they have been readily noticed; the solid, soaring, pushing shapes in art and architecture – all those towers, steeples and minarets. The symbol of women's life-giving energy, however, remained mostly hidden and mysterious. Yet they were all around us in textiles made by women in countries stretching from the Middle East to the Pacific.

The code is a diamond with four hooked projections. Often there is a cross-shaped figure or a smaller diamond inside it, representing the fetus. The shape may be stretched out, turned on its side, have extra hooks, or a whole lot of them may be strung together like beads to form a border. But the design is still basically the same.

It is first recorded in Anatolia in the form of a pottery die stamp 6,000 years before Christ. The diamond symbolises in geometric and abstract form the power of women as the source of all life. Perhaps it sprang originally from the W created by a woman's heavy, milk laden breasts and the M formed by the swelling pregnant abdomen between thighs which are spread wide apart.

A few years back I had seen an extraordinary exhibition of birth symbols from Eurasia and the Western Pacific in the Museum for Textiles in Toronto. Now I wanted to track down more of these symbols in all their brilliant colour and variety in Turkish carpets and woven wall hangings. And because the worship of the Mother Goddess which started in Anatolia manifested itself at different times in many different forms as it spread to other Mediterranean cultures – the Earth Mother, the Many Breasted One, the Queen of Night, the Moon Goddess, the Huntress – my search would also take me to museums to discover statues and carvings of her.

The Sumerians called the life-giving Goddess Ma and Marienna, the Hittites, Kubaba and Heba, the Syrians and Arabs Lat, the Cretans Rhoea, and the Phrygians, Cybele. The cult of Cybele, goddess of fertility and of all creation, spread from Anatolia to the whole of Greece. She reigned alone, lions on either side, until she took as her lover her son, the young God Attis. Later still, Zeus, the father god, entered the scene and a divine trinity was created of which she was the central figure. A mountain sanctuary on the slopes of Mount Panayir was from prehistoric times the shrine of this Earth Goddess and statues of Cybele were placed in niches in the rock. Eleven of them are in the beautiful little museum at Ephesus.

But Ephesus was above all the centre of the worship of Artemis, the greatest

Mother Goddess of them all, virgin queen, Goddess of Childbirth and of perilous ventures. She was the embodiment of the energy of creation, no nurturing mother, but the strength of birth itself. And though fertilised by semen offered through the castration and sacrifice of bulls, she belonged to no man. Beside her the statues of Priapus, each with an enormous erect penis weighing down his body, are like some Blackpool pier postcard, a grotesque caricature of sex, for she is the beauty and power of Life Incarnate.

Her first shrine was a hollow in a tree trunk with her statue just a block of wood inside it. Her most splendid was the temple at Ephesus which was four times larger than the Parthenon, with ceilings of cedar and gates of cypress.

The city of Ephesus was built in her honour and was the centre of the Ionian culture which formed the basis of the whole of western civilisation. It flourished seven centuries before Christ, until Athens, under Pericles, became ascendant.

The earliest surviving effigies of Artemis have an almost Egyptian stiffness typical of archaic Greek sculpture. There is in the museum at Selçuk a small gold statue, haunting in its simplicity, which shows a moon-faced young girl standing straight and tall with a secret smile on her lips. In full light her eyes are wide with amazement, but in gentle light her lids seem to lower and it appears that she withdraws into herself, in serene contemplation of her own feminine being.

The two statues of the Goddess dug from her temple still have a rigidity about them which owed more to her origin as a log than to any Egyptian influence. She reached out her arms to us. A triple row of breasts had budded and her whole body blossomed in a splendid exuberance of living things: acorns, pine cones, vines, roses, lions, griffins, deer and bees, which traditionally were her servants. She had all the sweetness, beauty, richness and power of life.

Yet the Goddess was not quite what she seems. Those breasts had no nipples. '*Pomegranates*' said one guide. But pomegranates are not that shape. '*Eggs*' said another. Nor are eggs. They are testicles. For originally the priest in her shrine had to castrate himself and offer his seed to the Goddess. The sacrifice of bulls to the Goddess goes back more than 6,000 years and perhaps it was a priest who suggested that bulls' testicles would be better still. Originally they were embalmed and hung round her neck. Later they were immortalised in marble.

Artemis is no comfortable Goddess and though women stand staring at her, I noticed some men turned quickly away. There are those who are disappointed in her because she does not conform to the conventional idea of feminine beauty. '*I much prefer Aphrodite rising from the waves*', one man told me. For

Aphrodite is all curves and gentleness. She is a sex object. Artemis is the energy and ripeness of creation.

Later Artemis became the Greek Diana, Goddess of the Womb and the Hunt, who controls the rhythms of menstruation. And later still her countenance changed to become the Virgin Mary. Legend has it that after Jesus' death St John brought Mary to live in his house on the mountains of Ephesus, and that she died here.

It was in Ephesus that the Ecumenical Council was held in 431AD at the Basilica of St John when Mary was first proclaimed the Mother of God. And it was here that the Pope knelt and worshipped at the feet of the Goddess who has for thousands of years been the Great Earth Mother, and whose prehistoric origin was the geometric code of the hooked diamond denoting female power and fertility.

This is the shape still woven by women into cloth, rugs and carpets from Turkey to as far as the Western Pacific today. For weaving is above all *women's* business. In Turkey they spin and dye the wool and weave the carpets, though it is the men who sell them. In the isolated mountain villages girls must remain as daughters in the family until they are passed on to another man's family as wives. They have few recreations or other ways in which they can express themselves, and into these rugs, which form their dowry, they weave all their hopes and dreams.

Men don't understand these symbols and when I asked, seem vaguely uneasy about them. They suggested they are *'rams' horns'*, *'stars'* or *'flowers'*, or that they were there to *'keep away the evil eye'*. Occasionally one would say that the symbols are *'about the family'* or putting it in the context of Muslim religion, point to a border with a key pattern or snake-like curves in a design and say that it is *'the belt of Fatima'*. (She was Muhammad's daughter and women pray to her for fertility). The significance of the birth symbol was hidden.

But it isn't only spinning and weaving that women do. The whole peasant economy is built on female labour: and hard labour at that. Women are picking and sorting cotton, carrying heavy loads on the back of their necks, plaiting straw mats, digging ditches, trudging and toiling, as well as tending children, scrubbing laundry on bare rocks, sweeping and cleaning and preparing the family meal, while many men sit drinking in the cafes from morning till night. They only get stuck into work when it involves machinery, like tractors, or the excitement of selling carpets. The athletic contests of the

Hellenic era have been transferred to the streets of harbour towns, and the ancient songs and sagas changed to sales patter. Young men, nattily dressed, with gold chains around their swarthy necks and rings on their fingers, fresh for the fray as each ship docks, compete for the tourist trade and proclaim the wonders inside their emporiums.

Compared with that, women's work was very dull indeed. Yet all peasant societies have been based on woman's labour and while men are off doing the glamorous things, like hunting and shooting, they have developed survival techniques and shouldered responsibility for the basic provision of food. One writer, tracing the culture of the Anatolian village of Catal Huyuk 8,000 years ago, says, '*Women and children could collect enough grain in three weeks to feed a family for an entire year. The men would return from the hunting or fishing camp to find the home base filled and overflowing with grain ... If we wonder how easily men are threatened by women ... perhaps we would do well to think back on the origins of agriculture.*'[43] He believes that because woman was so formidable the origin of agriculture, instead of destroying the religion of the Great Goddess of the Upper Paleolithic, produced a new form of the Earth Mother.

A New Baby

The carpet merchant's wife had a baby five days ago. Ann was a Canadian he met when he was in charge of the firm's jewellery department and stopped her in the street to try and sell her a harem ring. For the birth she was provided with the best of everything, including a private obstetrician who drugged her senseless for the delivery, when she wanted to be awake and aware. Now she had breastfeeding difficulties and her nipples were sore and bleeding. Other women were telling her that her milk might not be good for the baby and her mother-in-law was worried that the baby's sucking is feeble. Her doctor had ordered her to give regular sugar water and to take the baby off the breast for 24 hours, but her breast was now swollen and hard and she was in pain. I offered to go to see her.

They lived with the husband's mother and his brother in a miniscule 'summer house' on the hill above Kusadasi. It must have been impossible to get any privacy or for the couple even to talk alone together. Whereas a Turkish bride might have resigned herself to this, it must have been hard on a Canadian woman.

But the mother was busy with the meal downstairs and Ann and I sorted out that the baby wasn't really '*fixed*' and was chewing on the end of her nipple, instead of getting a satisfying mouthful. Hence the soreness and pain, the desultory sucking and the mass of impacted milk. I explained that the baby needed to draw the nipple into the back of her mouth and she could tell if she had done this because when she sucked her ears wiggled! It was a joy to get the baby on. Ann said the sucking didn't hurt her at all now, and the baby was having a gorgeous feed.

It was not just a technical problem. Ann was anxious and torn between Turkish traditional ways of caring for new babies and her modern baby books. Babies in Turkey were tightly swaddled, arms as well as legs and body, for 40 days. The mother did not take the baby out of the home during this time. She must not be visited by any other woman who had recently had a baby or, later, go to see a new mother, lest the baby became ill. Ann would have liked to take her baby out of doors. This shocked the other women. Fear of the '*Evil Eye*' being set on a baby is an expression of the reality of the risk taken by babies in this culture. Two hundred and twenty-five out of every 1,000 babies died before they reached their first birthday, either at birth or in the months afterwards. Ann had to cope with the orders laid down by her doctor, too. He represented the modern '*scientific*' way of doing things. This not only conflicted with traditional Turkish ways but also with her spontaneous feelings as a mother. From what she told me of the doctor's advice I guessed that he had studied in the United States about 20 years ago. Aziz, the baby's father, had been told that he must not kiss his daughter in case he gave her '*microbes*'. Her mouth must be painted with antiseptic to prevent thrush. There was to be no unnecessary cuddling and, above all, the mother must not take the baby into bed with her.

There was a meal waiting: fish, green peppers, crisp cheese pastries, yoghurt and grapes. No wine, of course, because they were Muslim, but glasses of tea afterwards. In the little room there was Ann, Saki, her brother, the mother, my husband and me and the TV set on non-stop and dominating the conversation. It seemed a crowd. Ann had left the sleeping baby upstairs, but her mother-in-law was obviously anxious about this and fetched the child. She had wrapped her tightly in a blanket as if swaddled, so that there was now a stiff, solid little bundle which she could hold in the way she is used to handling babies. All attention was on the baby's eyes. The rest was motionless, like a wooden doll.

When the baby opened her eyes she immediately talked to her. Turkish babies and small children get a great deal of stimulation, lots of touching and handling. They are the most important part of family life and the community as a whole. I noticed that wherever we had seen babies and toddlers fathers and grandfathers carry and play with them and everyone obviously took great delight in children.

The mother-in-law didn't speak a word of English, so we smiled. I was worried that she disapproved of my influence on Ann, who was now critical of the 40 days seclusion. I suggested that in the life of women who labour in the fields, cook, clean, wash and carry heavy loads, a period when they don't have to work for everyone else and can concentrate on their babies may be a very good thing. It was a tradition which should not be jettisoned without much thought, but it might be modified. I hoped I discussed it so that Ann could be more sympathetic towards what her husband's mother was saying and that she, too, could understand Ann's thinking better. When I left the mother embraced me and, far from being resentful, seemed to be very glad that I came.

The conflicts that Ann was going through are those which more and more Turkish women would obviously experience too, as male-dominated Western professionalism and technology changed the traditional patterns of peasant societies.

One of the things I wanted to do in Turkey was to see belly dancing. This was originally an important part of sacred rites enacted by women at the time of birth and there was evidence that it was also part of the worship of the ancient Anatolian Earth Mother. Even today in some countries belly dancing is practised in preparation for birth and during labour the women present dance around the mother and encourage her to make similar movements. Wendy Bonaventura, in her book *The History of the Belly Dance* reports that in Hawaii the *hula* is used as preparation for birth as it also is among Maori women in New Zealand and in parts of the Caucasus, the Middle East and North Africa. And where women no longer dance during labour the association of rhythmic pelvic movements with fertility persists in countries where young women get ready for marriage, wearing part of their dowry in the form of gold coins decorating their clothing, and dance with a strong pelvic movement to show that they are ripe for sex and childbirth. She quotes Armen Ohinin, writing about the belly dance in Egypt, as saying that in her youth it was *'a poem of the mystery and pain of motherhood. In olden Asia which has kept the dance in its primitive purity, it represents maternity, the mysterious conception of life, the suffering and joy with which a new soul is brought into the world.'* Over the years this birth dance changed and was degraded to the belly dance of the modern cabaret. It is athletic but not sensuous. The only Turkish belly dancing I saw was, in fact, rather less erotic than the belly dancing I had seen in the Crazy Horse Saloon in Paris! And when I consulted experts on Turkish culture I learnt that the modern Turkish dancer is descended from the dancers who were in each Sultan's household and called on to delight, entertain and stimulate jaded appetites, rather than those who danced in worship of Artemis.

Nevertheless, there was still an element of fertility rite in the dancing which took place in celebration of a marriage in Turkey, when all the wedding guests, men as well as women, joined in belly dancing.

Thailand

I broke journeys to and from Australia and Japan in Thailand, and lectured and did research there, too in the late 80s and early 90s.

There were obstetric nurses, but no midwives. Many upper class women feared that they would lose sexual attractiveness with vaginal birth and opted for Caesarean section. Men still had minor wives, though polygamy was not legally recognised. When I was there the Crown Prince had a morganatic wife who bore him five children. She was an actress whom he had been in love with for many years.

Women feared pain and thought Caesareans were pain-free. Thailand had one of the highest rates of drug use in the world. Doctors didn't tell patients what the drugs were that they are prescribing. There was wide-spread use of antibiotics for minor conditions such as colds, and a resulting general resistance to antibiotics.

Fathers were not present during childbirth. They could look through the glass of the communal nurseries to see their babies. A woman who had had a Caesarean could not see her baby until she was well enough to travel to the nursery, which was on a different floor to the postnatal ward. She was also told that she would not be able to breastfeed for three days and that the baby must have formula. Bottles were brought out and stood in jugs of hot water to keep warm.

Induction was popular for social reasons. For example, a baby must be born on its grandfather's birthday, or because the horoscope gave an auspicious date.

Other medical interventions, including surgery, were decided on, and dates set, for largely social reasons. A woman opted to have her appendix out and be sterilised at the same time, for example, and get back to work in three days.

Doctors gave little explanation of what they were doing, not only concerning childbirth but also in dealing with infertility and miscarriage. This was because if the doctor could not do anything it would result in loss of face, which was very important in Thailand.

I also visited the museum in Bangkok to see the birthing figures there. These very simple figurines in clay from Sangaloq dating from the Sukothai period – the twelfth to fifteenth century – showed the woman sitting with one knee bent and the other knee rotated outwards on the ground with her heel guarding her perineum. There was one which showed the mother with her hand on the head as the baby was emerging. Clearly, at that time women actively gave birth and knew exactly what to do to deliver gently and slowly.

Grandmothers Of The Umbilical Cord

In Nicaragua, nurses and other health workers were working together to offer women education for childbirth. Nicaragua was a country torn by war and revolution, where deaths and kidnappings occurred every week. Health teams were struggling to bring not only good care for women in pregnancy and birth, but to help them get the information they needed in order to make choices, prepare themselves for birth and motherhood, and find a voice as women that would affect the social changes being made throughout the country.

When modern kinds of maternity care were introduced to Latin American countries they were invariably based on the US model, with obstetricians making the rules, high-tech machinery and ostracism and humiliation of the local traditional midwives. Brave efforts had been made to resist this. Since the revolution in 1979, a model of health care had been created by the Sandinistas based on the principle that health care was the right of all people, and that the best of traditional practices should be incorporated. In 1982 a national training programme for the midwives – *parteras* – was launched, and by the end of 1984 more than 3,000 had been incorporated into the National Health Care System.

Midwives are called the *'grandmothers of the umbilical cord'*. They have a lasting relationship with each child whose cord they have cut, are highly respected members of the community, and take an active part in planning women's health care.

In other Latin American countries I visited I was in huge maternity hospitals where I saw women lying petrified with fear, alone and completely unsupported emotionally. A doctor leaned heavily on the woman's abdomen to forcibly expel the baby as quickly as possible. Following delivery of the placenta, the routine practice was for him to push his fist up into the uterus and sweep his hand round to ensure that no placental fragments remained. All this was without anaesthesia, or even caring words. In these countries, white women had private obstetricians, American-style, and dark skinned and peasant women were treated like animals.

There were hospitals like this in Nicaragua, too. But the important and hopeful thing was that nurses and midwives had come in from other countries, including North America and Britain, and were working side by side with local midwives, learning from each other, and had developed a system where there was a strong emphasis on the voice of the people. A Chilean midwife, Susanna, moved to Nicaragua and trained midwives, helping them to ask searching questions about their practices, and consider alternatives to interventionist obstetrics.

Yeshi Newman, an American midwife who helped with this work, said, *'The job that women have done for centuries – guiding the entry of new life – has been recognised, and the dignity of the women who do this work shines like the sun'.*

In Leon, Sophia, a Colombian-born exile married to an Italian doctor, started working with women giving birth in the big hospital, but conditions were horrific, and she was so outspoken that she could not continue her job there. So she switched to the street markets, set up a screen and arranged benches prior to giving talks illustrated with slides to anyone who gathered round. These covered all aspects of women's health and sexuality, contraception, abortion and birth. It was ventures like these, going out to the people rather than expecting them to come to you, which were at the heart of the enormous social and political changes in Nicaragua.

Canada

In the 80s Canada was the only industrialised nation within the World Health Organisation not to recognise midwifery. Midwives were classed as amateurs, remnants of an old wives' past tainted with witchcraft and ancient herb lore, and potentially dangerous. I was active in campaigning for midwifery in the different provinces of Canada. I knew excellent midwives in Toronto, and we planned a march on the College of Physicians while I was on one of my lecture tours there. Official recognition of midwifery rested with doctors. The decision was in their hands.

Michael Dickson, Registrar of the Ontario College of Physicians and Surgeons, was reported in the *Toronto Globe* saying, '*I do not consider it proper for midwives to be involved in births, either at home or in a hospital. It would certainly be our position that midwifery is part of obstetrics and is therefore part of the practice scene of medicine.*'[44]

The police told us that our march must keep on the move and there should be no standing around and proclaiming. This presented no problems. I was leading the march and would give birth performing my own birth dance, followed by all the other marchers behind me. When the day came I swayed, rocked, walked, breathed, held my breath, grunted, panted, circled and swayed with excitement and passion, birthing a life-like flexible baby doll through my box pelvis and foam rubber vagina and through the vagina out into my cradling hands.

All this was recorded by TV cameras. We must have been fairly persuasive, since Ontario was the first Canadian province to register midwifery. The Midwifery Act was passed in 1991, and in 1993 the Baccalaureat in Midwifery started.

Birth In A Soviet Time Warp

In 1989 a group of us – doctors and other specialists in birth and babies – were invited by the UK-USSR Medical Exchange Programme to meet for the first time a group of Russian specialists in order to share ideas – *glasnost* in action. My friends Wendy Savage, who was Senior Lecturer in Obstetrics and Gynaecology at the London Hospital, and Professor Norman Morris of Charing Cross Hospital Medical School, were also members of that group.

Following the two-day conference, I found it easy to escape the official programme of visits to showplaces and instead discover what it was like to have a baby in two Moscow hospitals, one a high-risk centre and the other a district maternity unit.

Birth education had been initiated and was firmly controlled by professionals, whereas in the West it was started by lay women: and classes were run by independent childbirth organisations such as the International Childbirth Education Association in the United States and the Active Birth Movement and National Childbirth Trust in Britain. These organisations began to come into being in the 50s, first in Britain and then in the United States and other European countries, set up by women who were themselves mothers and who resisted the increasing medicalisation of birth. They sought to provide emotional support and friendship in pregnancy, information about non-pharmacological ways of handling pain, and preparation for childbirth in small, friendly groups.

When birth education was introduced in the USSR in the 1960s, attendance at antenatal classes was compulsory from the thirty-second week of pregnancy. Most Russian obstetricians were women, but there was still heavy emphasis on their role as birth technicians and employees of the State, rather than on their understanding of birth as women and mothers themselves. I discovered that in psychoprophylaxis classes they had to follow the rules set down by a central authority: *'Women must be ... immunised to labour pain. Physicians must normalise and reorganise the minds of women poisoned by erroneous ideas.'* The language was authoritarian and didactic. The objectives of birth education were *'to teach the pregnant woman proper conduct during labour so that she may follow instructions properly.' 'By understanding all the medical measures conducted in the institution the pregnant woman will be disciplined.' 'The physician should emotionally emphasise motherhood's high social virtues confirmed in the Soviet Union by the establishment of government awards – orders and medals – and honorary titles to mothers of many children.'*[45] Russian psychoprophylaxis stressed *control* over the mother and her correct behaviour as a patient.

Preparing Women And The Political System

I have found that wherever birth education is not under the control of women themselves, but is promoted by large hierarchical institutions, it is dogmatic, authoritarian, inflexible – even punitive – towards women who do not conform. Women were told, *'Here is what will happen to you.'* They were taught to relax so as not to be a nuisance. They were supposed to lie in bed tidily under the sheets, to be quiet so as not to frighten other women or interfere with the smooth running of the labour and delivery rooms, to breathe in order to suppress the desire to scream out in pain. What this adds up to is that the woman was taught to control herself so that she could be more effectively controlled by those caring for her.

Within the Communist system education for childbirth took the form of pregnancy gymnastics based on psychoprophylaxis, instruction about the Pavlonian psychology of conditioned reflexes, and basic anatomy and physiology. 'Breathe in, 1, 2, 3, 4 – stop – breathe out, 1, 2, 3, 4, 5, 6 – breathe in! Breathe out! Relax!' Commands were rapped out as if by a drill sergeant. None of it bore much relationship to what the woman actually feels during childbirth. The idea behind it was to control her behaviour so that she was quiet and disciplined. Communist values regulated women's behaviour in childbirth. This last bastion of individuality, the intimacies of psycho-sexual life, inter-relationships between a mother and her baby, and between the couple and their child was made to conform to norms which each woman attained or failed to fulfil.

Fifty years earlier in the English speaking world ritual cleansing had been the norm. In Exploring the Dirty Side of Women's Health two research midwives describe how, in 1920s New Zealand, 'the aseptic technique reinforced the focus on the vagina as a passage of dirt, requiring aseptic measures as stringent as for surgical operation. Midwives wore gloves, masks and sterilised overalls, and the woman's body was shaved, bathed, emptied by enema, daubed with disinfectant and swathed in sterile drapes.'[46] This was still the case in Russia in the 80s.

Being with a Russian woman in childbirth in the 80s was like being stuck in a time warp. No fathers were allowed inside the hospital, let alone in labour wards. A huge enema apparatus was on a stand just inside the labour ward door. First a ritual enema and shave transformed the woman into a patient. A complete pubic shave and enema were routine. The implicit message was that the mother was dirty and birth was polluting, so the entire pubis must be shaved bald as a hard-boiled egg and her bowels emptied of their filth.

Then she was left alone, lying on a hard, narrow, high bed to 'get on with it'. She was expected to be quiet and disciplined, and if she had attended psychoprophylaxis classes to use these techniques to control herself and not make a fuss. So she lay biting her lip, moaning quietly, or writhing in silent agony.

When the baby was about to arrive she had to climb on a table and there was a hurried, often violent delivery. She could not hold or often even see her baby, which was given vigorous resuscitation and whisked away to the nursery. Mothers were left on trolleys with ice-packs on their tummies in the corridor for two to three hours or more before they set eyes on their babies. In one hospital I noticed nurses nipping off for a quiet smoke in the rooms where the babies were lying *'under observation'*. It was firmly believed that mothers could harm and contaminate their newborns if they were allowed to be with them. Before a woman was permitted to touch her baby, her fingers had to be painted with iodine to avoid conveying germs to the cocooned infants.

Midwives, nurses and doctors did not have to undergo this rite, though in any hospital it is the staff who are mainly responsible for cross-infection, as Semmelweis, the doctor in Vienna who taught his colleagues to wash their hands, pointed out long ago.

Bacteria that mothers transferred to their babies were perceived as the primary source of the epidemics of infection in hospital nurseries. These in turn threatened the staff of the institution. One professor of neonatology told me, *'I can remember when other staff of maternity hospitals would not shake hands with neonatologists because they considered them a source of infection.'* In this way the medical system reflected the same dread of external contamination that was expressed in the Communist political system.

In Moscow babies were fed according to the clock, a regime that had been the rule in the West 30 years before, and which caused great misery for both mothers and babies.

Watching this, helpless to do anything to comfort women, I realised how dramatic the changes being made in Western hospitals since the 50s were because of the strong voice of the childbirth movement. I often felt that we were making no progress in humanising birth, but only had to see what Russian hospitals were like to be aware of advances.

For every birth in the USSR a woman had between two and six legal abortions. In the UK at that time there was one abortion for every five births and anaesthesia was used routinely. For every legal abortion in the USSR it was estimated that there was one illegal abortion, too. I don't know how they worked it out, but experts guess 30 per cent of the illegal abortions ended in the woman's death.

I got the impression that abortion was the model for childbirth. Birth was simply evacuation of the uterus. Women endured it in the same way they had to put up with all the other hardships – living in flats shared between three or four families with only one kitchen; having to queue for nearly all food;

sometimes having three jobs – doing demanding work, moonlighting (one of our interpreters turned out to be a neurologist) and stuck with all the housework without any help from the men. This is why pregnancy could be a disaster.

Abortion was on demand up to the twelfth week of pregnancy, usually consisting of dilation and curettage without anaesthesia. Contraceptives were often unobtainable, but there was a great deal of suspicion about them too. A young doctor said she would never take the pill because it was '*dangerous*', and condoms were '*horrible*'. Abortion she considered safer, cleaner and simpler. So that was the favourite method of birth control. Many Russian gynaecologists did nothing but abortions.

Some obstetricians were making efforts to give birth more personal significance for women. In one hospital I visited the admission room was like the entrance to an abattoir, with a huge enema apparatus, an open lavatory, and two women being '*prepped*' at the same time without any privacy. But in that hospital, too, there was a ceremonial room – it looked like a parlour in an American funeral home – where the new mother met her husband and family and introduced the baby to them before she was discharged. A whole wall of this room was a stained glass picture of a mother and child, lit from behind.

First the woman went to the adjoining swaddling room where she was taught how to bind her baby and the resulting package was tied with pink or blue ribbon. Then to the background of music she emerged and the father saw his child for the first time, flowers were presented to her, and photographs with the new baby were taken. The music softened and a lyrical female voice announced: '*Now the new life is in your hands. The baby is your dream and when you get home it will grow up and take care of you. Good luck little baby! We want your parents to take care of you so well that you will grow up to take care of them in the future. Good luck, little citizen!*' – and the national anthem blared out.

The meeting of a father and other members of a family with a newborn baby, treated as a private and intimate event in Western countries, was in Communist society a formal ritual entry into the culture, one in which the baby was symbolically exhorted to be a good citizen, and in which the parents were reminded of their duties to train the child well. Ceremonies of this kind served a similar function to those of baptism and christening for members of the Christian faith.

To enter another culture in the way I did is always to intrude and to risk violating deeply held beliefs. I was warned that when I lectured to doctors I should be methodical and unemotional, because that is what Russians like. Yet our interpreter was getting tired (he could not translate the word '*sex*' so I had to improvise in actions) and I felt I could only make the points I wanted about a non-violent, rhythmic way of conducting the second stage of labour by acting what happens when women are surrounded by cheer-leaders yelling, '*Push! Push! Push!*': how this makes muscles go tight, and eyes pop out, and results in exhaustion.

I demonstrated the difference between this and birth when there is no rush and no commanded pushing. I was amazed by the doctors' ready laughter. They understood exactly what I was saying and we discovered that we shared the same sense of humour. These women obstetricians turned out to be warm, funny and passionate.

The USSR was largely out of touch with what was going on in the rest of the world. Even so, it was on the brink of change and we had an opportunity to affect the way that took place. While we were there a Vice-Minister of Health signed an order that hospitals must allow visiting of patients. There was a fluttering in the dovecotes as staff worried about how they were going to cope with that, in the same way that years before it was thought in the UK that if fathers were allowed in the delivery room they would faint and cause chaos.

An experiment was reported in Riga, where husbands could accompany their wives to hospital and stay during labour and birth, and described in a popular weekly magazine illustrated in colour. The rate of infection did not rise, (the reason given for the exclusion of all visitors), and the Ministry of Health said that men should be allowed into maternity hospitals. '*Birth perestroika has begun!*' Wendy Savage exclaimed.

Other experimental projects held hope for the future too. I met a doctor who, in an effort to reduce the amount of cross-infection in hospitals, was giving antenatal and postnatal care to women at home, and who planned to do home births later.

I got to know the doctor responsible for all childbirth education in the USSR – a vivacious, glowing woman who was dissatisfied with their rigid methods of training for birth. It consisted mostly of lectures by obstetricians, paediatricians and even a lawyer, to obedient classes of listening women. We hoped to collaborate and she wanted to come over here to work with me. Unfortunately, she was never able to get permission to leave Russia.

Yet women were hungry for change. For the first time there was open criticism of maternity hospitals in lively correspondence in a Moscow newspaper. Obstetricians and paediatricians were shocked by what they saw as an attack on good practice.

Campaigning For Midwives

The Tao Te Ching described the midwife 2,500 years ago. '*Do good without show or fuss. Facilitate what is happening rather than what you think ought to be happening. If you must take the lead, lead so that the mother is helped, yet still free and in charge. When the baby is born, the mother will rightly say: "We did it ourselves!"*'[47]

Since the first recorded accounts of birth, and in countries all over the world, mothers and newborn babies have depended on midwives. They are the experts in normal childbirth, and giving care so that the abnormal does not develop. Midwives in traditional cultures describe their work to unblock, open up, release and free the woman so that she can give birth. '*Midwife*' is from the Anglo-Saxon meaning '*with woman*'. She is also the wise woman, the '*sage femme*' who has insight into women's rhythms and the mysteries of birth and death.

During the 80s I visited midwives in many different countries. We challenged the establishment across huge swathes of the world which had been heavily influenced either by Soviet or North American obstetrics.

By the end of the 80s midwifery had been reborn in Canada and midwives were winning the long struggle to give woman-centred care. In Western Europe, new EC directives ensured that midwives, rather than being handmaidens to obstetricians, were able to take responsibility for continuous care of the woman through pregnancy, birth and postpartum.

This renaissance grew from childbirth organisations, and as my books on birth were published in 23 countries I was part of that forward thrust. In Ontario, British Columbia and Alberta, as in New Zealand, mothers and midwives together successfully challenged the power of the medical system. Through the 80s the childbirth movement exercised growing influence in countries such as Germany, and seedling movements in Poland and Hungary for instance, to help free midwives from the constraints of authoritarian medical systems. On the other hand, this was all very patchy. While small groups of midwives in Northern Italy, for example, got together to improve care and provide genuine choices – home birth is a case in point – that was lacking for most women in Italy, and the majority of midwives there were trapped in a system they dared not try to change. It was much the same for midwives in Spain.

Lecturing in the United States and Eastern Europe, I have often found that assumptions are made about normal and 'alternative' birth that contrast dramatically with how childbirth had progressed in Britain today. In the United States, for example, midwifery as a profession has virtually died and been replaced by assistants to obstetricians who have to sign the case notes after delivery.

In the UK obstetricians know that they rely entirely on the skills of midwives to retain some continuity of care, and in something like 70 per cent of births to catch the baby. Our whole maternity system would collapse if midwifery became further downgraded. The danger here is that birth is increasingly treated as crisis management based on risk assessment, and more and more women are classified as high risk and managed by an obstetric team. Fragmentation of care means that a woman may never see the same person twice. Notes are often not passed on.

In Italy, Russia and other Eastern European countries – where there is an autocratic and often totalitarian system of medical control, birth is treated essentially as emptying of the uterus and the model for it is abortion. In fact, in many of these countries the dominant method of birth control is still abortion. It poses a problem for these countries as they entered the European Community which has directives about midwifery training, women getting information they need to make decisions, and midwives' right to move between European countries.[48] This means that midwives should have the same levels of skills, and confidence to work with autonomy wherever they are. The Czech Republic got rid of midwives and replaced them with 'women's nurses'. Since 1960 the midwife has been called a nurse, and could only care for a woman after she had been referred by a doctor. Home births were effectively outlawed. And in December 2014 the European Court of Human Rights found that Czech legislation prohibiting midwives from attending home births does not interfere with women's rights to private life![49]

There are far too many obstetricians. Birth in which a woman can do her own thing has gone underground. In Hungary home births were made illegal unless attended by both an obstetrician and a paediatrician. But not *all* home births, only *planned* home births, though it is no surprise that research shows that unplanned home births are far riskier.

The UK was ahead of most other European countries in rediscovering midwifery, largely because of our campaigns as childbirth educators and the partnership between midwives and mothers. At the end of the 80s and beginning of the 90s I worked with colleagues in the childbirth movement to lobby Parliament and get good coverage in the media. We provided evidence to the Health Committee of the House of Commons. In 1992 its report was published which stated: *'There is a strong desire among women for ... continuity of care and carer throughout pregnancy and childbirth and the majority of them regard midwives as a group best placed and equipped to provide this.*[50] It recommended the development of midwifery-managed units, in and outside hospitals, and best practice models of team midwifery care, and concluded that midwives should have a right to develop and audit their own professional standards. In fact, team midwifery failed to give women-centred care. It talked about *'grossly obese teams'* and recommended case-load midwifery and one-to-one care.

The romantic notion of the midwife in touch with earth's secret lore, gathering herbs at full moon and dispensing them to cure every ill – the way midwives have often been represented in California – gave way to a realistic perception of professionals who audit their own work, assess the quality of research relating to all aspects of care, and are responsible to increasingly well-informed and critical consumers.

In Britain the Midwives Information and Resource Service – I was on its Editorial Committee – made research much more accessible to midwives and students.

An important development was research by midwives themselves. In the UK and Scandinavian countries midwives were critically evaluating obstetric and midwifery interventions of all kinds, and demystifying ritual hospital practices. This had a direct effect on care. Enemas and shaves were discarded. For years pushing had been a strenuous exercise entailing commanded, prolonged breath-holding and heaving, enthusiastically encouraged as if by football team supporters.

By the end of the 90s a woman could have her partner with her, or anyone else with whom she wanted to share the birth experience, including family members, women friends, and her other children. This wasn't the case for Northern Ireland, which was still heavily obstetric-paternalistic, and protest was brewing there.

As the 2000s dawned, there were lower rates of induction for *'post-maturity'*

– because a woman was a week over her dates, for instance – episiotomy rates plummeted, and also as a direct consequence of midwife research, a more relaxed approach to pushing and the length of the second stage.

Internationally, outreach work was firmly in the hands of midwives, if only because most obstetricians were not eager to work with the poor and did not fancy being stuck in unsavoury urban areas or in rural outposts.

Aboriginal midwives were beginning to provide care in their own communities. In New Zealand I had already explored with Maori women their concern to rediscover traditional childbirth practices. This was increasingly accepted by Pakeha midwives, who discovered traditions of good midwife care that had been lost in modern hospitals.

In the 1990s midwives in the West started to develop a clearer view of where their strengths lay. They broke out of isolation, began to link with midwives in other countries, and realised that they faced common problems. Till then a midwife often had little idea of the power politics in the health care system in her country, and even less in other countries. A new direct entry education began to develop alongside instruction which saw midwifery as either a top-up to nurse training, an extension of caring for sick people, and a way of producing compliant workers who prepared patients for the obstetrician, kept them quiet, and cleared up afterwards.

Yet some midwives felt cheated by change. They accepted, like good little girls, their subordinate role in a hierarchical hospital system headed by obstetricians and gynaecologists. When Italian midwives were told that they must no longer attend home births and their role as community midwives was to be restricted to antenatal and mother and baby clinics, they did not resist. When obstetricians produced protocols for care, midwives' only way of protest was to falsify the records so that, for example, a woman who had been happily but slowly progressing in the second stage for three hours or more was recorded on the labour chart as having a much shorter expulsive stage. It was the same for Spain.

In the Middle Ages midwives fled to Holland because it was the only country to offer them a sanctuary. Everywhere else the midwife was at risk of being persecuted, even put to death, as a witch. Midwifery in Holland still retained its autonomy vis-à-vis the medical system more than in any other country. A third of births were at home, and midwives provided total care for normal pregnancies and births.

In Australia the first midwife-attended home births took place for which mothers did not have to pay. Pilot programmes, with Government funding, were initiated. But there was still a long way to go. In many countries the home birth midwife found herself outside the official system. In most states of the US, the only way she could work was as an underground midwife, risking suspension, litigation and imprisonment. For these midwives it is rather like Christians in the catacombs. There is a great story to be told of midwife heroines all over the world who have been marginalised by the medical system, outlawed and criminalised, for their commitment to childbearing women and families. In medieval Europe they were burned at the stake as witches. In California they were put on trial for practising medicine without a license.

A vital element in a midwife's work is to protect women from potentially harmful interventions, and to ensure, as far as possible, that birth is not treated as an accident waiting to happen or turned into a medical crisis.

Women suffer post-traumatic stress disorder when they have been powerless and denied choice. They endure births in which technology dictates everything that occurs, and where authority is vested in those who design the protocols.

In helping to bring a human being into the world midwives stand at the crossing-point of generations, and share a journey that is a major life transition. I believe that midwives are the guardians of physiological birth, and an important element in my work must be contributing to midwife education.

Human Rights And Midwifery

Dr Agnes Gereb, a qualified obstetrician, had her third child at home just before she held the first conference in Hungary in the late 1990s.

In 2003 a group of us attended and spoke at the second home birth conference she organised. This included Dr Marsden Wagner, previously Director of Maternal and Child Health for the European Region of the World Health Organisation (WHO). After the conference we met with Hungarian Ministry of Health officials and senior obstetricians, who did not accept the evidence that home birth was a safe option for healthy women with an uncomplicated pregnancy.

In 2007 Agnes was struck off the medical register for attending home births. As an EU member, Hungary accepts that women have the right to give birth at home. But no midwives had been given licences to practice outside hospital, so this right was effectively undermined.

Agnes had been struck off the obstetric list for helping at home births, and then studied to become a midwife in Semmelweis University, was certified in 2005, and gained a BSc in Midwifery in 2010. In October of that year she was detained in a high security prison in Budapest charged with '*negligent malpractice*' and assisting at home births without a licence. She was arrested and put in chains because she called an ambulance when a woman in the discussion group at her birth centre went into preterm precipitous labour and Agnes caught the baby. She had advised this woman not to have a home birth. Both mother and baby were doing well.

In Hungary, while all birth outcomes in hospital were subject simply to an internal investigation, if it is considered necessary, out-of-hospital incidents are automatically treated as crimes. Agnes was remanded in custody for 30 days, her appeals were rejected, and though she had not been found guilty of any of the charges against her, her imprisonment was extended on 23 November 2010 by another 60 days. She was locked in a 6 m x 6 m cell with three other women for 23 hours out of the 24, forbidden to see her young children, strip-searched, and her body orifices probed before and after every visit in full view of visitors – including those from human rights MPs and her own lawyer.

The Hungarian Independent Midwives, a very small group, issued a statement of support, but midwives internationally were slow to follow since she was not registered, and the rumour went round that she was an obstetrician masquerading as a midwife. I explained to these organisations that she could not register as a midwife in Hungary *because* she did home births. She worked with 14 independent midwives who were also unable to register. I briefed the Royal College of Midwives in the UK, who later issued a statement calling for her release.

Wendy Savage and I produced a petition calling on everyone concerned about this to contact their Euro MP to put pressure on the Hungarian parliament to act so that women had the right to give birth at home with a trained midwife.

Petition on Behalf of Dr Agnes Gereb

We, the undersigned, object:

- *To the failure of successive Hungarian governments to regulate out-of-hospital birth in Hungary for the last 22 years, and thus failing to provide a legal framework to support and ensure Hungarian women's constitutional right to choose the place and manner of their birth.*
- *To the arrest of Dr Agnes Gereb.*
- *To the criminalisation of out-of-hospital midwifery services in Hungary due to a lack of government regulation.*
- *To the treatment of Dr Gereb in prison.*

We respectfully demand:
- *That the Hungarian authorities release Dr Gereb immediately.*
- *That the Hungarian authorities suspend all current criminal cases against midwives until out-of-hospital birth regulation come into effect.*
- *That the Hungarian authorities involve international and/or Hungarian experts with experience in the field of out-of-hospital birth to participate in the drafting of the regulations concerning planned, out-of-hospital birth in Hungary.*

We maintain that incorporating the option of planned out-of-hospital birth into the range of options offered by the Hungarian health care system will also improve the quality of hospital births in Hungary, for the greater safety and satisfaction of mothers and babies.

Dr Gereb's arrest and its implications for the institution of out-of-hospital birth in Hungary directly affect the right of Hungarian women to choose their place of birth. Hungarian women now need the Government's assistance to be able to take advantage of this right accorded to them under Hungarian and European law. We urge the Hungarian government to act swiftly in addressing this human rights issue for the women of Hungary.

We feel strongly that the conditions of imprisonment for Dr Agnes Gereb are both excessive and unnecessary. We wish to express our grave concern over these conditions and the treatment of Dr Gereb in prison, including the denial of the visitation rights of Parliamentary representatives. We urge the Hungarian government to act swiftly to bring to an end this unlawful and undignified treatment, in the full knowledge that the international community is watching Hungary's handling of Dr Agenes Gereb's case.

I took on the task of keeping the Royal College of Midwives fully informed and linking them up with midwifery organisations in other countries who were unaware that Agnes was a qualified midwife. So this was an important issue concerning midwifery rights in the EU.

There is a historical background to this midwifery crisis. In 1944 the Nazis had deported and killed 540,000 Hungarian Jews. Many midwives were Jewish. As a result there was an acute midwife shortage. In 1951 the Hungarian government passed a law that all women must give birth in hospital and be delivered by a doctor. Hungarian mother Anna Ternovszky, pregnant with her second child in 2010, took her country to the European Court of Human Rights to defend the right to home birth. The court ruled that women have the right to decide where they give birth and that meaningful choice in childbirth is a human rights issue.[51] More recently, though, in what Birthrights describes as '*a blow to women's reproductive rights in Europe*' the Court found that Czech legislation prohibiting midwives' attendance at home births did not interfere with women's right to private life[52] – meaning that the governments' obligations to pregnant women are now unclear. Ms Dubská is appealing the decision.

Agnes had always been a rebel. In 1977 she was charged with smuggling fathers into a hospital labour ward. Her punishment was to be banned from practice for six months. Some years later the head of that clinic declared proudly that his institute was the first to allow fathers into the labour room.[53]

Agnes had come to the first International Home Birth Conference we held in London in 1986. After that she set up the Alternatal Foundation and organised an International Home Birth Conference in Szeged in 1992. Dr Beverley Chalmers, WHO Consultant, and I were joint patrons, and speakers included Wendy Savage, Marsden Wagner, Michel Odent, and feminist midwife campaigner Lesley Page.

International protest prodded the Hungarian government into stating that Agnes was not registered as a midwife and that in future the government would control home births.[54] The Freebirth Support Group responded that she was not registered because no one offering home birth services was allowed to be.[55]

Free Agnes Gereb
Jailed for helping women give birth

- *Dr Agnes Gereb, a qualified Hungarian obstetrician and midwife, and international homebirth expert, was taken into police custody on 5th October – minutes after attending to a woman who had unexpectedly gone into labour at Dr Gereb's homebirth centre in Budapest.*
- *Dr Gereb is respected worldwide for her work on behalf of pregnant women. She has championed the right of women to choose how they give birth and had herself attended many thousands of successful home births.*
- *She has been held in prison since 8th October and her imprisonment has recently been extended for a further 60 days. Under Hungarian law she can be held without trial for up to a year.*
- *Agnes has been charged with 'reckless endangerment committed in the line of duty' and could face imprisonment for between one to five years.*
- *She is confined to her four-woman cell for 23 hours a day, and has been subject to strip searches, is allowed one 10-minute phone call every week and is limited to one hour of access to two of her family per month.*
- *She recently appeared at a court hearing shackled and bleeding from a wound caused by her restraints.*
- *Her lawyers have lodged an appeal against her continued detention and a complaint has been made to the European Court of Human Rights about her mistreatment in prison.*
- *Dr Gereb's case highlights the wider issue of the criminalisation of independent midwives – Hungarian law protects a woman's right to decide where she gives birth but in practice midwives assisting home births are denied licences by the Hungarian authorities. Midwives who do attend home births can be fined or sanctioned.*
- *This situation is profoundly disturbing in an EU member state that professes to respect human rights and the rule of law.*
- ***We are campaigning for Dr Gereb's immediate release.***

With a track record of 3,500 successful home births, Agnes is internationally recognised as one of the most experienced midwives in the world.

Home birth was not illegal in Hungary but anybody assisting one committed a criminal offence. This included simply crossing the threshold of a woman's home with the intention of discussing the option of home birth and sitting in her home while she was giving birth, without intervening. The Hungarian government worked on new regulations for maternity care. The law stated that after 24 weeks of pregnancy a woman had no right to refuse medical treatment, and that for 24 hours after birth she was '*out of her mind*', and so could not refuse treatment either. Those of us fighting this midwifery campaign considered it crucially important that any new regulations established midwifery as a separate profession with its own protocols.

The State Secretary for Social Inclusion, Zoltan Balog, who was also a Lutheran pastor, visited Agnes in prison and reported that, thanks to international pressure, she was no longer strip searched and was allowed pen and paper.

Agnes told him that she didn't trust the liaison between the medical parties and the Hungarian government. She was working for the establishment in law of an independent profession of midwifery free of obstetric control. The message she sent to her family and supporters was: '*I have not been broken. I will not be broken.*'

A vigil took place outside the Chief Prosecutor's in Budapest to run until the following January when Agnes's second detention was supposed to end. In fact, it was extended.

I arranged for Professor Lesley Page, then at King's College, London, to fly to Budapest at the end of November to lecture at the Academy of Science on the regulation of maternity services, and meet with parliamentarians and obstetricians. She had been deeply involved in the rebirth of midwifery in Canada. There a midwife could not remain registered unless she had a regular proportion of home births – the complete opposite to Hungary.

Lesley called for a National Register of Midwives in Hungary to give information and guidance and handle professional misconduct complaints. The criminal justice system should not deal with professional matters. Midwives in Hungary were registered only at the hospitals where they worked. Lesley stressed that registration must be at a national level.

Yet the registration of midwives was not enough. We both emphasised that the guiding principle of midwifery must be women-centred and community-based and respect the individuality of each woman and her family.

Neither home nor hospital birth can be completely safe. All women need a midwife. Some need a doctor, too. Most studies of perinatal mortality show that there is no difference between home and hospital births. But best evidence on perinatal outcomes reveals that with home births there are lower rates of epidurals and analgesics, fewer inductions and augmented labours, and fewer Caesareans, episiotomies and instrumental deliveries.

A wave of change mounted in Eastern European countries. This started in Poland and the Czech Republic in 2010. Women in Bulgaria resisted an obstetric system in which they were told they had birth choices but actually did not. That protest was part of a wider cultural revolution and the rise of a vigorous civil rights movement.[56]

CHAPTER ELEVEN

THE GOOD BIRTH GUIDE – TEN YEARS ON

For *The New Good Birth Guide* edition of 1989 I analysed 773 detailed reports from women about their care over a three year period between September 1985 and September 1988. I asked about their general impression of the hospital, their experiences of antenatal, intrapartum and postnatal care, to tell me how things could be improved, and to say what was the best thing about the hospital. The information they gave me revealed changes in practice and in the environment for birth which had been welcomed by women. Many of these cost little. Some – those that reduced obstetric interventions and instrumental delivery and Caesarean rates – cut costs.

More pregnant women wanted to think ahead about the kind of experience they would like, the setting, the people involved, and how they wished to welcome the baby. The search for information and choice between alternatives that started with educated women had fanned out to include those women who were previously less articulate about what they wanted.

Acceptance of responsibility is part of the transition to becoming a mother, and prepares her for responsibility once the baby is born. We learn responsibility by exercising it. We learn how to be adults by being *treated* as adults.

The response to this on the part of many hospitals had been to try and find a new formula that would satisfy consumer demands. However, generalisations about what women want are often made as if it were a matter of discovering a magic formula which can then become a standard part of institutional practice. As a result, in many hospitals a system – well-intentioned, but rigid – had been introduced without sensitivity to individual women's needs.

Some obstetricians still condemned consumerism as *'just another fad'*, and a dangerous one at that. One consultant obstetrician, Harold Francis, said, 'Some patients no longer accept advice ... They insist on dictating their own treatment. No other discipline in medicine has this treatment. Neurosurgeons do not have to contend with the "Good Neurosurgery Guide".'

Women were being encouraged to be mobile in labour. In a handful of hospitals they could move about freely, change position whenever they wished, and find positions and explore movements which were comfortable and which might help labour progress. But this depended still on individual caregivers, and it was often a matter of luck; 'When I told the midwife I wanted an active birth she went off and changed into trousers. The bed was removed from the room and replaced by a mattress, pillows and a beanbag.' 'I walked, rocked on all fours, knelt. I could move around as I wished. I spent most of the time walking round.'

Immersion in water was suggested by midwives who felt confident about this. At the time pools were not yet installed in many hospitals and an ordinary bathtub was used. 'I could have as many baths as I liked.' 'I wallowed in a deep, warm bath and was encouraged to stay in it as long as I wanted.' One woman described how she 'spent seven hours in the bath.'

Intervention had been reduced. Shaves, enemas and suppositories were no longer given routinely. In some teaching hospitals rates of induction had gone down. For example, in St Bartholomew's the induction rate fell from 20 per cent in 1983 to 9 per cent in 1984.

In some hospitals syntocinon stimulus of the uterus in labour had also decreased. John Hare, Senior Consultant at Hinchingbrooke Hospital, Cambridge, where active birth was encouraged, told me that women could be mobile right through childbirth, and 97% of women who chose active birth moved around throughout labour. Five times more women who did not choose active birth required artificial uterine stimulation. Women who lay in bed were more than twice as likely to have meconium-stained liquor and disturbing fetal heart patterns. The mid-cavity forceps rate had been much reduced by upright positions, and there were no severe perineal lacerations.

In some hospitals, too, women described squatting, kneeling or standing births, to put their hands down and receive their babies. A woman who had a forceps delivery told me, 'I was invited to lift my baby out when the head and shoulders were delivered.'

The ban on eating and drinking in labour had been lifted in many hospitals and women could eat and drink if and when they wished. Food might be encouraged to avoid ketosis, as it was in Hinchingbrooke, where hot chocolate, toast and honey were offered.

More hospitals were striving for flexibility of care and to respect personal preferences: *'I was asked whether I wanted the waters broken at 4 cm, so I chose not to have this done. I also stated that I didn't want an episiotomy, nor analgesics if I felt I was coping. These decisions were supported by the midwife. I refused the fetal scalp monitor because the baby's heart rate was coming back up at the end of each contraction.'*

One important element in this was the introduction of birth plans in a third of all hospitals. Pregnant women were given booklets with information and spaces in which to write questions they wanted to raise at each visit, and there was a section in which they could express what kind of postnatal care they wanted.

There was also genuine concern to give continuity of care where possible. At that time it had been estimated that the average woman in a British maternity unit saw between 35 and 45 different members of staff in the course of antenatal, intrapartum and postpartum care. The effect was confusion, bewilderment, disorientation, failures of communication and unnecessary risk, for to have a multiplicity of caregivers, however skilled and dedicated they are, can be dangerous. Organisational changes had occurred so that small midwifery teams working with doctors were giving total care. It is rewarding for a midwife to get to know the mother during pregnancy, as in the *'Know Your Midwife'* scheme at St George's, London, where there were teams of four or five midwives. Pregnant women were linked to these teams, not to the consultants.

Caroline Flint's research project on the *'Know Your Midwife'* scheme revealed that 51 per cent of mothers in the scheme needed no drugs for pain relief compared to 38 per cent of women who were not in it. It was financially viable. Costs were 10 per cent higher for the care of women outside the scheme. In one midwife's words, *'The system recreates a kind of village atmosphere, where a midwife works in a small area and knows everyone well.'*

It probably also resulted in safer care. Midwives were more accountable and examined their practice reflectively in small groups, exploring where they did things well and where they needed to improve the quality of care.

My earlier research had revealed that women often lacked privacy. They described people wandering in and out of the delivery room, and did not know who most of them were. One woman said, *'I felt like an animal with so many people present during the vaginal examination'*, and another, *'There was a succession of nurses and midwives, none of whom I had ever seen before or saw again after the birth.'*

This had changed: *'My partner and I were shown to our labour/delivery room and it was made our own by a midwife knocking and waiting to be asked to enter. There was no breezing in and out.' 'Little things mattered so much, like midwives leaving the room when I was using the bedpan.'*

Thought had been given to providing tranquil birthing rooms in many hospitals: *'No beds, lights dimmed, a mirror to see the birth, provision of bean bags, birthing stools, bathroom and toilet en suite, tape cassette, hot tub, rocking chair, valence chair, floor mats or mattresses. Free coffee and meals for the partner and a reclining chair to rest if labour is slow.' 'I took in two lemon balm plants, my own sheets, a tape recorder and music tapes, herb pillow, pictures on which to focus. The staff didn't even blink! I was shown straight into the birthing room with a futon on a carpeted floor, curtains, no lights, a valence chair, large cushions, and squatting bars.'*

More Cosmetic Changes

Ten years before I had discovered that time was a central issue – time given by doctors and midwives for discussion with a mother, as well as time for her to feel that she could work with her body instead of battling against it to get the baby born. Many women felt they had been on a conveyor belt in a baby-producing factory.

Particularly in the second stage, they often found that their own rhythms were ignored and they were coaxed or commanded to push. They used words like *'rushed'* and *'harried'*. Women were sometimes told it was the rule that they should be in the second stage no longer than one hour, and otherwise it would be a forceps or ventouse delivery. Occasionally time was restricted to 45 minutes. The disadvantages of this commanded pushing and prolonged breath-holding were demonstrated by Roberto Caldeyro-Barcia and his colleagues. The Valsalva manoeuvre can lead to cardio-vascular malfunction and pronounced dips in the fetal heart.

By the mid 80s in a handful of hospitals there were no restrictions on the duration of the second stage provided the mother and baby were in good condition. Sometimes women described second stages lasting two or three hours, or longer. A woman who gave birth in the Royal Maternity Hospital, Glasgow, told me,' *My cervix was completely dilated, but I had no strong urge to push. Sister said, "Just take things easy. The baby has plenty of room, so don't push unnecessarily".'* One woman, at Dulwich Hospital, described a second stage which lasted seven hours, a record for that particular hospital, and said, *'I never felt scared or out of my depth. The attitude was, "It's your birth. We're here if you need or want us". They kept telling my husband that he was doing a good job, too.'* They often laboured upright, squatting, kneeling and standing positions, and sometimes on birth chairs.

A typical description of the second stage was, *'The lighting was dimmed. I had one midwife. My husband sat on the bed at my side and the midwife sat on the end of the bed. Throughout, she maintained a relaxed, calm, almost casual atmosphere, and gave me immense confidence in myself and in my ability to give birth.'* Another woman said, *'As soon as the head was born the midwife placed my hands on his head and with the next contraction I lifted him out onto my tummy myself.'*

There had been a striking decrease in the rate of episiotomies, and more women had an intact perineum after birth. This came because of pressure by women and their anger at this ritual mutilation. In the 70s episiotomy statistics were not kept in many hospitals. Episiotomy was to be expected. In 1981 the National Childbirth Trust published the results of my research on women's experiences of routine episiotomy which revealed that it often caused unnecessary pain at birth and in the weeks after. It used to be claimed that it prevented a tear, that *'a nice, straight cut'* was better than *'a jagged tear'*, and that it saved pelvic musculature from trauma. None of these claims were true. It does not avoid laceration, or improve the condition of the perineum or pelvic floor, may intrude on the mother's relationship with her baby, adversely affect the start of breastfeeding, and result in dispareunia and stress in a couple's relationship for many months afterwards.

When I did research for the first edition of that book I found that protocols were produced by consultants who insisted on episiotomy for every primigravida after 30 minutes in the second stage. This was often interpreted as the half hour following full dilatation of the cervix, and some women hadn't even started to push spontaneously at all. Postnatal wards were filled with women sitting uncomfortably on episiotomy wounds and trying to breastfeed their babies while shifting in acute pain from one buttock to the other.

Following media focus, practice started to change immediately in many hospitals – especially teaching hospitals – and episiotomy rates were often halved within a matter of months. Research projects were initiated in several maternity units, and as soon as questions started to be raised about routine episiotomy, its incidence decreased, even before the results of randomised controlled trials were published. In the Royal Berkshire Hospital, Reading, for example, research was started, but the researcher told me that the rate was reduced by between half and two thirds even among women in the control group in whom the routine practice of doing an episiotomy to avoid a tear, however small that tear might be, was supposed to be continued. By the 80s women having second and third babies often described how everyone was walking about normally on postnatal wards and could feed their babies without getting into contortions.

I realised that I must have made a mark when at the British Congress of Gynaecologists in 1989 James Owen Drife, then a Senior Lecturer in Obstetrics at Leicester University and later Professor of Obstetrics and Gynaecology at Leeds and a witty columnist in the *British Medical Journal* put on a sketch with Walter Nimmo, the Director of Medical Research in Edinburgh at the piano, which was a parody of my *Good Birth Guide* – the *Good Patient Guide*.

The duo had made their name as young doctors at the Edinburgh Fringe, where they introduced the Fallopian Tuba with their student band, Unbelievable Brass. According to the *Sunday Times* the *Good Patient Guide* left the members of the Congress laughing so much that they were '*fighting for breath*'.

Each patient was identified by symbols in the margin; a black square, for example, signified that the woman had to be delivered in total darkness, a fur coat, that she was an accountant's wife, a stethoscope, a doctor's wife, half a stethoscope, a psychiatrist's wife. Capital 'O' obese. 'OO' she intends to breastfeed, 'OO7' she wants to bond. Thumbs up, member of BUPA, oil well gushing, a sheik's wife, oil well gushing down a sheikh's wife who is a member of BUPA, a notebook, a journalist, and a little notebook with a black hat, a journalist from the *Guardian* Woman's Page. '*Difficult patients*', Drife told his audience, '*explained why so many intelligent, middle-class obstetricians were forming self-help groups and practising "natural obstetrics". This was a method of doing without patients altogether* (loud applause) ... *now being pioneered by a London teaching hospital* (more loud applause).'

Repercussions In Australia

The publication in 1979 of *The Good Birth Guide* stimulated research and enquiries into health services and birth rights. In 1989, Health Ministers in New South Wales, Western Australia and Victoria commissioned reviews that included consultations with women who used the services as well as those who provided them. Women were sent questionnaires six to eight months after they had given birth.

Immediately after birth many women did not criticise care, and it was not until the second half of the year after the baby was born that they reflected more critically.

Over half the women who took part in the study had seen the same caregiver throughout their pregnancy, but in labour almost all women, whether public or private patients, had encountered midwives and sometimes doctors, students and other personnel whom they had never met before. With changing shifts they might also have met another new set of faces, and if they experienced complications or a long labour, as we have seen, they sometimes found themselves surrounded by multiple extra personnel while their partner was pushed to the back of the room. The challenge for maternity-service providers was to find ways of overcoming the current level of discontinuity and fragmentation in the way that care is provided.[57]

Close on 40 per cent who attended a public clinic said they saw a different caregiver at each visit: '*I sometimes felt that I had to remind clinic staff of tests required, for example that I had Rhesus negative blood, that I hadn't seen a doctor when they said I would. It just seemed a bit haphazard at times. The doctor (female) was too impersonal.*'[58]

What women wanted most was the recognition that someone was listening. The Chinese ideogram for '*listening*' is composed from the four signs for ear, eyes, heart and undivided attention. '*Such listening enfolds us in a silence in which at last we begin to hear what we are meant to be.*' (Lao-Tze, Tao Te Ching).

Jo Garcia summarised women's comments on studies in the UK as thick with '*recurrent images ... of cattle markets and conveyor belts*'.[59]

But the evidence is that change does not come, or does not come fast enough, when an expectant mother has a quiet talk with an obstetrician – only when there is open and public protest. There is a place for quiet talks, but we need more than that if our culture of birth is to see any radical transformation. The task calls for knowledge and understanding, the courage to question assumptions, and the energy to work together to create a way of birth in which women are recognised as adults and active birth-givers.

It is understandable that a woman on her own feels she cannot make any effective protest. But there's more to it than that. New mothers often tell me they don't like to write complaining in case someone at the hospital 'takes it out' on them or the baby next time. Anyway, they are grateful to have the baby and pre-occupied with the new challenges and 24-hour work of being a mother. There may even be an element of Stockholm Syndrome. That's what happens when a kidnap victim living right through the 24-hours with her captors, identifies – or even falls in love – with them. It's often only much later that a woman looks back at her labour and realises that she was robbed of any right to make decisions about her own body and her baby, and was treated like a naughty little girl – and feels helpless anger.

On the other hand, we cannot close our eyes to the epidemic of Caesarean sections throughout the Western world. In the United States one woman in five has a Caesarean. This is happening partly because of clock-watched labour – each patient is forced to conform to a time norm. It is also because doctors often no longer know how to deliver a breech baby vaginally, and because of unnecessary obstetric interference – induction, for example, when the uterus wasn't ready to contract, so there has to be surgery to get the baby born.

It's more difficult, too, for any woman in a high-tech hospital – even one with a simple, normal labour if she exceeds the time allotted – to avoid being festooned with tubes and wires and connected to boxes with flashing lights and reels of paper. Caregivers may assume that a patient's wishes are identical to their own management plan. When one woman said she did not agree to have her labour induced the midwife protested, '*Oh, but you wouldn't want to have your baby in the middle of the night, would you?*'

Women themselves may be convinced that the medical team have got it all streamlined. One mother told me, '*Induction is the only civilised way.*' The technological take-over of birth could be justified only if randomised research showed clearly that it saved babies' lives. No proof of this kind exists for routine electronic fetal monitoring, induction, and many other interventions in labour.

But when I feel most disheartened I look at what we have gained. In hospitals all over the country women are no longer given drugs for pain relief without being consulted first. Doctors and midwives now usually hand the newborn baby straight to the mother and parents have some time alone with their baby. In most hospitals nurseries for babies who are not labeled '*at risk*' have been eradicated. Rows of newborns yelling their heads off in boxes are a thing of the past. Instead mothers have their babies with them and with any luck can cuddle them close and feed them when they're hungry.

Yet we must face up to it. Many doctors are so star-struck with high-tech ways of controlling the uterus and detecting what is going on inside it that they don't watch and learn from what a woman can tell them. When technology fails, that's a recipe for disaster. '*Even God cannot sink this ship*', announced the Captain of the *Titanic*.

The Place of Birth, published in 1979 by Oxford University Press, stimulated research in the United States too. Writing to me from The Boston Women's Health Book Collective conference, Norma Swenson said that Iain Chalmers waved a copy of the book at the audience: '*Has a book ever been so much and so reverently handled … in three days? He would scarce let it out of his sight, so we all contented ourselves with fondling it.*'

She went on to prepare me for a NAPSAC conference in Atlanta: '*A feminist controversy has arisen about participating in the meetings, which derives from the fact that Georgia is a state which has not ratified the ERA (Equal Rights Amendment, a constitutional amendment guaranteeing that women may not be discriminated against because of their sex). Several groups of feminists, notably NOW (the National Organisation for Women, the largest and most popular of the groups) decided to apply an economic boycott against all states which have failed to ratify the ERA, by persuading national organisations to relocate expensive, revenue producing conventions to other states.*' She described it as '*a strange turf where left meet right, and feminists meet anti-feminists, but where the leading edge of change in childbirth in America is today.*'

More About Birth Plans

When I was thinking through the idea of constructing birth plans, I asked myself: how do you plan for a whirlwind? And does a woman get an entirely false sense of control over a force that is often unpredictable, elemental and passionate if she has made a plan? Plans can twist the birth experience into a juridical and confrontational mind-set.

A birth activist and one of my closest colleagues, Penny Simkin, lives thousands of miles away, in Seattle. We both believed that it was vital to discover women's experiences and to record them in their own words. Listening to women was the basis for research that led to understanding how to improve the environment for birth and help them afterwards.

In spite of being a physical therapist and incorporating Lamaze techniques, Penny focused on birth as an experience rather than an energetic physical activity or an ordeal to be faced. She modified Lamaze teaching and founded the Childbirth Education Association of Seattle.[60]

For each of us the Quaker spiritual ethos of making space for listening and learning was the basis of our work. She focused on birth as a life transition, not just a process that must be survived with exercises for breathing and neuro-muscular co-ordination.

When she introduced the birth plan in the United States, she did so in a way to avoid antagonism between a woman and her caregivers and 'enhance co-operation and trust'. I introduced it in the UK following this, so that women could work out what they wanted, make it clear to their caregivers, and also make choices if birth was not straightforward. I designed it as a basis for discussion during pregnancy to which caregivers should refer when a woman went into labour. For both of us the birth plan included conclusions about procedures such as shave and enema – routine in the 60s and early 70s – drugs for pain relief, drugs to stimulate the uterus, time-limits on different phases of labour, mobility in labour up to and including the second stage, pelvic exams, intravenous hydration, monitoring of the baby's heart, directed or spontaneous pushing, episiotomy, assisted vaginal delivery (forceps or vacuum suction) and the management of Caesarean birth, cutting the cord, rooming in with the baby or having it put in the nursery, care of the baby, breast or bottle feeding, and whether feeding should be timed or responsive to the baby's behaviour. At that time babies were still being routinely removed to the nursery. Another important element was the father's role. Was he to be there? An onlooker, or actively involved?

Birth plans came in for a lot of criticism from some midwives who complained that women were presenting them like 'laundry lists' and with ultimatums that were unrealistic. They claimed that they ignored or undervalued midwifery skills. I made the point that making decisions about birth in advance was a bit like going out on a picnic in English weather when it might rain or snow. Plans had to be realistic with a section for choices if birth did not turn out just as a woman would like it to be.

Later, like me, Penny founded a doula movement, Doulas of North America, so that women could have support from another woman through childbirth, and worked to educate midwives and reinforce their contribution to birth in a culture where obstetricians were professionally dominant over midwives. I went to speak at the Seattle Midwifery School, which opened in 1973, and became one of its patrons.

My survey of 1,795 women about their experiences of episiotomy was published by the NCT in 1981 and in 1984 Penny started her own small publishing firm and issued a book I had edited, *Episiotomy and the Second Stage of Labour*, revising it for the American market because practice was so different. For one thing, midwives had been more or less eradicated through North America and mid-line episiotomy was a standard part of normal birth, whereas in the UK episiotomy was less standard, and when it was performed it was done in a hockey-stick shape rather than mid-line straight down to the anus. The book sold well and rapidly went into new editions. She also published my book of batik paintings and poems, *A Celebration of Birth*. The International Childbirth Education Association (ICEA) bought the rights to this and produced cards of the pictures.

Penny introduced birth plans with some colleagues of hers in the mid-eighties, and I did the same in the UK a couple of years later. Plans turned up in different guises, and often made caregivers anxious. It is claimed that a pregnant woman arrived at an American hospital with a list of demands she'd signed with a lawyer. They started: '*I, Doris Smith, being of sound mind …*' and she signed it in his presence. '*That's why birth plans make me anxious,*' one midwife told me.

On the other hand, there were still women who relied on professionals to make all the decisions, saying '*I leave it to you Doctor. You are the expert. Whatever you say!*' Some obstetricians preferred women to think through what they want and make choices.

Others took it for granted that women are ignorant. Ann Oakley records an interchange between a doctor and patient:

'DOCTOR (reading case notes): *Ah, I see you've got a boy and a girl.*
PATIENT: *No, two girls.*
DOCTOR: *Really, are you sure? I thought it said* ... (checks in case notes)
oh no, you're quite right, two girls.[61]

Doctors and midwives do not have to be burdened with patients' total reverence. I was starting to meet some who realised that when women got utterly dependent on them it could be more threatening than open confrontation, for when things go wrong and a baby is damaged or dies, total faith may turn to litigation.

In the United States, where obstetricians may offer a woman everything she wants if she will trust them completely, insurance malpractice premiums are sky-high and some doctors are going out of business because it is all too costly. It is almost invariably those who put unquestioning trust in the doctor who sue for malpractice – not women who accept responsibility, weigh up the pros and cons of different kinds of care and make decisions themselves.

The paradox is that in the United States where midwifery was not recognised, and midwives were working outside the law, they were far less concerned about prosecution than obstetricians who had all the power of the establishment behind them.

Birth plans are a way for a woman to work out the kind of setting in which she wants to have her baby – teaching hospital or GP unit for example – and the general style of birth she prefers – high-tech and an epidural or drug-free and moving about.

Home birth is one option. Perinatal mortality statistics for planned (as distinct from accidental) home births in Britain are among the lowest in the world.[62] With a home birth a woman herself controls the setting for birth and doctors and midwives are her guests.

The sort of requests women make are: '*Please consult me beforehand about everything that is done to me and my baby*'; '*I should welcome the midwife's support to give birth actively, moving about and changing position in whichever way I am comfortable*'; '*I should appreciate help with the relaxation and breathing I've learnt in National Childbirth Trust classes*', and '*I'd prefer a second stage with no commanded pushing*'.

Those opposed to birth plans often urge women to be nice to their doctors to get what they want. Being nice is not enough. The kind of doctor who brushes aside a request saying, '*Of course you can give birth naturally. All birth is natural*', and who tells the woman: '*You can hang from a chandelier as far as I'm concerned*', is likely to be induction-happy, hooked on electronic fetal monitoring, and possibly knife-happy too.

Many doctors feel threatened by birth plans. I have heard an obstetrician dismiss them because, he says, he '*can't stand backseat drivers*'. Birth plans are not set in tablets of stone. At best, a birth plan is part of a good working relationship.

There are hospitals where women feel physically and psychologically assaulted in childbirth. In these hospitals, I hoped that a reminder that a birth plan was in the notes would give a signal that the woman was not prepared to acquiesce to conveyer-belt obstetrics, and knew what she wanted.

The challenge is to use them so that they become part of a developing dialogue between each pregnant woman and the people caring for her.

CHAPTER TWELVE

LENTILS TO DUBROVNIK

Lurid pictures of Dubrovnik in flames at night had been on the front pages. The beautiful port was besieged by land and sea. The areas around it were overrun by the Yugoslav National Army and gangs of irregulars. The city itself and the Dalmatian islands near it were flooded with refugees. Uwe kept his boat in a small fishing harbour on Korčula and had close friends there, and the local Caritas and Red Cross faxed us a plea for help: *'Last night the only remaining bakery in Dubrovnik was blown up. There is no bread, no flour, no lentils …'*

We appealed to the big charities – Oxfam, Save the Children and others – but they were already too busy in other parts of the world, especially Africa, and the Balkans were not their primary concern.

So we decided to do what we could as a family and start a relief agency from our home. I drew on what I knew as an anthropologist about Balkan cultures to work out what supplies would be most useful. One food we could send would be lentils, since they were familiar, nutritious and cheap, could be stored easily, combined with other protein and herbs and spices, and, when mashed, fed to small children and used as a weaning food. We started *Lentils for Dubrovnik*, long before any of the existing relief agencies were ready to make a contribution, on 6 November 1991. Our first load with nine tonnes of lentils, 50 kilos of chocolate, clothing and blankets arrived by lorry two weeks later.

Though 'Lentils' was the name, it wasn't just about lentils. We added many other foods, together with toilet, sanitary and cleaning materials. We wanted to supply the basic needs of women and children, and in January 1992 introduced gift boxes, woman-to-woman, baby-to-baby, child-to-child, and even island-to-island. Our daughter Tess took on the task of being Planning and Transport

Manager and was very skilled at this. Uwe managed the political end of it and sought help from big-wigs. He reckoned his talent was lunches! We found patrons in the Chancellor of Oxford University, the Bishop of Oxford and the Lord Mayor of Oxford.

I undertook publicity and contacted firms that produced food and everything else the refugees needed. Firms often approached others on our behalf when they knew the quantity of goods available. For example, a company that manufactured labels for clothing sought help from firms which used their labels and as a result we had a bulk supply of tracksuits by Alexon, trousers, t-shirts and other garments.

Transport was vital. In the 15 months that followed we sent 33 loads, 500 or 600 tonnes in 43ft lorries, and some in shipping containers on Croatian merchant ships. We used volunteer drivers and lorries that were either lent to us or, if necessary, hired for the occasion. The first lorry was ferried to the Continent by P&O free of charge. Covering all administrative costs ourselves, we sent our supplies by reliable routes to the twin Korčula charities Caritas and Red Cross. They were run from a tiny office by friends with whom we were in almost daily contact by fax or phone. They set out their precise needs. Our friends distributed the supplies with a multi-ethnic team of volunteers, helping people in every religious and ethnic group. (Father Josip distributed woman-to-woman parcels in Ston oblivious of the condoms thoughtful British women had included in their boxes. But then, he was the sort who would have laughed if he had learned about it afterwards.)

All that winter and spring Dubrovnik was completely cut off by road and basic supplies got into the city by sea at night. Around 85 per cent of the buildings suffered damage by shells or fire. Living mainly on bread and pasta, people were hungry and their currency almost worthless. Often no clean water was available because pipes had been blown up, so the only way to get fresh water was to put buckets out in the street and hope it rained. Eye infections were common. I was able to get water purification tablets from one company. It was cold at night and I managed to obtain thousands of blankets, too, and sent them out there fast. It was tremendously exciting when news came in from a firm giving something we really needed.

My Report on the Situation in Dubrovnik – January 3rd 1992

The Croatian member of parliament Matko Medo, a resident of Dubrovnik, rang me today to give up-to-date information on the situation there. This is the gist of what he told me: Eighty per cent of houses in Dubrovnik have been affected. Shops and houses have been sacked by marauding soldiers. In the old city the Franciscan monastery received 23 direct hits, although the library has been saved. There have been 17 direct hits on the Dominican monastery and 176 on the lane leading between the monasteries, with damage to the roof of the synagogue. The church of St Blaise has been hit, the cathedral and the museums. The Domus Christi, the oldest hospice in Europe, has had 10 direct hits, the oldest orphanage in Europe, the monastery St Clara, has been damaged, and the hospital on the island of Lokrum. He says one can stand and count with ease roofs which are undamaged.

For more than three months there has been a severe shortage of fresh food, no fishing has been possible, and there have been no milk or milk products.

20,000 people are living in camps outside the city. This includes refugees who came to Dubrovnik to seek shelter and those in Dubrovnik itself whose houses are destroyed. An attack on one camp resulted in 50 dead.

Altogether, there are 20,000 refugees to be cared for. Two thousand are in hotels without heat or running water, and 'the standard of living is that of the sixteenth century'. Water is rationed to one litre a day and the whole of the old city 'is a septic tank'.

Many people have stoves which depend on coal or wood for fuel, neither of which is available. At Christmas parts of Dubrovnik had their electricity reconnected, but it is only functioning at 35 per cent of normal capacity. There is no street lighting. A blackout is necessary because soldiers are shooting from the hills above Dubrovnik once night falls. At the moment the temperature in the morning is around zero, and babies and old people are at risk of hypothermia.

We were successful in getting supplies in quickly, so when I sought donations from food firms I asked if they had anything nearing the end of its date code, as well as anything in packaging that was about to be changed. We arranged next day pickups of goods on pallets. This worked especially well for Christmas puddings and mince pies. Since they were both unfamiliar foods in this part of the world, I wrote a leaflet about their history and significance that was distributed with the festive parcels. When alcohol is poured over the puddings and set alight the flame signifies the triumph of good over evil, light over darkness. There was still plenty of slivovitz around, so Christmas puddings were introduced into the culture, with information about their spiritual symbolism.

A local farmshop, Millets, with the enthusiastic support of one of its managers, Brenda Standen, sent a truck load of potatoes, and a local flourmill 11 tons of flour in huge bags. Eian Riddiford, a racing driver, generously drove lorries. On one of his trips he was shot at. Other drivers took in many tonnes of lentils, sweet foods from Lyons Bakeries and Jacobs, canned foods, rice, dried mashed potatoes, chocolates from Rowntree, biscuits (782 cases in one load), beans, soups, canned and dried milk, fruit juice, jam, fruit pies, eggs, candles, bedding, warm clothes, nappies (100,000 in a single load), children's shoes, big boxes of toys, analgesics and antibiotics given by Oxfordshire GPs (samples from pharmaceutical companies), other medical supplies from Parke-Davis, artificial limbs, zimmer frames, oxygen equipment, hospital lighting, 60,000 sanitary towels from Kimberly-Clark, laundry and other detergents, soap, shampoo, dried spices from Bart Spices (3,000 jars), and felt tips, paper, pencils, crayons and painting books for children.

A Child's View Of A Terrible War

In July 1992 Uwe went into Dubrovnik on the first of our lorries to be allowed in. The devastation around the city was appalling. Evidence of widespread obscene atrocities was abundant. In the city old people were still sleeping in the underground Aquarium within inches of the glass that separated them from the sharks. From Korčula he delivered some of the boxes that had crammed our house a few weeks earlier to the smaller island of Lastovoon on his boat. He brought back pictures by refugee children in playgroups and primary schools to which we had sent drawing and painting equipment. They were encouraged to draw and paint their experiences as refugees and what was happening in the world around them – wounded parents, planes and guns, ruined buildings and rubble – as a way to come to terms with their experiences of violence and death.

* * *

Korčula's usual population of 16,000 had been overwhelmed by 12,000 refugees, most of them women and children from southern Croatia and – since by then the war over Bosnia-Herzegovina had begun and now Sarajevo was coming under siege – from there as well. Priests, nuns and Red Cross workers who distributed the aid were giving all the love and care they could but the children were unhappy and anxious. Crouched in fetid underground shelters, these children had endured night after night of shelling and weeks of hunger and thirst. Families had been split up and many did not know if their relatives were alive or dead. Some children had seen their mothers raped, their fathers' throats cut, and their homes burned down. One three-year-old drew a picture of his mother and painted blood pouring out of an abdominal wound.

The killers were often not strangers, but neighbours – men living in a previously close, intermarrying community who turned into murderers. The four-year-old who said, *'Do not kill me, Uncle! I will be good!'* spoke to the killer as a well-known and trusted adult he was used to calling *'uncle'*. It is as though the child believed that, if only he were good enough, the violence would stop. Some of these children had lost both parents and, like many children, thought the death of those they loved was because they had been naughty. It was a terrible burden of guilt for any child to bear.

Yet many pictures were vigorous and positive. Houses, even when burning, looked astonishingly solid. The tombs visited by one little girl's mother are drawn with a monumental permanence which suggests that the ritual of mourning, and its public recognition, helps to heal. Planes dropping bombs are mixed with jolly-looking birds and coloured flags. The image of the ship occurs often in the paintings of the over-fives – ships which bring food, and, above all, hope. Many children drew the *Zlarin* bringing in canned baby food.

Most of these pictures were done by pre-school children, but we also have ones from older children. In these, there were obvious gender differences. The girls drew flowers, women in frilly dresses and people busy collecting water for cleaning and cooking – somehow conveying a reassuring sense of normality. The older boys, however, focused on the fighting. They drew strutting warriors, men firing guns, bayonets and tanks with intricate detail and precision, often cramming in every weapon of destruction they could. The greatest danger is that children who live with the reality of violence grow up to become violent in their turn. We ought to ask *'What are we doing to our children's minds?'* While boys cherish an image of manhood like this, can the killing ever stop?

From January 1992 onwards child-to-child personal gift boxes were organised through schools. I suggested that each of these should be packed with presents for a child of the same age – things like a doll, always some chocolate, a toy car, a construction kit, soap, a hair brush, bright woollen socks, a warm scarf, a teddy bear – and a photograph of the child giving them.

The novelist, Susan Hill, offered help and went round Oxfordshire schools. As a result children became enthused about the project and eagerly got together gift shoe boxes full of the kind of things they would want themselves if they were forced to leave home in the middle of the night with only one bag containing all their belongings. It was an exercise in creative imagination, social understanding, emotional intelligence, as well as international history, geography, and, because the children often wrote letters to the recipients, in English composition. Teachers welcomed the project because it also represented new ways of teaching that cut across formal classes and stimulated children's eager co-operation.

Our dining hall was piled with filled shoe boxes under the great oak table and in every gap and cranny, and when the lorry drew up outside our grandson Sam, still a pre-schooler, worked with us enthusiastically to load it. Yvonne Moore, who trained Active Birth Teachers in London, joined in with gusto and collected hundreds of shoe boxes. Her eight-year-old complained at breakfast time, *'Mummy, I can't reach the cereal cupboard!'* That's when she loaded a van and drove her boxes to add to those already in our dining room!

We had sent 800 gift boxes in our first load and, with publicity from Worldwide Television News, 3,000 in the next one. In April 1992 the shoe box scheme was taken over by some Clarks shoe shops and BBC Greater Manchester radio, administered by Sheila Faulkner's *'Who Cares?'* programme. 136 shoe shops gave out boxes and welcomed them back packed full of goodies. Then this scheme was expanded to Clarks shops in the London area. Subsequently 12,000 filled boxes were sent to Dubrovnik each week. There were so many that we could also send loads to Zagreb and Split, where there were large number of refugees, and even into areas still under attack – Mostar, Travnik and Sarajevo.

News came from Korčula that private initiatives like ours succeeded in providing 75 per cent of the refugees' food on the island. Nothing was going to waste, no money was going into administration, and theft was rare. Most relief agencies have to allow for theft. It is expected. But because Tess, our daughter, followed our loads right through to the consumers, we could keep tight control and see exactly what was happening to everything. When the Christmas puddings arrived, for example, a group of soldiers scooped some up and went home to their families each with a pudding under his arm. We were happy about that. The only other theft we discovered was by a priest who stole some packed shoe boxes for the children in an orphanage he ran. We wish he had asked, because we would have earmarked some for them, and he could have re-ordered regularly.

I faced an ethical dilemma when asked by local charities in Croatia to get hold of artificial baby milk from big international firms like SMA and Cow & Gate. From one point of view, introducing large quantities of their products was bound to serve as advertising, increase sales, and undermine women's attempts at breastfeeding. Yet we couldn't leave babies to go hungry, and when a mother was not lactating, either because she had suppressed her milk supply or because it had not built up or had dwindled, there was no alternative to feeding a baby on a breast milk substitute.

I was strongly criticised by some breastfeeding organisations in the UK who believed it was wrong to provide any artificial milk and in this way lend support to firms manufacturing and promoting it. But we could not leave babies to be fed unsuitable food like water thickened with flour (it was white and looked like milk) or to starve. So we introduced Chloe Fisher, a skilled and passionately committed lactation counsellor and midwife, to promote the benefits of breastfeeding with doctors, nurses, midwives and mothers, and simultaneously made artificial milk available for those babies who needed it.

Bosnian mothers in rural areas usually breastfed without problems. Muslim mothers expected to breastfeed for at least two years. This certainly saved many babies' lives. But those in the towns and women in Croatia were more accustomed to breastfeed, if at all, for six weeks or so, and then wean their babies on to the bottle. Many paediatricians had been trained in Germany, where this was the norm. We were challenged by a European culture that was basically anti-breastfeeding.

I researched promotional material about breastfeeding, found a good booklet based on cartoons that gave sound and simple advice, had it translated into Serbo-Croat, and UNICEF covered the cost of mass-producing and distributing it free of charge all around the country to every maternity unit and clinic. At the same time Chloe ran workshops for medical personnel and started up mothers' breastfeeding groups.

Advocates of breastfeeding, especially the mothers, sparkled with enthusiasm, and it turned out to be a very positive, joyful and successful campaign. We were not only saving lives in a country in a state of catastrophe. We were helping to create healthier babies now and in the future.

The astonishing result was that when Nina Smith of the National Childbirth Trust was invited to visit Bosnia 10 years later she told me, *'They are streets ahead of this country with breastfeeding.'* I got Nina and Chloe together to talk about what had happened, as Chloe was not aware that this had triggered a revolution. When she first arrived in Bosnia, Serbia and Macedonia, mothers without access to artificial baby milk were trying to feed babies on bread and water and sweetened black tea. Only peasants and the Roma breastfed, because it was considered *'primitive'.* Now in Sarajevo, for example, there were drop-in centres where mothers could go with their babies and stay all day, a cartoon leaflet to help them breastfeed based on a snazzy one published by the Royal College of Midwives that I had introduced with UNICEF, and Nina told Chloe *'They are still using the knitted breasts you took them'* (i.e. to demonstrate how to get babies latched on correctly.)

But back in the early 90s it had bothered me that even if we managed to help mothers and babies breastfeed, they had a difficult start in hospitals that still treated babies as the property of the hospital and kept them away from their mothers except for allotted feeding times. In response to a newspaper photograph of babies in a hospital lined up like sardines in a can, I wrote:

'The photograph of the newborn babies in a Sarajevo hospital with a nurse trying to warm them with hot water bottles was distressing. The sensible way to keep babies warm is for them to be with their mothers. The risk of artificial heating is that a newborn gets overheated and becomes dehydrated. Crowding babies together in a central nursery also leads to cross-infection.

'The Sarajevo women who are deprived of their babies because of outdated hospital rules are probably not only cold themselves, but miserable without their babies, and find it difficult to get breastfeeding off to a good start. Bottle feeding is bound to kill babies in a city where there is no electricity, clean water or regular, cheap supplies of dried artificial milk.

'This year the World Health Organisation and UNICEF launched the Baby Friendly Hospital Initiative; mothers and babies should be able to be together

day and night. A hospital environment should support breastfeeding and babies should be free to suckle whenever and for as long as they want. This is impossible when mothers and babies are segregated. Many women long to have their babies with them. A baby-friendly hospital must also be a woman-friendly hospital.'

I learned that moving into a country to provide aid entails action at different levels – practical and administrative, negotiation with national and multi-national firms, cultural understanding: personal relationships, media management and political enterprise. It was a great education for me.

We wound up the operation in early 1993, when the big agencies got going. Our remaining cash went to the Korčula Red Cross with permission to distribute it to local families in need who by then felt neglected in favour of the refugees.

CHAPTER THIRTEEN

LECTURES AND WORKSHOPS

In the 80s and 90s I was offering a wide range of lectures and workshop topics for the international tours which I undertook – that included the United States, European countries and the Antipodes. To give some examples:

Creating the best environment for birth
I ask what kind of setting is needed to support the spontaneous process of birth. I illustrated this with slides of my grandson's birth in water in the family home.

Birth and the transition to motherhood
Birth is not just the delivery of a baby. It is a major emotional and social life transition for a woman and for a couple. This can be obstructed by insensitive and authoritarian patterns of care. An exploration of how women are nurtured during and after childbirth in different traditional cultures, and the relevance of these for our own society.

Getting in touch with the baby during pregnancy
The unborn baby is often seen as a mysterious package, a doll hidden in the toy cupboard, and today, as already a patient. An exploration of how a woman can learn more about the baby inside her, and the benefits of this prenatal bonding.

Postnatal counselling
Any woman who has had a bad birth experience needs a friend who can offer non-directive counselling. We explore together how to listen in a way that is active, reflective and validating, and can help a woman integrate this negative experience in her life, and find strength within herself to cope.

The non-violent second stage
The expulsion of a baby is often treated as a race against time. It is stressful, uncoordinated and violent. In this workshop we explore ways of respecting the rhythms of the second stage and achieving a gentle birth.

The benefits and risks of birth plans
What birth plans are and common misconceptions about them. Midwives' and obstetricians' criticisms of birth plans as mere shopping lists made by anxious women. How the creation of a birth plan can be an important element in education for birth stimulating discussion and negotiation with caregivers, and help those attending the mother as well as the woman herself.

Midwives and mothers working together towards change
An account of the changes taking place in British hospitals as a result of concerted ventures by midwives and mothers. Discussion of how midwives and mothers can be most effective in working together, and the challenges and opportunities in the future.

Women's experiences of episiotomy
What episiotomy is, how it came to be a standard part of an obstetric delivery, its benefits and risks as a routine practice, and women's accounts of episiotomy and its short and long term effects. A discussion on how routine episiotomy can be avoided, and of how more women can be enabled to give birth without perineal trauma.

Traditional rites and symbols in childbirth
The implicit meanings of ceremonies and symbols in traditional birth practices, and the relevance of these to childbirth today.

Change in childbirth
Recent developments in childbirth, how these are perceived by childbearing women, and how birth may be in the future.

Instinct and culture in childbirth
The relationship between biological and social elements in childbirth, and how the physiological process may be affected by the psycho-social context within which birth takes place.

Sex in pregnancy and after childbirth
The woman's changing body, emotions and relationships.

The psychology of breastfeeding

How a woman's ability to breastfeed spontaneously and in a satisfying way for both her and her baby is influenced by emotional factors, by social pressures, and the importance that the help and advice she is given should be empowering rather than lowering her self-esteem.

The rebirth of midwifery

How obstetrics has changed the role of the midwife and the way in which midwives perceive themselves. The rise of the childbirth movement and the midwife's reclaimed identity: an international view. A discussion of what will be needed for the midwifery renaissance to become a reality.

New Zealand – Maori Birth Traditions

When I go to other countries to lecture, there may be book promotion as well, and I fit in a period of research if I possibly can. I did this with the Maori in New Zealand in 1990 when I was invited by seven women elders to learn at first hand about Maori traditions of childbirth, which are '*tapu*' (the Maori word for taboo which has a layer of supernatural meaning). Younger Maori women are not allowed to learn about them. I had been with the Maori before, and it was as a result of this that they invited me to come and be initiated into the secrets. They said that then I would have responsibility to write and speak about them. Traditions differ between the North and South islands, but are very similar to those in the islands of the Pacific, in Fiji, for example. These people travelled in their boats all over the Pacific – and the Maori are part of the greater Pacific culture.

Carved over the entrance to every '*marae*' (place of worship) is a vagina. Access to the Maori culture and to the values of Maoridom is only through a woman. In the same way, in formal religious rites a man speaks only when called by a woman. Women are the '*callers*'. They enable men to express themselves.

The *marae* itself is constructed in the form of the human body. The lintel over the door depicts the way into the womb of an ancestor through the body of a woman who conceives the Maori members, nourishes them during gestation and gives birth to them. She is the portal to birth, life and death. Any person stepping over the threshold under this lintel becomes ritually cleansed.

I entered the *marae* of Papakura through a door that depicted a woman with carvings of people of the northern tribe on her left and right side. Her arms were raised to either side of her as if clutching beams and she squatted, feet firmly planted on the ground, whilst two carvings of the people of the tribes fanned out on either side of her.

Traditionally, at sunrise a Maori pregnant woman gets up, faces east and breathes slowly and fully as the sun rises. At sunset she turns to face west, and breathes slowly as the sun sinks

The God of the Universe formed human beings, and afterwards created the lesser gods, including Kamaro the God of the Sea, who in turn created marine life. Uemoko shaped the plates of the earth, then shifted them, moving America away from South Africa and New Zealand away from Australia, for example. Pakeamarktir was the God of the elements, wind, rain, lightning, thunder and storms.

When a woman gave birth she went with other women into the bush and they made a warm nest. It is called 'Korama'. She often delivered the baby using another person to support her as she knelt forward. This might be one of her other children. A man told me, with pride, *'I myself helped to bring my sister into this world when my mother was giving birth. I went before her and knelt down and she leant over me.'*

Patient Advocates

I met the first patient advocate to work at a large women's hospital in New Zealand, Lynda Williams. Her brief was to give all women using the hospital information about their rights, help them understand how the medical system works, ensure that they had access to their medical records, deal with complaints, and be readily available to listen to them. She was independent of the Area Health Board and directly responsible to the Health Commissioner (like our ombudsman) and so could be effective.

Her appointment followed a scandal that rocked the country in the 80s. In 1988 the Minister of Health revealed that for more than 20 years women at the National Women's Hospital had been used as guinea pigs in research on cancer of the cervix. This type of cancer was not treated, in spite of the fact that since the early 60s it had been known to be a precursor of invasive cancer. Judge

Silvia Cartwright said that Professor Herbert Green had ignored virtually all the existing research by withholding treatment from women with early changes in cervical cells.

These women did not know they were being used as research material, had no opportunity of withdrawing from the study or of giving informed consent to it, and believed the many investigations and the surgery they had for research purposes were actually methods of treatment. In fact, even when malignant cells were multiplying quickly, some women were told there was nothing wrong with them.[63]

The judge called for the appointment of a patient advocate in the hospital to be a voice for patients on ethical committees and in the development of information about treatment protocols, make sure that information was available in a woman's own language, and heighten awareness of emotional, cultural and social needs. She called for a *'human link between the medical and administrative services and the patient'*. In a damning indictment of the medical system, she said, *'I accept that individual doctors, nurses as a group and the medical superintendent all believed that they put the patient first. But I also have ample evidence that this is not always the case. Nurses have been conditioned to protect patients by stealth. They cannot, therefore, be effective advocates who will act bravely and independently.'*

Lynda had been a childbirth educator for 12 years, was on the Auckland Women's Health Council, and had four children herself. *'One of my main goals,'* she told me, *'is to empower women in a system that is continually disempowering us. I don't want to become yet another crutch to be leaned on, but to empower women to take back control of their own health care.'* She said it was hard not to be worn down by hospital bureaucracy, *'In an institution like this the rights of the patients get lost in other kinds of issues such as staffing, which assumes more importance than the needs of individual women.'*

Her appointment led to the development of a system in which advocates had the difficult task of confronting and challenging an entrenched medical position. Some members of staff believed that the advocates' job was really to make work easier by getting patients to obey instructions. They expected her to sweet-talk women into believing what had been done to them must be for the best because doctors are experts.

At that time there were some patient advocates in the UK in places like Hackney, where there was a large immigrant population. They helped women who did not speak English. The patient advocate in Leeds told me that in theory she could help anyone, but in practice her work was limited to ethnic minorities.

A real patient advocate is quite different from interpreters employed in hospitals. Interpreters translate what doctors and nurses are saying, helping women to conform to hospital protocols. Advocates take an active part in policy-making.

I believe that women need patient advocates in every maternity unit and every hospital where gynaecological surgery is performed. Women's health issues were still controlled by a group of senior consultant gynaecologists. Having a patient advocate right there in the hospital, yet independent of it, enabled women to speak out about what they want and negotiate changes in the system. So I started to write about this in newspaper and magazine articles.

Since that time advocacy has become established as vital wherever power is unequal – in mental hospitals and the mental health services, for example. My daughter Polly was actively involved in the training of advocates for users of the mental health services and in setting up services.

In the 90s Polly worked voluntarily with Rape Crisis and with Lesbian Line in Oxford, and out of this grew wider advocacy work and her appointment as Co-ordinator of Volunteers in the Oxford area for women with mental health problems, most of whom had been sexually abused. Then she went to Wales and was responsible for co-ordinating all statutory and voluntary mental health organisations in the South Wales valleys, Merthyr Tydfil, the Rhondda and Cynon Taff – an area where there was extreme social deprivation since the closing of the mines, and where services were severely underfunded. Her task was described as 'service user involvement and development', making sure that routine services took into account the needs of people to be involved in the design and working of all agencies, and ensuring that individual voices were heard. Mental health patients need help with building confidence and self-esteem, but were often considered unable to make choices for themselves and were simply treated with drugs, and stigmatised when they did not comply with plans made for them.

Islands Of The Pacific

On my first visit to Fiji in 1993 Uwe joined me from Harvard, where he was a Visiting Scholar from then until 2003. We stayed in a beautiful hotel on the tiny island of Vatulele. There was a communal table in the restaurant, a personal pool through the glass wall of our room onto the heath that stretched to the sea edge, and wild horses galloping free. I met a waiter who took me to his village to learn from the local midwives and talk to women.

Talking to the traditional village midwife in the open just outside the village, we were discussing her work. You couldn't interview anyone without a crowd gathering and taking part – a definite advantage – more to be learned. So every question I asked, every subject I raised, stimulated a response from the women who stood around us. At first the midwife was keen to show that she conformed with the bio-medical standards imposed by the hospital system. She sought approval. I represented, whether I wanted to or not, the American technocratic way of birth. It was difficult for me to make it clear that I was not testing her. So I talked about birth ways of women around the world – having other women to help them, for instance. It was quite hard going. She couldn't trust me yet. The conversation got more lively and the bystanders helped. Then she started to explain how she managed the second stage of birth: '*When the woman lies down ...*' she said. My eyebrows shot up and I exclaimed, '*Oh, they lie down! In many countries women don't like to lie down. They kneel or squat or stand.*' At that point the crowd of women suddenly burst into activity. '*Of course we don't lie down!*' They exclaimed. '*We stand. We stand. We swing-along!*' First one, then another, then all of them broke into a pelvic dance, slowly rotating and rocking their hips. The midwife laughed and danced, too, and I joined them. We understood each other exactly. The children joined in. It was an instinctive birth dance shared across cultures. We didn't have to talk about it. We *knew*. Birth is movement. Birth is a dance!

An invitation to lecture and do research in Hawaii in 2003 presented an opportunity to interview midwives and mothers and explore childbirth for the second time on the islands of the South Pacific.

On this visit we stayed on the island of Maui. It was a good base from which to fly in a single engine plane to the scattered islands and get an idea of birth traditions and the problems presented by a medicalised birth system in which heavily pregnant women were directed to fly to the big hospital, either already in labour, or to wait, isolated from family and friends, until labour could be induced. This is a model similar to that in the Canadian far north when in late pregnancy women were flown to a hospital in Winnipeg, and where at that time midwifery units had not yet been created on the reservations. As a result important birth rites were not enacted and the children born far from home were deprived of tribal membership.

Fiji has a rich birth culture. When the Chief's wife gives birth members of the community blew on conch shells four days after to welcome the baby and the mother and baby's first week are passed in complete seclusion. The mother and maternal grandmother massage the newborn baby with coconut oil, a tradition that continues now.

Adiseru was a 52-year-old Fijian midwife who had been working for 33 years, and was apprenticed with her mother. She learned from her how to massage the pregnant woman with oil twice a week from when she was two months pregnant. She gave her advice. She should never wear tight clothing around her neck, or a necklace, lest the cord twists round the baby's neck. In the second stage of labour she told the woman, 'Slowly, slowly, ... Gently, gently.' Native midwives never did episiotomies, and might guard the perineum with the flat or side of their hands when they thought it necessary. She told me she could tell in pregnancy whether a baby is a boy or a girl, because girls are on the left. Then she slapped me on the shoulders and roared with laughter. Other women joined in. How gullible can you be?

Research in Hawaii was preceded by my addressing a large gathering of US-trained midwives in Honolulu, in dazzling light facing huge windows and brilliantly sunny gardens, when the air conditioning had failed. Unfortunately I passed out at the podium. The result was dramatic. I came to with midwives surrounding me offering a wide range of skills. They massaged my feet, shoulders, head and back, gave instructions about breathing, and engaged in meditation and chanting. I felt in safe hands, though there were rather too many of them! An incident like this has an amazing uniting effect on a crowd, and we became very merry afterwards. We all moved out into the garden and sat on the grass, where the meeting continued.

These midwives were a lively lot, with sympathy for local cultural traditions that had proved their value, and I enjoyed learning from them. In the nineteenth century Hawaii was Japanese and until the Second World War Japanese midwives gave childbirth care and worked alongside native midwives. On the rural western side of Kauai and Lanai the old language was still spoken, and native midwives used the hula during childbirth to 'help move these babies down'. Yet on the small islands women were flown to deliver in hospital in Honolulu and this was mandatory for first babies. Midwives say that many refused to go to the hospital because '*birth is easier with midwives at home*'. On Tara, where there was no doctor, nurses – not midwives – delivered most babies, but I discovered that there were four traditional midwives, who used touch and massage, and placed women in warm water to treat pain.

Grandmothers are enormously important in this culture, as in Fiji, where the first baby is given to the maternal grandmother, or sometimes an aunt, to raise. Grandmothers have the right to choose any child of a daughter. A woman who is barren can ask for a child, too. The practice of surrogacy is traditionally well established and if a woman cannot conceive by her husband she can select another man to be the biological father, while her husband remains the social father.

Pele is the grandmother goddess, *Tutu*, and Mother Earth is the goddess *Papa*, representing the female principal. Grandmothers sing sacred chants and lullabies to the baby, so that the child starts to learn cultural values early. A traditional midwife tells me, '*We share. What is mine is yours. What is yours is mine. We all care for each other.*'

Talking with Hawaiian midwives, I learned that before American missionaries came a man's parents chose his wife, but that this changed with American influence.

As the time of birth approached the family gathered to help by pooling their *mana* (vital life force). The mother knelt for the birth, with one or more female companions supporting her back, while the *kahama*, a male healer, or the midwife, knelt in front of her. '*Men are always put away during birth.*'

I talked to a fifteen-year-old Kauai woman who told me that her maternal grandmother massaged and rotated the baby into the right position at the end of her pregnancy, '*So I had no troubles*'. After the birth she said she went straight back to work. I said, '*Oh, really?*' and told her that in most countries other women cared for the new mother, and she then quickly amended what she was telling me, and said that at first there was a 30 day period in which she was nurtured by women and no men were allowed in the house.

A midwife aged 86, who had started midwifery when she was 25 and retired at 70 because her sight was failing and her arms were no longer strong enough to hold a woman up in a good position for birth, described how she spread coconut leaves or grass on the ground and women helpers supported the mother's shoulders and arms from behind. The mother held onto a stake in the earth. In pregnancy she advised women to have regular exercise and eat plenty of vegetables, special vegetable jelly, and hibiscus leaves, and avoid drinking much tea. Instead she should have tea made out of lemon leaves. She should not eat red foods, including crabs and lobsters, which 'make the baby have tumours' or any long fish such as barracuda. If labour was very slow she gave the mother herbs that were rich in natural oxytocin. One thing that these traditional midwives did not do was to inject synthetic oxytocins, a major cause of fetal death, uterine rupture and maternal death in countries where traditional midwives have adulterated their practice with powerful drugs that have been introduced by professional obstetricians and midwives. Oxytocin is useful in controlling haemorrhage, but when generally available at pharmacies in rural areas, and used in labour, it can be very dangerous.

This elderly midwife buried the placenta outside the hut or dropped it in water, and advised the mother to drink taro and cassava, either boiled or as juices, and eat vegetables and fish. She gave the mother herbs when a newborn baby was not thriving, the essence of which would be conveyed to her baby in the breastmilk. She told me that sex while a woman was lactating 'spoils the breastmilk'.

Sweden

Janette Brandt, a bright spark in the Swedish birth movement, came from Abergavenny and first met me at the NCT in London, in 1962, when I gave a talk on breast feeding. She writes in a series of emails to me in 2014: 'There you were, up front, with breast milk oozing through your bra, leaving damp patches on your bust and so rapturously happy that women can nurture their babies without having to rely on the bottle!'

'When I arrived birth preparation was stagnant! Dick-Read's method had been adopted – but not modified over 20 years.' Janette started groups in Adult Education Schools (AES), but a year later the Government reduced financial support to all AES.

'Psychoprophylaxsis was introduced in Sweden in 1969 and presented as "Learn to Give Birth"! Defined levels of breathing had to be … used systematically, all with the purpose of blocking pain sensations. Another issue was that there were too few anaesthetists to provide adequate pain relief when necessary. This situation gave rise to pressure groups. Some wanted the right to "pain-free birth" *using epidurals. Others … claimed the right to give birth with little if any pain relief medication, using PPM (Psychoprophylactic Method).'*

'In 1970, Sheila Ljungren (an English NCT Member in Gothenberg) and I publicised the need for a Swedish counterpart to the NCT. We contacted Bonniers, and in 1977 your 'Experience of Childbirth' was translated and published as 'Aktiv Forlossning' (Active Birth).'

'Comments have been made to me over the years that I must have had a tough time dealing with all the back-biting talk that was directed at me, but in all honesty it didn't have the impact because I didn't perceive the irony/criticism, due to my poor understanding of Swedish! I was happy teaching and encouraged by what the parents had to say concerning the value of prepared birth. Through close contact with the parents after birth, I learned what to improve upon.'

Janette says that now Sweden is on a *'collision course for conflict! … An example is the manufacture and sale of weapons that bring in huge amounts of money to the arms industry in a country that is supposedly neutral! Sweden had developed from a small country, isolated from Europe, into becoming a part of Europe. She is still influenced by America and at this present time in politics is deep into Thatcherism … People are aware that privatisation has gone too far endangering Sweden's long established Social Welfare system … There are lots of complaints from patients and parents concerning the National Health Service … There are an increasing number of people turning to the fascist party Swedish Democrats.'*

'I think all this and the huge impact of IT technology (Sweden has the largest usage per person for its population, in Europe) has an effect on birth. It becomes impersonal and theoretical.'

American TV programmes are horror documentaries increasing the fear of birth and being prepared for the worst. She went on to say: *'Parents want a 'short course' where time for reflection and thought is not catered for! Some find the subject of birth too confusing and become anxious about right/wrong choices, sadly leading them to making no choices at all!'*

First Water Birth Conference

In 1995 the first International Water Birth Conference took place at the Wembley Conference Centre, with mothers and birth professionals from around the world.

The Active Birth Movement, the Association for Improvements in the Maternity Services and Splash Down water birth services worked together to present data from a new environment for birth.

Researchers, midwives, obstetricians, neonatologists, general practitioners, birth educators, obstetric physiotherapists, sociologists and parents with the experience of water birth came from 19 countries.

Speakers included Dianne Garland, a pioneer of water birth and a midwife supervisor who designed the first under-water Doppler; paediatrician Dr Marsden Wagner; Dr Michel Odent; Dr Paul Johnson, Consultant Clinical Physiologist at the John Radcliffe Hospital in Oxford; Caroline Flint, midwife at the Birth Centre in South London and President of the Royal College of Midwives; Cass Nightingale, Manager at Hillingdon Hospital; Dr Josie Muscat, part of a team that introduced water birth in Malta; Dr Piera Maghella, who founded the Active Birth Centre in Modena; Dr Yehudi Gordon; Dr Faith Haddad; midwife Lesley Page and Jayne Ingrey, the founder of Splash Down. It was a brilliant occasion.

Marsden Wagner said that water birth was branded as dangerous mainly because obstetricians did not have control over it. It represented the social model of birth.

Michel Odent discussed accusations against water birth on the grounds that it was 'not natural' and also mentioned that birth under water was reported in a French medical journal in 1804.

Paul Johnson said that if the onset of labour is spontaneous and no drugs are administered a fetus is born with its cord intact into warm, fresh water and does not breathe until it surfaces into cool air.

Jayne Ingrey said that women must have choice. Information is power.

Beverley Beech, one of the organisers of the conference, said that water birth was an alternative to dangerous drugs, and makes it more difficult to intervene in labour. It needed proper evaluation.

Caroline Flint spoke of the birth pool providing a 'watery cocoon' for a woman, it affects the balance of power, 'the woman is in charge', she is more mobile and 'inviolate'.

Cass Nightingale stressed the importance of midwives being well trained for water birth and able to deal with any emergencies. In 1994 there were 3,505 births at Hillingdon, and 60 per cent of women used water at some time during labour. It was the primary method of pain relief. 'Women basically deliver *themselves, therefore the midwife should only need to lean over the bath on one or two occasions – to feel for the umbilical cord and to lift the baby out.'*

Dr Josie Muscat analysed the results of the first thousand births in water. Perception of pain was on average 50 per cent less in water.

Faith Haddad presented results from a pilot study of water births at the Garden Hospital in London. Most women giving birth in the pool had an intact perineum or only a first degree tear.

Piera Maghella said that Italy had the highest rate of Caesareans in Europe and most doctors per inhabitants.

Yehudi Gordon focused on issues of safety and stressed the need for a complete audit: *'The enthusiasts are confident that water birth will continue to maintain the safety record which has emerged in the studies.'*

Lesley Page talked about surviving the *'onslaught of the uninformed ... Far too many people today assume that more technology has improved the quality and safety of birth.'*

Researching Midwifery

In the 1990s midwives in the West developed a clearer view of where their strengths lay. They broke out of isolation, began to link with midwives in other countries, and realised that they faced common problems. Till then a midwife often had little idea of the power politics in the health care system in her country, and even less of the politics in other countries. A direct entry education developed alongside out-dated instruction which saw midwifery as either a top-up to nurse training, an extension of caring for sick people, and a way of producing compliant workers who prepared patients for the obstetrician, kept them quiet, and cleared up afterwards.

In the countries of western Europe EC directives about midwifery training now lay down standards of midwifery. Rather than being handmaidens to obstetricians, midwives should have the education and status to take responsibility for the care of women through pregnancy, birth and post partum. That could never have happened without input from childbearing women, and their commitment to midwifery.

The UK was ahead of most other European countries, largely because of our collaboration as childbirth educators to forge a partnership between midwives and mothers. Through the 90s I taught midwives at universities in the UK and internationally and became Honorary Professor at Thames Valley University.

In Britain the Midwives Information and Resource Service made research much more accessible to midwives and students, and I served on their Editorial Committee.

An important development was research by midwives themselves. In the UK and Scandinavian countries midwives were critically evaluating obstetric and midwifery interventions of all kinds, and demystifying ritual hospital practices. This had a direct affect on care. Enemas and shaves were discarded. A woman could have her partner with her, or anyone else with whom she wanted to share the birth experience, including family members, women friends, and her other children. There were lower rates of induction for 'post-maturity', episiotomy rates plummeted, and a more relaxed approach to pushing and the length of the second stage. There was better understanding of women's emotions in childbirth, and how to provide optimal care for those of different ethnic and cultural groups. Internationally, outreach work was firmly in the hands of midwives, if only because most obstetricians were not eager to work with the poor and did not fancy going to rural outposts. In Australia I explored ways in which Aboriginal midwives were beginning to provide care in their own communities. In New Zealand I discussed with Maori women their concern to rediscover traditional childbirth practices, and incorporate that which was of value into contemporary practice. This was increasingly accepted by Pakeha midwives, who discovered traditions of good midwife care which had been lost in modern hospitals.

The new midwife takes responsibility with confidence, is an educator and advocate for women's right to make informed choices, and supports them in giving birth in whatever places they select as best for them and their babies. She attends women who give birth at home, and ensures that they have the best care possible. In some countries pilot programmes started up with Government funding. In Australia in 2005 the first midwife-attended home birth took place for which mothers did not have to pay. Yet in many countries the home birth midwife found herself outside the official system. In most states of the United States, the only way she could work was as an underground midwife, risking suspension, litigation and imprisonment

In the Middle Ages midwives had fled to Holland, the only country to offer them a sanctuary. Midwifery there still retains its autonomy vis-à-vis the medical system more than in any other country. A third of births take place at home, and midwives provide total care for normal pregnancies and births. This comprehensive service could not be provided without maternity home care assistants. They help midwives care for the mother, baby and family for up to 10 days after birth, give practical help with breastfeeding, and do the housekeeping and cooking. I learned that these care assistants helped during and after 73 per cent of all births. The Netherlands are the only place where women can rely on this.

Insurance for Independent Midwives is an important political issue for midwives internationally. These are midwives independent of established systems that keep midwives subordinate to obstetrics.

Science And Sensitivity

Lesley Page's book *The New Midwifery: Science and Sensitivity in Practice* came out in 2000.[64]

Midwives need to study the politics of maternity care, how institutional systems work, how power is exercised, and ways in which competing claims for territorial control operate. Then they will be able to join with childbearing women to create a system in which the new midwifery, described in detail in this ground-breaking book, develops and flourishes.

Throughout history and in cultures across the globe a midwife has never been just a technician, someone who manipulates a round object out of a small hole. This has always been recognised in traditional cultures, where the midwife uses her empirical skills, enacts prayers and rites that make the way safe, choreographs the birth drama and the interaction of everyone taking part in it. The midwife's tasks are multi-dimensional. They involve hands-on diagnosis, treatment, massage and giving comfort, together with understanding the psychology of pregnancy and birth and awareness of relationships and their effect on a woman's ability to open her body and give birth.

Today the midwife's role is multi-dimensional, too. She must have up-to-date knowledge of birth-related research and the knowledge to evaluate it. She needs to be reflective about midwifery and obstetric practice in the light of this research. Her practice should be evidence-based. She works not only in a bio-medical framework but with emotional and social aspects of birth. She needs the skills to meld the art and science of midwifery. She gives each woman not only her knowledge, but the personal warmth and caring of a skilled companion and friend.

Any woman who has had midwife care will tell you that it is not just a question of what she knows and how clever she is that matters, but who she is as a *person*. Research on women's birth experiences reveals that it is the quality of the relationship between a woman and her midwife that is the single most important factor looking back on birth as a satisfying experience.[65] All this research bears out a major theme in the pages of *The New Midwifery*,[66] and mothers' accounts of their feelings about their midwives are remarkably similar.

Albert Einstein once said, '*Not everything that can be counted counts, and not everything that counts can be counted*'. The quality of the relationship between a woman and her midwife is difficult to evaluate in numerical terms. But this is a vital element in a positive birth experience.

In all cultures the roots of midwifery lie in a one-to-one relationship between a woman and a midwife who is well known in the community and has a life-long relationship with the family, the mother and the child she has helped into the world. In Guatemala, for example, like Nicaragua, the midwife is the '*grandmother of the umbilical cord*' and, as in many other societies, by her participation in a major event in the life of the family she becomes, as it were, a member of that family. No one needs to plan for this in a peasant society. It just happens. It is much more difficult in post-industrial society, where contacts between people are constantly shifting, ephemeral and superficial, and where close bonds tend to be restricted to the nuclear family, immediate peer groups in a school or leisure activity, and, perhaps, a segment of the work-place.

My own research in a major English teaching hospital revealed that it is often difficult for a woman to get to know her midwife or for a midwife to get to know the woman for whom she is caring.[67] Fragmented care undermines their self-confidence. Some felt '*abandoned*': '*I was disappointed that the first midwife had to go off shift and leave 50 minutes before the baby was delivered, as I had built up trust in her and had a rapport with her. I didn't have the opportunity to do this with X in the second stage of labour.*' A woman who had a previous still-birth said: '*One midwife who knew my history might have made a great difference. They were complete strangers. You ought to know your midwife.*' Women who did not know the names of their midwives tended to have a more negative experience of birth, particularly when they had as many as five different ones. (This may be correlated with length of labour, and numbers are too small to come to definite conclusions.) Those who had a positive experience usually knew the names of their midwives. They said: '*It was great to have the midwife as my friend*'; '*A positive experience was dependent on having the midwife of my choice who I had built up a relationship with and had confidence in. This can be very hit or miss depending who is on call. I was lucky.*'

It is impossible for any midwife to give focused care when she has to rush from one patient to another and relies on an epidural and an electronic fetal monitor to take her place. Women said: '*We had one midwife covering four women, all close to delivery*'; '*I was left alone for 35 minutes plus while being monitored in the admission room. By the time the midwife returned I was nine centimetres dilated.*' One woman said that each time another midwife put in an appearance she did a vaginal examination: '*It was the worst and most traumatic aspect of the birth.*' Women commented on the lack of shared information between midwives and inadequate hand-over between shifts. They had to explain their priorities, if there was time and they had the courage to do so, to each different midwife.

In many hospitals there is a shortage of midwives. As a result, women encounter a wide range of '*team members*' and care is thinly spread between a vast number of staff: '*The room felt like Clapham Junction with people bursting in and out and a ward round coming in unannounced*'; '*There was a constant stream of registrars, consultant, house officers, anaesthetists and students in and out of the room all the time*'; '*I felt desperately the victim of the lack of communication. There were too many people.*'

Even women who had satisfying birth experiences were appalled at conditions on post-natal wards: '*All I ever kept hearing was, "Oh, sorry, we are just too busy at the moment".*' They had little help with breastfeeding and what there was often incorrect. Many received conflicting advice: '*I found it very confusing to have different advice from a huge number of midwives*'; '*I never saw the same midwife twice.*' A woman whose baby became severely dehydrated while with her on the ward said that the midwives had no time to help her. When conditions are like this women may be discharged without breastfeeding having been established, with low self-esteem and, in one woman's words, '*totally exhausted*'. One result is distress after childbirth increasingly recognised as post-traumatic stress disorder.[68]

Discussion about standards of midwifery care has to take place in the context of the pressures put on midwives within rigid hierarchical structures ill adapted not only to the needs of mothers and babies but also to those of the midwives.

Spiritual Midwifery

Ina May Gaskin in the United States rejected the emphasis on techniques to 'control' behaviour in labour.[69] *The Farm* midwives of Tennessee believe that feeling is more important than control. This expresses my own view that birth is potentially a profound psycho-sexual experience – not just for the mother, but for both parents. Birth Centres reflect this emphasis on emotional and relational aspects of birth and parenting.

Ina May writes: '*When birth first began to be shown on US television during the nineties, decisions were made in broadcaster's boardrooms that it would be acceptable for people to see an incision made in a woman's abdomen and uterus and a baby's head emerge through that incision, but not to clearly see a baby emerge from a woman's capable body, from her vagina.*'

She says she '*never made the obvious connection between sexual feelings and birth until I witnessed a laboring woman whose husband was sitting at her side pull him closer and passionately kiss him during a long contraction. Her relaxation during this intense part of labor was instant and impressive: I could feel it in my own body. A feeling of calm confidence pervaded the birth room. This was an "aha" moment for me, because I realised just then that my own social conditioning had prevented me from imagining how much a little making out might help not only to augment labor but to numb pain at the same time. The ecstatic and beautiful birth that resulted from this woman pulling her husband to her for a kiss – a real consciousness-changing kiss, mind you, not just a peck.*'[70]

Psychology To Promote Compliance And Persuasion

For some psychologists working in the field of childbirth exploring emotions in terms of an unfolding psycho-physical process throughout pregnancy, birth and after is primarily problem-oriented. The key to effective communication and counselling skills is to offer information, allay anxiety, promote '*compliance*' and '*persuade*'.[71] '*Persuasion*', Sherr writes, '*may be necessary at many stages:*

from the first decision about where to have the baby, to pain management, alcohol reduction, smoking cessation'. This statement set off alarm bells for me. Are women to be *'persuaded'* not to have a home birth, to agree to induction or to an epidural that they did not want! The terms *'compliance'* and *'non-compliance'* pepper the pages: *'The skilled performance of the initial contact interview is the factor which determines information flow, satisfaction and often compliance.'*[72]

Where there is *'communication proficiency'* this author claims that *'compliance and informed consent can be increased'*. Insufficient time for communication is *'false economy'* because *'dissatisfied clients often return and in the long term take up more time'*, and other effects are *'missed diagnosis, increased legal action, litigation or suing, poor knowledge transfer, limited future health education, non-compliance and failing to seek medical care'*.[73]

She argues that women must really like antenatal care or they would not turn up for it: *'The actual behaviour of most women demonstrates their respect for and belief in a system in their overwhelming attendance at antenatal clinics'*,[74] ignoring evidence that women fear that if they do *not* attend the baby may be harmed.

So psychologists don't seem to have all the answers. In fact, psychological counselling may be as dangerous as an intervention when unevaluated screening procedures and obstetric interventions are assumed to be beneficial. Just as PSYOP – that is propaganda by another name – is used in warfare, so psychology – again propaganda by another name – is used in hospitals to enhance patient satisfaction with the care already provided and to increase compliance. If this is really what clinical psychology is all about, it manipulates, exploits and traps women in a medical system dominated and controlled by professionals and reinforces the power of the professionals, rather than serving the needs of the women for whom the service is supposed to exist.

Couples need information to ask further questions, understand the answers, and be in satisfying partnership with caregivers. This aspect of childbirth education is vital as obstetrics gets more technically complex.

Some obstetricians feel uncomfortable about it, because they see all the decision-making as their responsibility alone. But whose baby is it? Pregnancy is a tremendous opportunity to prepare the couple for the responsibilities and decision-making of parenthood.

CHAPTER FOURTEEN

BECOMING A GRANDMOTHER

When Tess made me a grandmother I faced a major life transition without any understanding of what it entailed and what the challenges might be, or what my daughter wanted. I had a picture of what I *did not* want to be – interfering, know-it-all, bossy or sentimental, and neither Uwe nor I saw ourselves as what Stephen Spender called in one of his poems, '*Cardboard cut-outs of grandparents*', eagerly waiting for grandchildren to visit, but peripheral and largely irrelevant to their lives, with the real action taking place elsewhere. I wanted to go on being *me* and not have to fit a stereotype. I did not need, even particularly want, my daughters to have babies. Partly because I had committed myself to motherhood with gusto, and had gone on from there to do research and be involved everyday with mothers and babies, my life was richly satisfying and I was unlikely to romanticise grandmotherhood.

When I visited Tess in the United States where she was living with her husband and working as an electronic engineer she quietly announced, '*I'm pregnant.*' It was all very low-key. So low-key that I asked her whether she wanted the baby. She did. And then she said, '*I didn't think you would approve.*' That was a shock. She said I was so approving of her academic sisters that when she chose motherhood she feared that I might think it was second best, a waste of her potential. I felt rather ashamed about that.

The truth was that I was thrilled that this was something – becoming a mother, with all its joy and problems – that had been an important life passage for me and one that I could share with her now.

Daughters make all sorts of assumptions about how their mothers will respond to being told that they are pregnant. The same goes for daughters-in-law and mothers-in-law. It is worth asking, '*Why does she expect that reaction of me? What is she telling me about what I have said and done, and also the unspoken messages I have sent her?*' I think Tess's doubts about my reaction to her pregnancy pointed to the struggle I had experienced as the wife of an Oxford don and the mother of five to make space for myself and to be able to achieve anything apart from motherhood. I used to write in the early mornings before the children were awake. There were many times when a child came into the room and I said, '*Wait a moment. Let me finish this sentence.*' We communicate to our children the things that matter the most to us, often without even knowing that we are doing so. It is not only a matter of struggling to build a career while at the same time being a homemaker and mother, but helping people outside the family as well as inside it, from personal moral commitment, and in my case, wanting my children to grow up ready in their turn to challenge social injustice, inequality and the abuse of power. But we may also be saying that everything must be clean and tidy in the house, that children should always be polite and well-behaved, putting particular stress on religion or politics, on keeping up with the neighbours, or our grandchildren's academic achievement, social skills or being good at sport.

For me, having grandchildren was a bonus. My identity was not encased in the grandmother model. In this research I discovered women who were exuberant in their role as grandmother. But many others were troubled. Some felt burdened with all the problems and none of the joys. Becoming a grandmother can reveal new aspects of the self, bring opportunities to develop and learn as a person, and see the world with freshness and vitality through the eyes of a child.

Though there are classes to prepare for birth, grandmothers are left to cope on their own. Occasionally you come across newsletters with titles like '*Creative Grandparenting*' containing articles describing how '*hugging can improve your health*', and text books used in adult education classes '*on achieving grandparent potential*'. But in general grandmothers have to pick up ideas of how they should be, what they ought to do, and what it is normal to feel, by sheer chance from other women who have been through the same astonishing, bewildering transition.

For many women becoming a grandmother is something more. It is a symbol of ageing, of being '*past it*', just a spectator on the touch-line, the invisible older woman.

Grandmother care is under-valued and often despised. But to become a grandmother gives us the chance to rediscover ourselves as mothers. When I was in New York I sat in a playground in Central Park for an interview with the *New York Times* journalist who wanted children to be in the scene. You don't see children in the streets of New York. The only place to go is where kids are corralled. There were few mothers with their children, only one granny, and the other dozen or so children were being supervised by nannies. There are many warm and wonderful nannies but these were bored, detached, their faces slack and expressionless. Childcare was obviously a tedious chore that somehow had to be endured. They did not talk to the children. They just gave orders. They often did not even look at them. When children cried, they did not comfort them. When a child did something that made him happy – reached the top of a climbing-frame, for instance – they did not join in this or even acknowledge it. A two-year-old was distressed and had been crying non-stop for half an hour. I learned later that he was one of twins and had never been separated from his twin before. He had been plonked in a swing, and screamed until I thought he was going to vomit. The woman in charge of him stood at the side of the swing, pushing it back and forwards, ignoring him while she continued a desultory conversation with friends. Meanwhile the single granny was running around bright-eyed and sharing in the excitement of her grandchild's discoveries and achievements. Here was one-to-one child-centred care given by a woman who was enjoying it. It provided a dramatic contrast.

As I've watched babies and small children with nannies and au pairs, with minders and day-care providers in many countries I have come to the conclusion that grandmother care is often among the best kinds of childcare, even if that is only possible for a few hours at a time and mothers at work must rely on other people to be the primary care providers.

A book came out of this – *Becoming a Grandmother*, and was published by Simon and Schuster in 1997.

Grandchildren

When Tess had Sam, her first baby, I was impressed by her strength and had utter confidence in her. She chose to give birth at home relaxing in a pool of water until the baby was about to pop out, when she moved to dry land. They lived at the end of the Manor garden in a bungalow built for them in 1993 and we were an extended family. The children were an integral part of my life. A new baby was often plonked on my bed in the morning as Tess had to get Sam dressed for school or do a school run. I was more relaxed about being a grandmother than I was about motherhood, especially the first time round. The first baby is highly experimental. You wonder whether you can possibly do it and if the child will survive. When I saw little Laura, nearly a year old, picking up beads and carefully putting them in her mouth, I didn't get alarmed. She was not going to choke on them, because she knew she must not swallow beads. The important thing was not to startle her or trigger conflict.

For *Becoming a Grandmother*, I did research in Australia and the UK, with further material about women's experiences of their own grandmothers from Israel and Poland, for example. There have been marked changes in the lives of grandmothers over the last 100 years – and the last 50 years- and many feel alienated from daughters and daughters-in-law, especially daughters-in-law, because the whole culture of child-rearing has altered, and they don't know what they can say that will be relevant. They told me, '*I bite my tongue*', '*I've learned to keep quiet*' and '*I never give advice*'.

My personal experience witnessing Tess giving birth in water inspired me to work with other birth activists to organise the first International Water Birth Conference. I was amazed watching her, the way pain melted away when her body was submerged, and how she moved so easily. She could almost somersault. She was spreadeagled like a frog, on her back, semi-squatting, and got in all sorts of positions, without any difficulty. When she stood up she was uncomfortable and sank down into the water again. I gave a birth pool to the John Radcliffe hospital in thanksgiving for Sam's birth.

Then we had the International Water Birth Conference in 1987. Four of us got together and hired the Wembley Conference Centre, which seats 2,000. It was crowded. It was important to find out what was happening around the world. There were many questions to be answered. People were doing research who were completely out of touch with other researchers, and I was surprised as the abstracts came in at the number of randomised controlled trials that were being undertaken. We also wanted to hear from the practitioners of water birth, midwives – usually midwives because most doctors didn't like sitting on the floor waiting – and other researchers and parents. We needed to form a network and put them in touch with each other.

Diary Of A Week In 1996: An Appetite For Life

Sunday

Enjoy craft fair with daughter Tess (electronic engineer and website specialist), Laura (the baby), Sam (six) and Polly (sailing and youth worker daughter). Meet up first with Celia (psychologist daughter) and Sue (her partner) for lunch at restaurant in Kenilworth with gorgeous vegetarian food, where disposable nappies are produced when Tess runs out. She cradles Laura at the breast, wrapped in a capacious shawl knotted over her shoulder. Wish more restaurants were baby-friendly. Laura slurps and smacks her lips to show what a delight breastfeeding is, but table of business men behind us don't notice, thank heavens!

Monday

Work on my new book, *Becoming a Grandmother*, to chorus of morning bird-song which livens it up no end. Editorial comments have been faxed for chapter I've written for American anthropological book – most tedious part of writing academic paper: further citations, counter-arguments, explanations, clarifications.

Early morning is my best writing time – an oasis of peace. I often start around 5.00 a.m. If I work through the evening, especially if it entails writing, I can't sleep at night. So I must chill out.

It could be some quick crosswords or reading a detective story. I soak up Morse, in his familiar Oxford setting. Even Poirot, who dates from 1920 – a gentle contrast to the crazy violence and sadism of contemporary sleuths like Montalbano. They probably improve my writing style, too, making it snappier and steering me away from academic jargon. Certainly if I read a lot of foreign research I get to the point where I can no longer produce a simple sentence. If this happens in my memoirs, I apologise. I have worked too hard.

Today I start later and slog away from 6 a.m. till mid-afternoon.

Whenever I get down to writing concentration is punctuated by a ringing phone, including Birth Crisis Network calls. Today a woman still not completely continent, and with no clitoral sensation, after botched episiotomy and catastrophic repair. Then another, from Germany, who had failed prostaglandin induction for '*fetal growth retardation*' over three days followed by emergency Caesarean section, and 3.6 kilo brain-damaged baby. She says birth was like rape. It sounds as if medical-surgical management was disastrous. It is vital that these women have a warm and immediate response. They have had to sum up a lot of courage in order to ring me.

Then I find time to read *The Enchanted Horse* to Sam and give Laura lavender oil massage. Admire his painting of a Shetland pony and himself in '*pooey field*'.

Tuesday
Masses of stuff on dictation machine for my secretary to put on the computer. I get on with painting old school desk for Sam. Hen with chicks, owl, goose, rabbits, frogs on chair, and underwater scene inside. We go through second and third drafts.

Acrylics dry out while I deal with umpteen phone calls about publicity for my new book, *The Year After Childbirth*. *Woman's Hour*, breakfast TV and arrangements for lecture tour in United States September/October when it's published there. Mix fresh yellow, scarlet, pink for sun.

Uwe, still in Harvard, phones to fix holiday dates and his sailing trips, so we have a diary session. Thinking of Bali holiday on my way back round world in autumn. Mix paints again. Phone rings – woman considering home birth and wants help getting it. Then another who wants elective Caesarean section. Listen – discuss. Mention that occasionally when a woman has been sexually abused as a child this may seem only way she can give birth that she can tolerate. Then flood-gates open and her distress pours out. She describes the abuse which she has never told anyone about. She has been blaming herself and believes that she must have been responsible for causing it. Tell her she is being reasonable and I'll support her any way I can. She is happy for me to ring obstetrician, whom I know and admire, as she can't put it into words to him.

At lunch-time committee meeting to plan International Water Birth Conference next April. We've hired Wembley Conference Centre – big commitment. We lunch in conservatory on salads and daughter Nell's tasty tomato and olive bread. She enjoys cooking and turns out everyday dishes with a special touch: stuffed potatoes with mushrooms and cheese, sweet and savoury scones and pizzas.

Vine is flourishing at last, and has overtaken one I stencilled on wall to encourage it while it was sickly. How many of water birth research projects on risks and benefits will be at the stage where there can be at least preliminary reports? Janet Balaskas is organising posters, as she did for Active Birth Conference.

Plan small exhibition crafts – garden statues, pots, painted children's furniture – by Creative Women in the Manor for September and wine evening to open it. That will be fun. To London overnight because TV early morning. They put me up in Forte Crest Hotel – never again! Public rooms flashy but bedroom grubby and falling to bits, and food inedible.

Wednesday

TV chat show am. Then meet Celia to choose vivid peacock de Morgan tiles for her fireplace and ship tiles for Uwe's (late) birthday present. Free hour, and buy beautifully cut and sewn Japanese swinging loose linen coat at Egg.

Back home, write lecture notes on sexuality and breast feeding for Vienna conference. Organisers want everything in advance. Midwife on our MA course at Thames Valley University and Queen Charlotte's – the only midwifery MA – has written to ask me to be her supervisor for dissertation, so I read work she's already done on mother goddesses and midwifery arts compared with medical management. Propose that, since she is moving to New Zealand, she interviews Maori women. I can help with fieldwork I have already done there and my discussions with Maori women aged 80–104 about tribal birth traditions and their personal experiences.

Thursday

Sun blazing – try to turn courtyard into scene more suited to house that was modernised in 1492 (when they put in ceilings and fireplaces). Heave old bricks around and make base for pots of lavender, rosemary and lilies, and plant herbs. Nell guides me. She was trained as a gardener at Pershore College. Looks like elaborate oriental grave. What do I do about exposed plastic drains? Have another go.

Swedish midwives' workshop here tomorrow. I always offer a buffet lunch. I roast some vegetables, enjoying their different shapes, colour and aroma. Sandwich this work in kitchen with reading some research papers in garden. Earth warm in sun, leaves a singing green, wild flowers starring the paddock – the England of John Clare.

Mr Lay, macho village elder who is our gardener, is on ride-on mower on a search and destroy mission. He is wonderful at training roses and fruit trees, stone walling, and disciplining nature, but this is supposed to be our wild flower garden. I rush up, wave my arms like windmills above roar of machinery, '*Please don't cut down the flowers!*' He thinks I'm mad, mutters, '*Blumin weeds! What do you want them for?*'

Into kitchen to chill Somerset cider. Fridge over-crowded. Full milk bottle crashes to tiled floor. Phone rings. Breathe out, drop shoulders and relax! Good! Jenny, social anthropologist daughter, is lecturing in London on sexual abuse and the media and will stay Friday night. I clear up mess in kitchen, then go to farm shop and pick luscious strawberries. Buy their home-grown wonderful mauve and pale green asparagus. I mix hollandaise with orange juice to make a sauce Maltaise for tomorrow.

Friday
On dot of 10 a.m. coach releases 30 midwives from hospitals and universities all over Sweden, armed with cameras, and I stand at door shaking hands and smiling, while Jean – stalwart National Childbirth Trust colleague from long ago who has come to live near – serves coffee and cake. They want to take pictures first, and I present a little patter about history of house. Then down to hard work. I'm lecturing on god-sibs – the women who came to support a woman in childbirth in medieval Europe, '*turnabout*' care by North American pioneers, nurturing women in birth in diverse cultures, and contrasting this with social isolation and male control over women in techno-childbirth today. They eat an enormous lunch. Not a crumb of apple-almond tart left. Afternoon topic, discussion of language in childbirth: medical – '*the uterus*' as if it were not part of a woman; engineering elements – '*birth canal*'; woman-blaming – '*incompetent cervix*', '*lazy uterus*', '*failure to progress*'. In Swedish and some other northern languages nipples are '*breast warts*'; sado-masochist brutal – '*fetal head battering perineum*', and in Swedish '*exploding*' perineum.

Wave them off to John Radcliffe Hospital where midwife Ethel Burns will tell them about birth pool and midwives' and women's experiences of it there. Jenny arrives and we relax in garden over champagne cocktails. Laura lies under sunshade on grass, kicking, cooing and laughing. We indulge in asparagus, artichoke and strawberry feast.

Children At Birth

At age five, my grandson, Sam was invited to witness the birth of his sister. Tess had decided on a home birth in a pool. Sam made it clear that his place was right where the action was going to be. He knew more about birth than many pregnant women do. He had seen his own birth photographs, and all his questions had been answered candidly. He had recently pressed the button on the slide projector as I spoke to one of my groups of midwives and doctors who regularly visit my house for workshops. He had heard Tess talk to them about her physical and emotional feelings at each phase of labour.

During Tess's pregnancy, my picture book, *Being Born*, was Sam's favourite during quiet times together. He knew how the baby developed in the uterus and what it could do at each stage of pregnancy. Equally important, he had seen and held babies and knew that they couldn't play with him, though they could communicate through gaze and the sounds they made. He realised that they needed to be handled with consideration and gentleness. Sam was present at each antenatal exam, which took place in the familiar environment of home. He watched the midwife palpate Tess's uterus, heard the baby's heartbeat with the hand-held Doppler ultrasound, and felt the baby's movements.

Tess talked with Sam about her birth plan and suggested that he might make a birth plan, too, listing the things that were important to him. So, with help, he wrote carefully:

> *If Tess has to go to hospital, I want to go, too.*
> *I want to take the birth photographs.*
> *I want to cut the cord.*
> *If she needs a Caesarean operation, I want to see it.*
> *Tess can hold the baby first, then Sheila, then me.*

When the great day came, Sam and his father, Jon, settled in the kitchen with felt-tips and paper, while Tess floated in the pool set up in the sitting room. Sam wandered in and out, obviously aware that something momentous was happening but not anxious about it.

He was in the room as the baby was born, sharing his mother's excitement and anticipation as she pushed. Afterwards, he sat on the rug by the log fire, cradling his baby sister tenderly in his arms. She looked up into his eyes, and he spoke softly to her. They were friends already.

When Tess had Josh in 1996 there were three midwives and me as well. It was like a party. Jon and Sam popped in and out and Laura slept until she woke just as the baby's head crowned. We laughed a lot and Tess was enjoying herself! Sam made a chocolate cake to go with the champagne to celebrate the new baby. He burned the first attempt and Tess had to labour through the awful smell of burnt chocolate. He made a second cake, and waited until Tess had finished a push before coming in and announcing that he had made this cake 15 minutes ago. *'Where was the baby?'* he demanded. That spurred her on and with two more pushes Joshua tumbled out.

Victorian children – at least, members of the middle classes – believed the doctor brought the baby in his little black bag, or that it had been picked from under a gooseberry bush. Girls grew up utterly ignorant about where babies came from or how they got out.

Death, however, was considered highly suitable for children and morally uplifting. Children joined the mourning circle around a death bed, viewed the corpse and made mourning cards. However, shielding them from any knowledge about birth was a sign of social status. While the poor lived in crowded hovels, where death and birth were open to everybody, those who had more money could shroud birth in secrecy.

It wasn't always like that. In the Middle Ages, Florentine and Siennese painting of the birth of Mary, the mother of Jesus, and of St John sometimes showed children present, either playing or helping the god-sibs, the women friends who attended birth to care for the mother and baby. There are German woodcuts from the sixteenth century which show children at birth, too.

Until the time when most births in Britain took place in hospital, following the Second World War, children were often quite naturally around when a baby was born. They were sometimes sent off to Granny when delivery was imminent but often Granny would come to care for them in their own home. They were always involved with the preparations, and often had a cuddle from Mummy during labour. Sometimes children just happened to be present at the birth, although their parents did not necessarily plan this, and they climbed onto the bed to hold the new baby when only a few minutes old. They did not get much education or preparation for what to expect during the birth, but it was a normal part of life.

In many cultures it is not only considered natural for children to be present at a family birth, but an important part of their education. When I was learning about traditional ways of birth in South Africa, a Zulu chief told me how young girls would prepare the birth hut and make it beautiful with wood carvings and beads. Children attended both birth and death, he said, *'because it teaches them to respect life.'*

In most peasant societies in southern and far Eastern countries, women have always given birth surrounded by female friends who offer practical help and emotional support, often bringing small children with them. When birth is moved to hospital, the woman becomes a patient and birth is rarely an experience for the whole family.

In Britain today most babies are born in hospital and children learn about birth from TV. They see a woman suddenly doubling over in pain, and then there is a mad dash to hospital. It is often a drama in which the baby's life is at risk and, sometimes, the mother's too, and they are saved by a high-powered medical team performing an emergency Caesarean in the nick of time.

We condition our children to think of birth as a medical emergency, like a road accident or a heart attack. It is scary. It is not surprising that many mothers (especially first-timers) are afraid of birth and want to make sure they have an epidural as soon as they step through the hospital doors. But having your children there for the birth can have positive benefits for the mother, because it demedicalises birth.

In my research with parents and children in Britain, Australia and the United States, children who were there often communicated a sense of awe and wonder. The children's pictures for me usually showed Mummy smiling. Sometimes she was even a Queen wearing a crown. There was often a big cake and it looked like a party. They are pictures of Happy Birthdays!

Carcassonne Ramparts

Laura was five months old and Tess flew out to Carcassonne with Sam and Laura to meet us for a short break. We went up into the old city for supper and then wandered round the alleyways up to the ramparts. We found a puppeteer there with a marionette exactly the same size as Laura. The stars were sparkling in the night sky, he was playing rollicking music, and a group had collected to watch. So that the children could see, we went up close until Laura was right in front of the dancing puppet. She was entranced. She became restless and pushed away from Tess's arms. Then, intently observing, she started to dance too, keeping every movement identical. Marionette and child moved in unison. In mirror image, she copied each gesture, each step, minutely, in time with the lively music. I had not realised that at that age such a young child could observe, interpret and comment this expertly. I became aware of Laura's talents in communication and recording and understanding behaviour.

Episiotomy

By the 1970s routine episiotomy and forceps to deliver the baby had become standard practice on the grounds that women could not stand the agonising struggle to give birth and this would shorten the second stage of labour. Women were stereotyped as *'inherently frail'*, *'predisposed to insanity'*[75] and *'the nervous inefficient products of modern civilisation'*.[76] Active Management seemed to solve the problem by making birth the gynaecologist's responsibility, not the mother's.

DeLee compared the stress of delivery to that of falling on a pitchfork that cut through a woman's perineum and the effect on the baby as like having one's head crushed in a door. He went on to say: *'Labour is pathogenic, disease producing, and anything pathogenic is pathologic or abnormal.'* So birth was not, and could not be, a normal human activity.

Chloe Fisher was a community midwife with whom I have worked closely over the years. In 1980 she pointed out that even in the 1950s Constance Beynon showed that women who were not told to push had a *'much higher rate of spontaneous deliveries than those who were chivvied'*.[77] Chloe commented, *'A major reason for the increase in episiotomies ... has been the midwife's attempt to enable the woman in her care to achieve a spontaneous delivery in the limited time allowed – knowing that otherwise she must hand her delivery over to the obstetrician to be delivered by forceps. Simultaneously, there has been much discussion about the merits of episiotomies as a measure to prevent future pelvic floor problems – though there has been no evidence to support this. We have now reached the stage where a small tear is considered evidence of poor delivery technique but to perform an episiotomy is absolutely acceptable.'*[78]

Chloe had been the midwife at the birth of my first grandchild, Sam. He

was a nine and a half pound baby. Tess did not require an episiotomy and her
perineum was intact. As he slid out he looked up at her and smiled.

CHAPTER FIFTEEN

WHEN THERE IS NO BIRTHPLACE

There are women for whom there is no place to give birth.

In war, ethnic conflict and under military occupation – and wherever any social group is perceived as inferior – mothers and children are the most vulnerable and become victims of the dominant power.

This happened in rural areas in the ex-Russian republics. My friend Dr Ethel Burns, a midwife, who works with midwives in Vietnam and the ex-Russian republics, described how Nagorno-Karabakh, a self-declared independent state in the early 2000s, faced the bitter aftermath of a war between Armenia and Azerbaijan. Shushi, once the capital of Armenia, and Lachin both lie in what local people call *'no-man's land'*, and inhabitants have even less access to healthcare resources than in other parts of this impoverished country. With a barely functioning phone system, no railway or civilian airfield, and often no electricity or running water, the only public transport was an erratic bus service, and pregnant women not only had great difficulty in getting to the hospital in the main town, Stepanakert, but were sometimes treated as outcasts if they did manage to get there. They needed money to bribe caregivers for access, and staff and other women might ostracize them.

Examples could be multiplied from almost every continent. The Gaza Strip is described by the Israeli Information Center for Human Rights in the Occupied Territories, as *'one gigantic prison'*.[79] Checkpoint tragedies have occurred when women trying to get to the hospital across the border with Israel from villages in the Occupied Territories were held up by the army. The hospital may be only a few kilometres away, but they were barred from reaching it because of fear that any Palestinian, including a heavily pregnant woman, might be carrying explosives. Between September 2000 and October 2004, 61 women gave birth at checkpoints and 36 of these were stillbirths.[80] Amnesty International stated: '*The practice by Israeli soldiers of delaying or denying passage to women in labour at checkpoints … constitutes cruel, inhuman and degrading treatment*'.[81]

Fortunately there exists a new spirit where Israeli and Palestinian midwives are trying to work together to integrate members of all religions and ethnic groups into the maternity care system. Wendy Blumfield, who founded the Israel Childbirth Education Centre, says:

'*Our organisation is totally apolitical … Every new group starting a training course includes Arabs and Jews, Moslems, Christians, religious, secular and representatives of the many different immigrant groups. So today we can offer our services in Arabic, Hebrew, English, Russian, French and Spanish. We opened up the entire area of the Arab villages in the Galilee because of our connection with the Scottish hospital in Nazareth. We ran courses for their midwives and for the nurses of the well-baby clinics in that rural area. Today Miriam Shibli, a Bedouin midwife who is head of the Nazareth maternity ward, is also the academic co-ordinator of our organisation*'.

She went on to tell me, '*So much of our national budget is spent on defence that our health and education systems are stretched to the limits and there is more poverty than there has ever been.*'

Pregnant Israeli and Palestinian women suffer from the constant threat of violence. Women in the Gaza Strip know that they may not be able to reach the nearest Israeli hospital if they are haemorrhaging or go into pre-term labour, because of barriers at checkpoints. Home birth rates have gone up, not because women want them, but because there is no safe alternative. Elective Caesarean section rates have risen for the same reason. Intense anxiety is a powerful element in the experience of pregnancy for the whole family. Mary McNabb, a British midwife, who visited Palestinian communities under military occupation, says, '*During pregnancy, women live in fear of a variety of threats to themselves and their unborn children: exposure to gunfire; effects of poisonous gases used by security forces; going into labour during prolonged curfews; and getting trapped in a car or ambulance at IDS checkpoints on the way to hospital*'.[82] Rita Giacaman, Associate Professor and Research and Programs Co-ordinator at the Institute of Community and Public Health of Birzeit University was quoted in the Amnesty report as saying that women are very fearful of childbirth under these circumstances. '*The result is a tendency towards over-medicalisation of the process of giving birth, which is that women feel that they need to be able to control the time when they go into labour to ensure a safe delivery and see Caesarian and induced delivery as the only way to do so.*'[83]

Women have given birth in ambulances, hospital elevators, and sometimes on the ground at checkpoints, watched by Israeli soldiers. A woman in labour may be told to strip so that the soldiers can satisfy themselves that she is really pregnant, and is not carrying explosives under her bump. Amnesty International reported a checkpoint tragedy in which a woman, Maysoon Saleh Nayef al-Hayek, was trying to reach the hospital in Nablus from her village 10 miles away. Her husband drove her and her father-in-law to a checkpoint and they were all ordered out of the car.

'We told the soldiers I had to go to hospital to give birth as soon as possible, that I was in severe pain. They first refused, then told me to uncover my belly, so they could see I was telling the truth. All this lasted about an hour and we were told to go ahead. We drove on and after a few hundred meters I heard shots from the front of the car.

'The car stopped and I saw that my husband ... had been shot in the throat and upper body, and was bleeding heavily ... Soldiers came and pulled me out of the car. They made me take off all my clothes to examine me. Then they left me on the ground, bleeding from the wounds and in labour. I asked for something to cover myself with but they didn't give me anything.' Her husband was dead and she gave birth in a hospital lift.

Amnesty International also cited the case of Rula Ashtiya who was forced to give birth on a dirt road at the Beit Furik checkpoint after she was refused passage in August 2003. She went into labour in the eighth month of pregnancy and her husband called an ambulance. They were instructed to go to the checkpoint because the ambulance could not get past, and it would wait for them on the other side.

'We took a taxi and got off before the checkpoint because cars are not allowed near the checkpoint and we walked the rest of the way; I was in pain. At the checkpoint there were several soldiers; they were drinking coffee and tea and ignored us. Daoud approached to speak to the soldiers and one of them threatened him with his weapon. Daoud spoke to them in Hebrew; I was in pain and felt I was going to give birth there and then; I told Daoud who translated what I said to the soldiers but they did not let us pass. I was lying on the ground in the dust and I *crawled behind a concrete block by the checkpoint to have some privacy and gave birth there, in the dust, like an animal. I held the baby in my arms and she moved a little but after a few minutes she died in my arms.'* Her husband said, *'She was holding the baby in her arms, covered in blood and the umbilical cord was on the ground, in the dust and still attached and I had to cut it with a stone; I didn't have anything else to cut it with. And I picked up Rula in my arms and she was holding the baby and I carried her to the car and we went to the hospital.*[84]

The United Nations calls on Israel *'to ensure the protection and safety of Palestinian women as well as their unconditional access to crucial services in health, nutrition, education and employment'*. It called on the Palestinian Authority to legislate to ensure *'equality and equity between men and women in respect to all their human rights, in line with the Convention of the Elimination of All Forms of Discrimination Against Women'.*[85]

Pregnant Asylum Seekers And Mothers

Women and children form most of the casualties of war in the world today and it is estimated that many of these women have been raped. Rape is used as an instrument of torture. For liberating troops it is the spoils of war.

Women who state that they have been raped are frequently not believed in courts of law. This struggle for justice often starts in the country from which they flee. One woman was told by a judge that she could not have been raped because she was not a virgin, and men only want to rape virgins. Other women have been told that they could not possibly have been raped because they were too old.

In Britain, women and children suffer most from the way the authorities deal with asylum seekers. These women often speak little English, have no family or friends to support them, suffer immense psychological damage from what they are going through, have paid vast sums of money to get here, and come expecting to find freedom. Instead, they encounter persecution, are put into custody with their babies, or have them taken from them by the Social Services on the grounds that they are destitute and therefore unable to care for them. To be a refugee is to be criminalised.

This is happening in a country that has always been a sanctuary for people seeking freedom from oppression, and whose economy has relied on their skills for many hundreds of years.

Many of the women had no documents to show the authorities, because they had been snatched from their beds, put into custody, and socially isolated. A law passed in 2004, the Asylum and Immigration (Treatment of Claimants) Act, deprives failed asylum seekers with children of all support and then takes the children away with the aim of encouraging their mothers to return to the countries from which they have fled. Women are also transported to the airport to be removed even after removal instructions have been cancelled. The whole situation is chaotic.

To be of any help to a failed asylum seeker who is pregnant and can't find a doctor or midwife to give her care, has a baby taken from her, or who is put on a plane to be forcibly returned to a country where she was raped, entails instant and decisive action. It can't be left to committees. Crossroads Women's Centre does this superbly, and is one of the organisations I have worked with closely.

Legal Action for Women (LAW) is a grassroots anti-sexist, anti-racist legal service for all women based at the Crossroads Women's Centre. They have told me how they can sometimes only get action from the authorities, lawyers and professionals, when someone from their organisation rings up with an English accent. If an African worker calls the request to speak to a woman may be turned down. When an educated English voice is heard, the response to the same request is positive.

In 2004 many women who had escaped from Eritrea and Uganda, where there are systematic human rights violations and torture is endemic, had their claims for asylum turned down by the Home Office. The result was that they were no longer entitled to housing or support and were made destitute. Some were offered a floor to sleep on by men who then raped them and hired them out to other men. Some were offered help by unscrupulous solicitors, or people who posed as solicitors, who demanded money or sex and did nothing about their claims.

Organisations like Amnesty International publicised asylum issues and, Liberty, Legal Action for Women, Women Against Rape, Black Women's Rape Action Project, and some MPs took up the cases of individual women. I often served as an expert witness, a specialist in the anthropology of birth and motherhood, and always focused on the rights of the child, since legally this gave us most chance of keeping the mother and baby together, prevent them from being expelled from the UK, or free them from detention. I stated that women as mothers and caregivers are discriminated against, as defined by the Convention on the Elimination of All Forms of Discrimination Against Women. I claimed that mothers and their babies are treated in a cruel, inhuman and degrading manner, as defined by Article 37 of the UN Convention on the Rights of the Child, and according to the European Court of Human Rights' statement concerning the Rights of the Child.

Sometimes I needed specific knowledge about the situation in the country from which a woman had escaped. It was often difficult to get up-to-date information about a particular country.

Lily (not her real name) was from the Gambia. Her mother died when she was two, and her father when she was five. She was sent to live with a paternal uncle who, she alleges, raped her from that time on. She was discriminated against, abused and beaten by 20 or more male relatives as well as her uncle. When she was 14 she was married against her will to a 70-year-old man, who beat and raped her. She was treated in this way because her mother was from Senegal, a very different culture in which girls are not 'circumcised', and the men of the family said that she was the bastard child of a prostitute. Sometimes older women in the village helped bind her wounds. One woman paid for her to go to a herbalist and treat a fracture in her arm as a result of beating. If she was returned to the Gambia she believed that her husband would abuse her for running away, and her uncle might kill her, because he had always told her he could have her killed like her mother. There was no one else to whom she could return and she had no way of earning a living.

I wrote: 'Being forced to return to the Gambia is bound to deepen her trauma. From my understanding of precept and tradition among the Mandingo, social pressures in the community, and perception of her duty to her uncle as the father of her child, will cause her suffering. If she does not conform, she will be treated as a social outcast.

'The Gambian record on women's rights is inferior to that of many other African cultures and progress toward outlawing clitoridectomy and infibulation is very slow. In a jointly commissioned report, A Situation Analysis of FGM in the Gambia, three UN Agencies, WHO, UNFPA and UNICEF, expressed concern in 2003 that 80 per cent of girls and women are at risk of genital mutilation. Activists are banned from using the public media for their anti-FGM campaigns. The UN has urged governments to take action to provide an enabling environment to pave the way for protecting girls from the practice and its negative repercussions.

'Though I cannot comment on Gambian prejudice against women from Senegal and the stereotyped view that they are prostitutes, Senegal has an active health and human rights programme to end female genital mutilation recognised by the WHO as groundbreaking, and it is planned to eradicate female genital mutilation entirely in the next few years. This may accentuate different values in relation to women's bodies in Senegal and the Gambia.

'Lily is very unlikely to be able to find counselling and support if she returns to the Gambia, or to receive state protection, especially as there is no law against family rape.'

Rose, from the Cameroons, aged 24, and speaking very little English, arrived in England on her cousin's passport and eight months pregnant. She was immediately imprisoned and was facing deportation in a few days. I learned from her that she had two previous children by her father who abused her, and who abducted the first child when two years old, and either sold or killed him. Her aunt sought a reconciliation with her father, but he beat her up and made her pregnant again. The aunt took the baby and told the father that it had died. Then she again sought reconciliation at a family get-together, after which Rose was forcibly returned to him. He sold her to a friend of his own age who already had three wives. This was when she escaped to England with the false passport.

Her great fear was that if she was returned to the Cameroons her father would kill her. She had found a solicitor, whom I contacted, who had not yet had time to study the papers, and asked Immigration to defer her removal on the grounds that she would not get the care she needed as a pregnant woman in the Cameroons.

Meanwhile she was taken to the airport, but refused to get on the plane. She was put in Gatwick Detention Centre.

I had to go abroad, and my daughter Tess took over. She rang the director of the airline to point out that this pregnant woman was at risk of going into pre-term labour if she was forced onto a plane, and that his airline would be acting against international law. The airline refused to carry her. The Immigration Authority relented after she had already been made to board the plane. She was taken off just before it flew. From that point on the solicitor built a strong case, and she was granted asylum.

* * *

Yasmin was also from the Cameroons and had been in detention for three months. Her son was born prematurely at 34 weeks. I talked to her in May 2002 when he was four months old and what she told me is typical of women's experiences in detention when they have a baby: *'I was in hospital for three weeks and then went home. After one week there was a knock on the door at 7 a.m. They said, "Your case is over. You are going into detention." They put my things into bags. I could not tell the midwives or health visitor where we went.*

'My baby has not had his immunisations. Every day I ask and they say, "We are looking into it." I am really worried about him. There are many people here, many children, from many different countries, who may have diseases. What will happen if he catches a disease? The rooms are very cold. My baby has eczema. For three months the medical centre wouldn't give me anything for it. They said it was dry skin. They don't do nothing, just speak, speak. I am depressed. If I was outside and my baby was sick I would go to hospital, or buy medicine. Here you go to the medical centre and you have to wait two weeks to get one cream. Every day wait, wait. They give you a few baby things and clothes, but you have to give them back when you leave. I have nothing. When I was at the Bedford Detention Centre they told me to leave my things at Reception and then they burnt them. My baby's birth certificate was burnt. How can I show that he is my baby? My friend has brought me some clothes. You have to go to the office every time you need nappies or milk. Sometimes the office is closed. They only give out three nappies at a time. One time when his milk was finished I asked for a new tin and they said they wouldn't give me a tin, just enough for one bottle, so I should go to the office every time he needs a bottle. But he needs a bottle every two hours! So I prefer to use the milk which my friends bring me from outside. But sometimes they refuse to give me milk which my friend has brought.

'Today, when I came back from church, my room had been searched. They went into my cupboard and took away all the milk and baby food my friend had brought me. I went and told them it was mine. They said, "Do you have a receipt?" So I showed them the receipt. They should wait until we are there before checking the rooms. What would happen if they left the door open and someone else went in and took something?

'This place is not for children. Here they don't even weigh the baby. They do nothing to protect him, even though he was born premature.

'When I arrived in August last year I was detained at Oakington. There was no care there for my pregnancy. Then I was released and they sent me to an address in Leeds. But that address was full so they sent me to another place. But they sent the court papers to the first address and so I missed the court hearing, and when I did not come they dismissed the case. The solicitor has said, "Your case is closed." They think I am a person whose heart knows my case is over. But how can they remove me when they have not heard my case? I can't back down, because I have a baby. What will happen to him if I go back? I have no money, no family.

'They tried to remove me, but they didn't tell me. They came to me and said, "Give your baby to the nurse. We need to weigh him." I said, "No, I'll come to the medical centre with him if he needs attention." When I was there, they took him from me and put me in the van to the airport. They only gave him back to me when I was in the van. It was a trick. But in the end there was no place for me on that aeroplane, so they brought me back here.

'Because they came to take my baby I'm worried all the time, whenever I hear keys. I can't sleep at night – a small noise and I'm awake. I walk around at night – just walk, walk.

'They have a library here and a church, but suddenly they say you can't take your baby with you into the church. I want to go to pray, to forget this place. But I'm nervous of leaving the baby, being separated from him.

'We don't eat good here. Sometimes I eat just once a day. Every day rice, chicken, rice, chicken, and they give very little. I can't breastfeed him as I don't eat well.

'I'm alone in this place. You don't trust anyone. I've lots of friends outside, but in here I have nobody to ask advice or tell my worries. The medical staff just say, "It's OK. It's nothing." They don't listen. They should listen to me. I am the mother and I know when something is wrong.

'You don't have any information about when you will be moved. People disappear. You don't know if tomorrow you are going to be here. In the night neighbours disappear.

'Sometimes the staff ignore you when you come to speak to them. But the conditions here are better than Bedford. It was like a prison. I was there with a premature baby and the midwives had given me vitamin K to give to the baby every day. They took away the vitamin K. You had to ask to go to the health centre, but the officers would never bring me to there. They always said, "Later, we are busy." So he only got vitamin K for the first month. Babies here – is not good. They *tell me detention is not prison, but it is. The baby is closed up in one place. You can't do anything, see people, get fresh air. You can't enjoy your baby.*

'Tell me, why should they keep us here? How can I run away when I have a baby and no money? Where can I go?'

Gloria was from Vietnam, aged 25 with a baby three months old. She did not speak much English. Her benefits were removed when her application for asylum was turned down, she had no legal representation, and no interpreter had been provided. The Bureau for Immigration Detainees asked if I could help her. She was in Campsfield House, an immigration removal centre outside Oxford, had been served a deportation order, and was terrified of being sent back, since her father, a senior police officer, had been murdered and all her family were missing. She had a heart problem, had been unable to get registered with a GP, and had stopped eating.

GPs often turn down failed asylum seekers. Kate, for example, was from Romania, a music student who was married and pregnant with her second baby, now two days past her expected date of delivery. She had been trying to find a GP to accept her for two weeks, but no-one would take her on because, though she had a valid passport, she had no visa. I acted swiftly and found her immediate midwife care at a hospital with a freestanding Birth Centre.

Anna, a 20-year-old Nigerian woman and 21 weeks pregnant with her first baby, did not realise she was pregnant when she fled from the country. Her partner was a British citizen and lived in London. She was very stressed, vomiting more or less non-stop, and had no antenatal care. The detention centre staff would not take her to hospital for a scan because they told her she might try to abscond, and by the time they got around to it, it was too late. When she arrived in England immigration officials instructed her to claim asylum in Ireland, so she went there, could not get it, and was then told that she could not claim asylum in England because she had already tried to do so in another country.

Giving Birth In Prison

After a prisoner gave birth in chains in Wythenshawe Hospital, South Manchester in 1995, her solicitors contacted me and it was then that I first realised the sheer cruelty with which prisoners were treated in childbirth. I took up the prisoner's cause, achieved wide media coverage, and, among other things, had an article on the subject published in the journal *Birth*. One result was that a new midwifery service was developed to enable women in Styal prison to have top midwifery care. The aim is *'to provide midwifery care which is woman-centred, recognises and is sensitive to the needs of each individual woman with the emphasis on choice, continuity and control throughout the pregnancy continuum, at the same time ensuring accessibility of all services.'*

Briefing of parliamentarians and a media campaign were necessary and a group of us in childbirth organisations started to work together to free women from their chains. Beverley Lawrence Beech, Chair of the Association for Improvements in the Maternity Services (AIMS), was fitted with a secret camera by Channel 4 News, and filmed a new mother in hospital manacled. The result of our campaign was that the Government announced a change in policy and practice: chains must come off. Until January 1996, women in British prisons were still giving birth shackled.

Chains stayed on, however, when women went to and from hospital, and even in hospital until *'treatment'* started. Prisoners with loops of chains clanking beneath their coats, handcuffed to prison officers, were still a common sight in some antenatal clinics in 2008.

A great deal remained to be done. I explored the possibilities with National Childbirth Trust teachers in the area of Holloway of setting up a doula scheme, to offer woman-to woman support in late pregnancy, during birth and afterwards. There was already an NCT breastfeeding counsellor working in the prison and she became one of our doula group, who were renamed *'Birth Companions'*. They help women handle birth physiologically by moving around, breathing and being massaged, and to breastfeed. They also support a woman who opts for an epidural or is having a Caesarean section.

One problem is that a woman cannot know until the last five or six weeks of pregnancy whether she will be permitted to keep the baby. She may not allow herself to bond with it. Women sometimes tell their families, *'Don't buy any clothes for the baby.'* They are in an emotional limbo. This is because towards the end of pregnancy the Admissions Board of the Mother and Baby Unit decides whether a woman will be allowed in the unit. If she does not get a place she is separated from her child, who then goes into the care of the social services and is fostered or looked after by relatives (most often the woman's mother).

Women were rejected for the Mother and Baby Unit if they talked back to prison officers, were in conflict with other prisoners, or did not obey orders.

Holloway is the largest women's prison in Europe. A 24-year-old psychology student whom I shall call 'J', in prison on a five year sentence for slashing a friend's face with a craft knife in an argument over a man, was told that her baby would be taken away at birth. She decided to challenge the decision. I learned about this soon after the Admissions Board meeting, obtained the minutes of the meeting from the solicitor, contacted the woman's mother and the woman herself, and determined to fight this to the end. (I had already tried to help seven other prison mothers and only been successful with one, a 17-year-old from whom a judge had ordered her baby to be removed for two weeks after her due date in order 'to punish her'.)

A decision of the Admissions Board had never been challenged before. Most of the accusations against 'J' were unsubstantiated and petty: she took a carton of milk that was not hers; she had made 'snide remarks' to a woman who was reduced to tears; she picked quarrels; she did not get up in the morning. (This happened after she had been told that her AFP level – Alpha-fetaprotein, screened with a blood test – suggested she had a Down's Syndrome baby, and then that amniocentesis revealed the baby had an extra chromosome, though not Down's.) One board member complained that she did not seem to be looking forward to her baby, implying that it should be removed from her for this reason. Another, a health visitor, said that to care for a baby 'you need to be able to co-operate with everyone. She didn't'.

I started to work with 'J's' solicitors. I asked John Davis, Emeritus Professor of Paediatrics at Cambridge University, to be an expert witness, and he readily agreed. With a statement from him they went to the Crown Court and were granted leave to appeal. I was concerned that there had been no independent psychological assessment. I asked Dr Suzie Orbach if she would do one free of charge and she did so immediately, pointing out in her report that 'J' was suffering from both shock and depression.

'J' had given birth on the day that the first appeal was turned down. She learned that the case had failed just after she delivered her baby daughter. She told me, 'If they take my baby away from me they might as well kill me.'

I rang journalists and there was lively interest. At the *Independent*, Jack O'Sullivan was magnificent and seemed the ideal person to interview 'J'. She gave me permission to let him have the number of the phone at her hospital bedside.

As far as her guards were concerned she was talking to a friend, though, of course, they listened to every word. The legal correspondents of the *Guardian* and the *Independent* were hot on the trail, too, and Andrew Marr wrote up the story in the *Express*. I kept in close touch with the press and TV, and Frances Crook of The Howard League threw her energy and detailed knowledge of the prison system into the campaign. The Maternity Alliance also became involved and, because 'J' was breastfeeding, I solicited help from breastfeeding organisations. Mothers, fathers and babies turned up outside the Crown Court when the appeal was heard with big notices saying, *'Remember the child'*.

On the first day of the appeal 'J's' barrister focused on the rights of the child. Counsel for Holloway asked for more time to prepare his case. When one of the three judges asked, *'Are you going to tear this baby from her mother's breast?'* those of us who were determined to keep mother and baby together felt the first flush of success.

The judges asked whether, if he was given the week for which he asked, he could assure the Court that the mother and baby would be kept together during that time. The barrister wheeled round and asked the representatives of Holloway whether that could be arranged. There was an awkward pause. He turned back, with obvious embarrassment, *'No, my Lord.'* The judges' eyebrows shot up into their wigs, and one said, *'You can't? Goodness me!'* They allowed him the weekend to get his act together, but insisted that mother and baby were not separated.

Over that weekend the solicitors for Holloway contacted 'J's' solicitors to try and arrange a settlement. When the court assembled on Monday morning it was agreed that the Admissions Board of the Mother and Baby Unit should sit again. It had to consist of different people, be chaired by someone from outside the prison, and none of the previous charges about her behaviour were to be considered, because none had been proved.

The judges ruled that in future, primary consideration must be given to the rights of the child.

This case created what the judges called a *'practical precedent'*, meaning that others should refer to this judgement when fighting similar court battles. Holloway had to honour the rules of the European Human Rights Convention and the United Nations Convention on the Rights of the Child. Holloway had neglected to comply with prison service regulations and in future the Board should be properly constituted, the correct protocols observed, and a prisoner should have the right to a legal representative.

Following this successful appeal, J was admitted to the Mother and Baby Unit at Styal prison, where she found the atmosphere surprisingly different from Holloway. She could keep her baby with her there for 18 months. She planned to resume her psychology studies in prison.

The Governor of Holloway resigned the day after the Appeal. A week later Richard Tilt, the Director General of the Prison Service, announced a review of principles, policies and procedures for mothers and babies and setting up of a working group to include professionals from health, social services, probation and relevant interest groups.

It is easy to remain ignorant of conditions in prisons. At that time in 1998 there were more than 3,000 women in British prisons, and 61 per cent were mothers of children under 18 or pregnant. There were only 64 places in Mother and Baby units throughout Britain. Between 1993 and 1997 the number of women in prison leapt by 76 per cent. I believe that any commitment to help childbearing women must extend to speaking out for the most vulnerable and voiceless in our own society. Women in prison are often the least educated, and victims of violence and sexual abuse. 33 per cent are first-time offenders, over half had their first child when they were teenagers, 27 per cent are single mothers and 34 per cent of prisoners in Holloway are black. Pregnancy can be an opportunity for development and change.[86]

CHAPTER SIXTEEN

IN THIS CENTURY

Romance Distorts Everything that is Real in Human Experience

An organisation called Family and Youth Concern produced a film for schools and youth clubs which was supposed to teach girls how to say '*No*' to sex and wait for their prince to come.

June, a good-time girl, gets pregnant, fails her exams, has an abortion and goes into a dead-end job. Linda, on the other hand, says '*No*', goes to college and has a white wedding with all the trimmings, while June watches, envious and miserable. The message is clear – good girls wait, virginity intact, until a ring is on their finger. Bad girls enjoy themselves, have abortions, and end up unloved and without a man.

The film was welcomed by some Fleet Street journalists who seemed to be missing out on romance in their own lives. '*I'm enraptured by the idea,*' breathed the *Daily Express*. '*Remember those wonderful ages we spent nibbling crisps and each other's ears … making plans for a thrilling virginal honeymoon?*' And the *Daily Mail* announced, '*The word "No" is the best contraceptive, the only true preventive of VD and a recipe for happy married life.*'

It was part of a backlash to the sexual revolution of the Sixties. It took its most exaggerated form in the United States, where a new Puritanism denounced all who did not conform to a rigid, restricted morality which claimed to be based on the Bible. My book on breastfeeding published in Britain with a lovely photograph of a mother and baby during a pause in breastfeeding, with her breast and nipple exposed, had to be changed in the United States to one with invisible nipples. Before many radio and TV shows I was warned not to be '*explicit*' and never, ever refer to the male member. On a popular Mid-West chat show the presenter, quivering with rage, denounced me for my '*disgusting*' beliefs about sexual relationships. Revivalist preachers in crowded stadiums whipped up hysteria against homosexuals and the mob roared for blood. These puritans, instead of lopping heads from religious statues and smashing stained glass windows, burned down abortion clinics and feminist book stores. This was the creed of the '*moral majority*', often obscene in its hatred, always bigoted and, in spite of its lip-service to the '*right of life*' – life-denying.

As for sex education, the idea seemed to be that if you dangle a frothy white wedding gown and a three-tiered cake in front of girls, they don't need any. Girls under 16 certainly would not require birth control, nor the abortion that, in practice, follows society's refusal to permit them contraceptive advice and counselling.

Teenage girls were offered once more a glittering fantasy, the tinsel and stardust of romance, and it was implied that once they've got their man everything will be happy ever after. Girls growing up are not short of this candy-floss, even without having lessons about it in school. There is a whole industry based on it. Publishing houses like Mills and Boon turn out titles like *Cinderella SRN*, offering a lotus land of romance in place of the boredom of life as an office junior or on the dole.

While women were reading romantic fiction, men read pornography. Neither romanticism nor pornography treats sex realistically, and neither acknowledges a woman as a person.

What bothers me about romance is not only that it conditions girls to be exploited by the first man who convinces them he's Prince Charming, but that it snuffs out a girl's potential to be herself and do what she wants. Self-worth becomes something that is conferred on a woman by a man and lasts only as long as he wants her.

Equally harmful was the romantic theme that a man '*awakens*' sex in a woman. Yet we are sexual beings from birth. You only have to watch a baby at the breast, little hands and feet curling in delight. Adults find it difficult to acknowledge that a girl is capable of having sexual experience with her own body and within herself. Passionate friendships with other girls or older women are treated as trivial and silly, because women aren't supposed to love other women, or get strength and support from them. Everything is supposed to come from the man. The candy-floss of romance is substituted for reality and the girls themselves enter into the conspiracy, seduced by its glamour. Teaching girls about romance therefore evades the main issue, which is that each of us needs to accept responsibility for the way in which we use our sexual energies.

Teenage girls are under enormous pressure to be sexually active. Many are very unsure of themselves and use sex to obtain some proof that they are of value and that somebody wants them. Teenage girls risk pregnancy because they think that at least a baby will be someone to love who in return will love them. They look to the baby to give them the sense of worth that's lacking in their lives.

There are all sorts of teenage myths about conception: it can't happen if you do it standing up, if the girl doesn't have an orgasm, or if the boy was drunk – and it certainly can't happen the first time. Even when contraception is available to boys in the form of condoms, girls often don't check whether a boy has them because they feel less guilt if sex if unpremeditated. It's the romantic image again. If you're carried away it's forgivable. Doing it with forethought is wrong.

The romantic nonsense with which society stuffs the heads of teenage girls is directly responsible for many unwanted pregnancies. If we really want to help young women avoid pregnancy and exposure to sexually transmitted diseases, teachers would do better to run assertiveness-training for girls and courses in how to respect girls for boys. When it comes to it, it's confidence in her own worth that enables a young woman to think through what she really wants, choose between alternatives with knowledge of the consequences, and make a decision that is right for her. And young men need to recognise and respect those decisions.

Marketing Pregnancy Ultrasound

A personal ultrasound scan that showed the moving fetus came on the market in 2002. It was advertised as promoting bonding between fathers and babies. The US company recommended that if a man invested in one of these machines he not only would get to see the baby for himself, but for the first time could touch its virtual image. A representative of the firm said that parents *'get a sense of security that you don't get without having an ultrasound … It's as if you were playing a video right through the womb'*.

BBC *Woman's Hour* interviewed me and Jim Thornton, Professor of

Obstetrics and Gynaecology at the University of Nottingham. Jim was really keen on it, while I was highly critical. I said, *'It's good advertising. It's another way men have found of invading and usurping women's bodies: "Anything you can do I can do better". There's a pregnancy belly around, too, a big silicone thing a man can strap onto himself so that he feels what it is like to be pregnant. And perhaps you could have silicone breasts filled with milk!'*

The presenter of the programme, Jenni Murray, protested, *'Hold on! Do you think this is more for fathers than mothers? Maybe mothers would like to be in touch with the baby, too.'* I replied, *'Mothers are in direct touch with the baby inside them and in an intimate relationship. They can feel the movements of the different parts.'* Jenni said, *'It seems to be a rather wonderful and lovely thing to have to at least pretend to touch your baby. There was an experiment in which pregnant women were divided into groups when they were having their ultrasound examination. With half they turned the screen away from the woman, and with half they turned it toward her. Just seeing her baby made parents less anxious and more happy, and helped them bond. It lasted through the pregnancy.'*

My reaction was, *'There are other ways of bonding with a baby. It's as if the baby is "out there", almost like an astronaut in space. It actually divides the mother and baby in their intimate relationship. In all our experiences in life we seek pictures, take snaps, record videos, but I think we need to evaluate what is happening with the introduction of this new technology.'*

I was also concerned that we did not know if there might be risks with the indiscriminate use of ultrasound. *'Pelvic x-rays were used for 50 years without recognition that they increased the rate of cancer in children under 10 years of age, and even after the research was published that demonstrated this pelvic x-rays continued to be performed.'*

Jim said, *'Sheila is right. You cannot absolutely prove that anything is safe. We have been using ultrasound in pregnancy for 30 years. It has been studied very closely and so far, there is no evidence of any adverse effects.'* Jenni Murray commented that *'Once the technology is there it may be you can't put that genie back in the bottle.'*

I concluded, *'This idea of obstetricians taking over bonding and companies producing technology to promote paternal bonding – I don't know – what is the evidence? I think the real question is, "Do these guys change more nappies?" That would be a wonderful randomised controlled trial.'* Jim said it would be a lovely trial and he would like to undertake it. I don't think he ever did!

Conversation analysis

In workshops for women preparing themselves for Birth Crisis counseling Celia and I used recordings (made with women's permission) of real interactions I've had with women calling me for help with trauma after childbirth.

A recording of one of my conversations with a woman suffering from post-traumatic stress disorder:

> FIONA: *'I just thought, oh I was just being – hysterical'.*
>
> CALL-TAKER: *'Well ... You ... it's a pity you blame yourself then.'*
>
> FIONA: *'I wish I'd been stronger.'*
>
> CALL-TAKER: *'Yes it's very, very easy looking back on situations to think 'I wish I'd been stronger, I wish I'd done that. The point is those things happened and you did whatever you could under the circumstances to the best of your ability.'*
>
> FIONA: *'You're right. And we always could have done more I suppose, everyone thinks.'*
>
> CALL-TAKER: *'Yes, yes and none of us are perfect and we all have ideals of behaviour don't we. And some of us sort of drive ourselves a bit about it and demand an awful lot of ourselves.'*
>
> FIONA: *'Thank you for saying that. Nobody else has said that.'*

Celia and I worked together to analyse more than 400 phone calls to the Birth Crisis help-line examining the interaction between Sheila and the callers and using what we learned for workshops with midwives and other caregivers.

We looked at ways in which they started and ended, for example, how a call-taker shows she is listening without interrupting, and the use of silence.

Members of the group form pairs and a call is played and then suddenly stops. Participants acting the part of call-takers are asked to follow this with what they would say next. The callers say how they felt about it and there is general discussion of the benefits and disadvantages of the way the conversation is going.

There is no script to follow. What matters is how the caller experiences what is said and not said.

A conversation includes sounds and exclamations as well as words. Story-prompts include, *'Okay, tell me what the problem is'*, *'Tell me about it'*, *'What happened?'* and reactions when a woman is choking in distress or breaks down weeping: *'You are feeling pretty rotten aren't you?'*

These contrast with call-takers' comments that demand answers, sometimes quite aggressively, *'Why are you crying?'*, *'Have you got PTSD?'* or *'What's wrong with you?'*

We noted ways in which a call-taker might show understanding. Saying *'I understand'* is just a claim to understand. But non-verbal reactions like a sharp intake of breath (to show understanding that a procedure was painful) or a long drawn out low-pitched *'ahhhhh'* to show empathetic understanding of a caller's disappointment displays understanding at an emotional level. And words can seem like interruptions whereas these 'reaction tokens' are often done in overlap with a woman's talk and encourage her to continue.

In the discussion with Fiona I use the terms *'we'*, *'us'* and *'our'*. Whilst telling Fiona that she is not to blame for what has happened to her, I take Fiona's *'we'* and include myself in the category of *'people who could have done more'* and who *'are not perfect'*. This treats Fiona's feelings as common to the human condition, shared by caller and call-taker, rather than being Fiona's idiosyncratic failing.

We believe that conversation analysis is a valuable resource for midwifery education.[87]

Australia, 2007

Keith Hartmann was a young registrar at the John Radcliffe Hospital who many years later, when I met up with him in Sydney, Australia, told me that Professor Alec Turnbull made the decision to stop inducing labours routinely when Iain Chalmers' research on oxytocin revealed that it had harmful side-effects, together with my writing about women's negative experiences of induction. I was surprised to learn that I had had any effect at all on his practice. But within a matter of days the induction rate was reduced.

Keith had taken over an old house in the Paddington area of Sydney when I was lecturing in Australia in 2007 and had established the Mothers' Retreat to give skilled and sensitive post-natal care and breastfeeding help to new mothers in hotel surroundings, with a superb chef and one-to-one midwifery care.

The Royals

Saying '*no*' to hospital, making an informed decision to give birth in a place of their own choosing, is vital for women to reclaim the experience.[88]

But there are signs that hospitals are changing. Diana brought fresh air to royalty, and Prince Charles continued to do the same. She was much criticised, but her contribution to reclaiming birth for women started radical changes in hospitals. During the pregnancy with her first baby, the private wing of St Mary's, Praed Street, rang me to ask what equipment I would advise so that she could give birth in an upright position. I said that Charles looked strong enough to hold her. And that is what happened. It was the first active royal birth – a contrast to the Queen's reflection that with modern anaesthesia birth had become '*a sleep and a forgetting*'.[89]

In 2013, Kate and William gave birth in the same hospital, and, using self-hypnosis to enable Kate to centre down, experienced it as a spontaneous process for which a woman's body is perfectly equipped.

Entertaining An Audience

After a series of operations on my hips and oesophageal tract and dental surgery I was anxious that I wouldn't have the energy or mental focus to give of my best at the Royal College of Midwives (RCM) Student Conference at Telford in November 2013.

It was quite a long journey to get there, I was walking with great difficulty, and worried that I might let down the crowded professional audience. In all my lectures I aim to engage, communicate and *act*.

In fact, it went well and I was pleasantly surprised at the reaction. At any rate, the conference report included an enthusiastic section about my contribution:

'*And then, the crème de la crème of speakers, Professor Sheila Kitzinger took to the stage. The RCM could hardly have chosen a more apt speaker. Professor Kitzinger is an activist for natural childbirth, a social anthropologist and an author, but more importantly she is a believer in women and nature and the power of the female body to create life. She described labour and birth using the most beautiful imagery and terms, allowing us all to join in her belief that labour and birth need not be painful and frightening but can instead be "awesome" and "thrilling" and "powerful". She painted a picture where women transcend and become one with the demands of their bodies, where they recognise the sensual aspect of the experience and allow it to become a natural part of labour and birth without shame or embarrassment. Because if the 84-year-old is not embarrassed to speak in frank terms about the beauty of birth, why should we be? And she was breathtakingly good. A hush fell over the room when she spoke and I think every student in attendance was captivated by her descriptions of labour and birth. I only hope I am privileged enough to see labour as she sees it and to end my career feeling as inspired as I do today.'*

Heterosexuality: A Challenge

I did not plan to be heterosexual, of course. If I had known my three radical lesbian feminist daughters then I'd probably never have made that decision. I just *was*. A child of patriarchy, I was shaped by it. I expected to love a man, and did. I married, made a home, had a family, established deep loyalties.

When our eldest daughter, Celia, turned 17 in the early 70s she was in her first term at Bryanston School in Dorset. It used to be a single sex school, for boys, one of those independent schools in which they opened up to girls in the sixth form quite simply to civilise the boys. She only managed three months there and then was expelled for suspected lesbianism.

Celia described herself in a paper in *Feminism and Psychology*[90] as *'of the generation growing up as Martin Luther King's impassioned "I have a dream" speech – a demand for freedom and justice for American "Negroes" – was broadcast on crackling radios across the world; as heated public debates raged about the international community's response to the massacre and starvation in Biafra; and as the Aldermaston protest launched to a powerful British nuclear disarmament movement. I was a teenager when the UK Government responded to feminist pressure by enacting a startling piece of legislation (the 1975 Sex Discrimination Act) requiring employers to give women "equal pay for equal work"; and – like everyone else I knew – I boycotted the products of apartheid South Africa and joined the protests against the killing of Steve Biko in police custody. These struggles against oppression and injustice were discussed over the family dinner table and raised in Quaker meetings for worship on Sundays. My collection of badges/buttons include "ban the bomb", "power to the people", "stuff the system", "silence is the voice of complicity" and "equal pay NOW!" But I knew nothing about lesbian and gay issues. Homosexuality was never discussed as a compelling issue of political justice.'*

In the 70s homosexuality was still seen as pathological – a condition to be remedied by treatment. Mothers were largely responsible for their children growing up *'abnormal'*. It came from having a weak mother and an overbearing father, or *'a severe domineering mother and a weak father, or an absent father and a mother trying to be both mother and father to a lonely child'*. Even an author who later came out gay himself claimed that homosexuals *'would like to be considered not seriously deviant, but healthy, harmless, and law-abiding until proven otherwise'*.[91]

As Celia says, *"'Healthy, harmless and law-abiding" was no kind of positive self-image for a teenage lesbian steeped in the moral and political values of civil disobedience and struggles for social justice.'*

Thirty years after she was expelled from Bryanston School the chaplain, Alan Shrimpton, wrote asking her for an entry to the school Year Book, by which time she had published four books and numerous articles on gender and society. She replied, *'Bryanston back in my life again? Wanting information about my books dealing with lesbian and gay issues?! Wow – hasn't the world changed in the last 30 years, and thank goodness for that!'*

The Chaplain responded saying he sympathised totally with her feelings about her treatment and treasured the image of me storming the Headmaster's study – *'WONDERFUL – and yes, please write a piece about it!'*

Uwe

My husband, Uwe, and I share fundamental values. Uwe's father was of Jewish lineage, so as a child Uwe was classified as a half-breed 'Mischling' in Nazi Germany and an enemy alien in Britain. I first encountered him (briefly) at a meeting exploring the problems and challenges of building a better society. We were anti-racist, anti-sexist, anti-discrimination of any kind. We called for World Government, international understanding, and peace.

We were trying to analyse society and understand human behaviour. When we married in the Quaker Meeting House at Oxford, we committed ourselves not only to each other, but to work for political and social change as equals, '*flying wing to wing*'. My relationship with him, and the discussions we have, help me define my feminism with more precision, in different ways, but just as powerfully, as my relationships with my daughters.

Uwe, too, is a campaigner. He is passionate about human rights, international peace and building strong supranational institutions both in Europe and world-wide. He loved his first job working with a band of dedicated idealists at the Council of Europe in Strasbourg where he was its first British economist. Those were the heady days of designing and constructing the European Community. In 1956, since Britain refused to join, he returned to Oxford, using his Fellowship at Nuffield College, his books and his frequent TV exposure as platforms to argue his case. And in January 1973, as soon as Britain did join, he was appointed Political Adviser to the first British Vice-president of the Brussels Commission, Churchill's larger-than-life son-in-law Christopher Soames. In fact for most of the 70s he worked on the continent – in Brussels, at the University of Paris and as Dean of the European Management Institute in Fontainebleau – flying home at weekends.

Having pioneered European Studies at Oxford in the 50s, in the 80s he returned to champion Management Studies. That was a subject much despised in Oxford. But he organised Templeton as a Management College of the University (and became its founding President). That prepared the way for the new Oxford Business School.

He always put a lot of energy and enthusiasm into voluntary work, particularly start-ups and reformist initiatives. He was founding Chairman of the Committee for Atlantic Studies, the Major Projects Association and, after the Yugoslav wars, the Campaign for Civil Courage based in Sarajevo. He served on the Councils of Oxfam, the European Movement and Chatham House, and – while at Harvard – of Institutes for Conflict Management and for Global Leadership. He was President of the British Alliances Françaises and is still Patron of Asylum Welcome. So, if we rarely flew wing to wing, we were and are still birds of a feather!

Of course, discussions with a man are different from those with women. I acknowledge that compromise with men can easily become treachery to women. I realise that I walk on a tight-rope. Yet I look at who I am and where I am and try to determine how I can use this creatively. Women are under constant pressure to service the men in their lives. When they give birth they are controlled by a male-dominated, autocratic, hierarchical medical system. Many remember birth as a kind of rape. In challenging the male model of childbirth and offering the knowledge they need if they are to make informed choices between alternatives, question medical authority and develop self-confidence, I strive towards reclaiming our bodies in childbirth – to take birth back for women.

My politics spring from powerful personal experience. But it is vital to go beyond the purely personal and specific. My own birth experiences were very positive, and it would be simple for me to talk only about the joy of birth. Yet I spend much of my time listening to women who have been subjected to violence in childbirth, and my political understanding has been sharpened by awareness of the abuse that many women suffer.

My starting point was women's satisfaction and fulfilment in the experience of birth. What I have learnt has opened my eyes to women's rights, rights to informed choice, humane care, the control of our own reproductive health. How we give birth is part of a much wider challenge that concerns our lives as a whole, women's lives everywhere in the world.

Maternal deaths are the second biggest killer of women of reproductive age (after HIV/AIDS). Every year, nearly 300,000 women die due to complications in pregnancy and childbirth – 99 per cent of them in developing countries.[92]

The concept of '*freedom*' in childbirth must mean more than freedom from pain, freedom from unnecessary intervention, or freedom to do our own thing. It means a whole range of reproductive freedoms for women everywhere: freedom to choose whether or not to have a child in the first place, the right to free contraception, safe abortion, freedom from compulsory sterilisation, the right to adequate health care, freedom from grinding poverty that causes stillbirth and neonatal death, and freedom from exploitation by multinational companies who dump drugs in the Third World and offer '*free gifts*' of formula milk to new mothers, with the result that lactation fails and babies die from dehydration and diarrhoea. In the same way, the concept of '*freedom*' as applied to heterosexuality and lesbianism is not simply a matter of personal choice, but the social and political structures within which choices are made.

I didn't plan my life. Instead, I have taken opportunities. It may even be that in challenging me heterosexuality has somehow also energised me.

Celia and Sue

Same Sex Marriage Legal, 29 March 2014
The legislation of same sex marriage was lavishly covered by the media. The *Sunday Times* reported this interview with Celia:

My Week: Celia Kitzinger
My wife and I are so glad I resisted the order to marry a horse[93]

Nuclear Threat
Last week the Marriage (Same Sex Couples) Act came into force, and my marriage to my wife of 11 years, Sue Wilkinson, was finally recognised by the British Government. It has been a long battle for legal recognition since we got married in Vancouver in August 2003, because when we came back to the UK in 2004 we were legal strangers.

We expressed concern to the government, but with the Civil Partnership Act about to pass, they told us our marriage would be recognised as a civil partnership. A heterosexual couple who married in Canada would have their marriage recognised in the UK, and it seemed unfair ours wasn't. We went to court, but the government intervened to say it thought our marriage shouldn't be accepted as a marriage. The judge rejected our application, saying it would threaten the nuclear family.

That was only eight years ago, though it did seem outdated at the time. I didn't think that in my lifetime I would be legally married.

Victory in Canada
Sue and I met in 1984 at a conference. We're both psychologists and we went to hear each other's papers and then got chatting in the bar. Soon we became friends, but it wasn't until 1990 that we became a couple. In 2003 Sue began a two year job at Simon Fraser University in Vancouver, and I used to visit her. It was a particularly exciting time, as the campaign was being fought to change the law in Canada during her first six months there. Campaigners were opposing civil partnerships, which they said were second best.

Whenever I returned to England, Stonewall would be campaigning for civil partnerships, saying marriage was a heterosexual institution. It was a strange experience shuttling between the gay movements in the two countries, because they had such different views. We didn't make the decision to get married until a few weeks before we did, but it was an amazing thing to be able to do.

Stonewalled

It was a struggle when we got back to the UK to fight what we saw as discrimination – that our marriage wasn't recognised. During the trial the judge agreed we were discriminated against, though he still ruled against us. We were supported a great deal by OutRage!, but Stonewall was a dead loss. We didn't have the gay movement solidly behind us – in fact it felt far from that. Stonewall at the time felt that civil partnerships were a special gay thing and that Sue and I were assimilating into a heterosexual model by wanting marriage. We were quite a visible anomaly. People felt more able to take potshots than they do now. We got some amazing stuff sent to us. One person claimed it was like marrying a horse. They said, 'If you can have gay marriage, why not bestiality?' My sister drew a wonderful cartoon of me in full bridal regalia marrying a horse. It was very funny.

Return of the Rings

That chapter of our lives was finally brought to a close with the passing of the same-sex marriage act in July. Sue and I had taken our rings off when the judge said we didn't have a marriage, because we didn't want to pretend that we did if it wasn't legal. The legislation came into force last week – and new marriages can take place from 29 March – and we escaped to the pub in the country on Wednesday night. One minute after midnight we popped a bottle of champagne and put our rings back on. It was quite lovely. It was a moment that was both personally important but also important for us as activists. In my lifetime homosexuality had been defined as an illness and it no longer is. Marriage was really the last bastion of inequality in the law for gay people in this country.

Equal At Last

I teach sociology at York University, and my students, along with friends and family, have been supportive and congratulatory. My students have been coming in with their essays saying, 'Ooh, you're going to be married this week.' Many of the students are from other countries and some are lesbian and gay. For some of them there is huge discrimination. We've had some very kind emails from students saying, 'Thank you for doing this.' We've had practically no opposition this time. The whole of my personal life and academic career has been shaped by the inequality to which I have been subject because I am a lesbian and have always been out as a lesbian. Now that my marriage to Sue is legally recognised, I can get on with my life and simply be an ordinary equal citizen along with everyone else.

All My Daughters

My daughter Nell makes wonderful sculptures, and she and I delight in colour, shape and construction, expressing joy through clay and paint. Only one daughter, Tess, had children. But many lesbians have children too, and many heterosexual women don't. So the question I was constantly being asked – 'Don't I want more grandchildren?' – was irrelevant.

I focused on childbirth, took the 'personal' and made it 'political', challenging accepted norms and practices around birth in much the same way that Celia and other feminist daughters did about women's relationships with men personally, politically and legally, and as my mother did in opposing male power that promoted violence and war.

It is exciting to work with my daughters, to share ideals, have my mind stretched by their insights, their searching questions, research and protest in a culture that, like others around the world, where individuals are slotted into place with assumptions about social class, gender, race and education. Polly led the way with her work for Rape Crisis.

Celia and Jenny have explored birth and have gone on to examine the other great life transition – death, making Advance Decisions and having rights in that part of the journey of life that none of us can escape. Understanding how culture shapes the major transitions in life, and similarities between patterns of birth and dying, impels us to think how we can make informed decisions about experiences when we may not be able to voice our concerns because we do not have full capacity. This is not only informed decisions, either, but informed refusals. After Polly's dreadful car crash she was was subject to a series of interventions to save her life, severely brain-damaged with no choice about whether or not this happened. This led to Jenny and Celia's study and a campaign for making legally effective Advanced Decisions, so that each of us can state ahead of time how we must be treated.

In an online resource dedicated to Polly and inspired by her work Jenny and Celia recorded the experience of 65 people whose loved ones were in a vegetative or minimally conscious state. Topics included hope, care, treatment, making decisions, impact on family and reflections.[94]

Jenny is a Professor of Media Studies at Cardiff University, and raises a lot of money for research.

They have also curated what they called a *'Death Festival'* but which they renamed *'Before I Die'* because of objections from some of those who might attend. It is about powers of attorney, organ donation, and other decisions to make before death.

Jenny and Celia write academic articles and seek to influence policy and public debate about how treatment decisions are taken on behalf of those who have lost the ability to decide for themselves.

This is something which is also important to us as a family. Jenny went to court to apply to become a welfare deputy for Polly – to ensure someone could represent her more effectively in day-to-day decisions about her care and Tess is utterly committed to practical issues relating to and helping Polly who is now fully conscious, but severely brain injured, and needs round the clock care in a neurological centre.

Vegetarian Hurdles

I became a vegetarian when I was nine years old and decided I did not want to cause unnecessary suffering to any living creatures. I announced that in future I would eat eggs and cheese, but not meat and fish. It was difficult for my mother, who hated fussing about meals and disliked cooking. So she relied on feeding me canned baked beans, with cheese when rations allowed it, and green vegetables and eggs when the chickens from the farm around the corner were laying and there were some spare. Father was a great cook in his family's Scottish tradition, but the dishes were limited. He made very good porridge and scrumptious potato scones.

Self Image In Pregnancy

In the 70s there was not much discussion about nutrition in pregnancy. You were supposed to have a *'good'* diet, and that was it. Teaching at NCT headquarters and in my house just outside Oxford, I encountered stars, celebs and women famous for their achievements.

One of the most glamorous who came to me when she was expecting her baby was a model whose pregnancy clothes were gorgeous, created especially for her by a top designer. The other women in the group were goggle-eyed! Her image was so important that she was determined to stay as slim as possible and dieted strictly. She ate almost exclusively *'health foods'* that were rich in vitamins and minerals, but was in fact starving herself. This worried her mother, who rang me.

The model's partner, a well-known fashion photographer, was anxious about the setting into which she was introducing her baby. The bedroom, she told me, was dramatic, dark, with isolated pools of light – not the kind of cuddly, soft pastel setting which most expectant mothers plan as a nest for their babies. I told her it sounded different, but was OK.

Perhaps I should have taken this as an opportunity to explore pregnancy and motherhood in terms of artistic expression. What is in the eyes of the beholder? What images are being projected? I failed to do that. Her baby was born prematurely and needed special care. And there were some worrying weeks in which it was not known whether she would survive. That baby is now a well-known photographer herself.

I learned from this experience. Pregnancy is also about the presentation of self. It can be very difficult for a woman whose self-esteem depends on the way she looks. With women and couples I explore feelings about the pregnant body – positive as well as negative emotions, and this always leads to lively, in-depth discussion.

Vegetarian Pregnancy

I enjoyed four vegetarian pregnancies (one with twins) and had easy, happy births. In spite of the warnings often given to women that vegetarian food may not provide essential vitamins and minerals in pregnancy, there seems to be no single ideal diet for pregnancy – and vegetarians don't have to eat special foods or take vitamin and mineral supplements unless their nutrition misses out on vital elements. Inuit women eat fish and whale blubber in pregnancy, African women millet and vegetables, Indian women rice, curry and ghee and Japanese women raw fish and tofu. Though their diets are very different, they all live on whole, fresh food which their bodies can make use of to build the cells of new life.

In spite of warnings that vegetarians are at risk of malnutrition from insufficient protein, vitamin B12, iron and calcium, a vegetarian diet can either be very good or very bad.

In the 70s a study was done of the nutrition of pregnant women and breastfeeding mothers on *The Farm* in Tennessee, a spiritual community whose members were vegan (but nowadays many are lacto-vegetarian). It is where the world famous midwife, my friend Ina May Gaskin, demonstrates her skills to visiting midwives from many countries, and where she wrote the book *Spiritual Midwifery*. That research revealed that women were found low in vitamin B12 and many were anaemic, so they were advised to fortify the soya milk they drank every day with vitamin B12 and to take supplementary iron and calcium. Another study compared mothers and children at *The Farm* with the general American population and revealed that *The Farm* women put on more weight during pregnancy, very few had pre-term babies, and only one woman out of 143 developed pre-eclampsia (a disease in which blood pressure is raised, fluid is retained under the skin, a woman puts on a lot of weight and the placenta is at risk of malfunction). Their babies weighed as much or more at birth and grew as well or faster than children generally. In fact, in each additional year that a woman had been a vegan, her baby's birth weight went up by 42 grams. The researchers concluded that a diet without animal protein is fine for pregnancy.

A cheese and egg-eating vegetarian, I enjoy my meals. Uwe eats fish and meat and chews away at dead bodies with relish, and frequent lip smacking comments about how good it is. It can put me off my food.

Sticking to being a vegetarian with good humour is not simple. On holiday in Normandy a distinguished chef, to whom we had travelled some distance, felt insulted by me asking if there was anything vegetarian on the menu, refused to serve either me or Uwe and turned us both off the premises.

In Taroudant, Morocco, we had a gorgeous holiday, but it was hard for me to get anything to eat except tossed salad. At one meal a concerned stranger at the next table intervened and tried to negotiate on my behalf. He sent a message to the chef and went into the kitchen to show him what he could do. But to no avail. It was Antonio Carluccio – one of the most exciting cooks of the age!

It has got easier over the years, but restaurateurs may still try to coax me to eat fish, 'or try a few thin slices of ham', and I often have to share a board of which only one ingredient is vegetarian.

In supermarkets it is important to read the small print, which is often minute for those whose sight is deteriorating, to detect animal gelatin, whey products, flavourings and other ingredients.

In delicatessens, assistants who may have just left school are inadequately supervised, do not know the ingredients, and often cannot find out from the kitchen, haven't a clue about what is in anything, or how to find an alternative, and go off poking along the shelves. So it's better to be safe than sorry.

The horse meat scandal triggered alarm about what is hidden in our food. It was a symptom of a larger challenge. Restaurants, cafeterias, supermarkets and delicatessens should be aware of what is in the food they offer and from where it comes, avoid discrimination against those with specific food wishes, whether this is based on health needs or stems from religion, social culture or personal conviction, and get their act together.

Vegetarian Gourmet

In TV programmes about culinary competition cooks and chefs refer to family recipes and childhood memories. They present 'my Mum's recipe', 'what I learned from my Nana', 'Godmother' or 'Grandpa' and with trembling hands, gasps, moans, wows – sometimes weeping and often with ecstasy – offer dishes inherited from beloved relatives.

Nothing could be further from my own experience. Mother hated cooking, despised it, and didn't want me 'wasting time and energy' on what she saw as a trivial activity imposed on women. She said sternly, 'We eat to live. We shouldn't live to eat.' She thought a daughter ought to be doing other things – not be trapped in the kitchen. So I never learnt to cook.

Some time during the 80s I worked out that I must have cooked 11,648 meals since I got married, and that does not take into account gooey delights for babies, toddlers' specials or the party where 60 people mill about chewing and slurping. For much of the time each meal was for seven people – all vegetarian except for a carnivorous husband.

Of course there was willing assistance: five pairs of eager little hands helping to knead and bake bread. Bread-making is much more fun as a communal activity, even if a fair quantity gets trodden in the coconut matting. Drop scones on my grandmother's Scottish griddle were quick and easy and there was the excitement of watching the bubbles come up and deftly flipping them over. And brushing the griddle with a flour-dipped feather to see if it was hot enough to flop on potato scones.

My basic educational principle was that my five daughters should learn how to do domestic tasks when they were very young, so they didn't have to *think* about them later when they had important things to do. We had a dreaded rota system which never worked and was the cause of constant quarrels. The first choice on the rota went to the first one up in the morning. In the early hours, my time for writing, I often tripped over a drowsy child sleeping outside our bedroom door, determined to be first.

Three-year-olds can be quite good at stacking the dishwasher. It is a far more sophisticated educational apparatus than all those shapes that are supposed to slot into each other at nursery school, even if the china does get chipped. The girls did not share my principles though and as they got older, acted as if they were a squad of slave labour.

I went in for *'good nutrition'* in a big way, wholemeal everything, kelp in the soup, wheatgerm thick on the muesli – which was proper Bircher-Benner style with lots of apples. This was interspersed, however, with phases of scrambled eggs, baked beans, and rice puddings straight out of a can, when time refused to be squeezed any further.

But I'm glad I don't have to make three meals a day any more. It's not just the cooking but the whole business of preparing food, clearing away, washing pans, planning ahead, making lists, checking what's in the fridge and the cupboards and the freezer, the trek through the supermarket and the limbo of waiting to get through check-out and then heaving the stuff into the boot of the car and heaving it out again. A repetitive, exhausting kind of servitude in which women are trapped day in day out, because that's what mothers are *supposed* to do. (Men help when they can, of course.)

In traditional cultures women did not question this role, but they were not alone with such tasks. They did them in the company of other women. I've seen

Caribbean women enjoying tedious things like shelling nuts or coffee beans, or stirring food in a big pot over the fire, while they talk, exchange news and laugh together, shooing away the chickens, nursing the babies and sharing out the chores. Compared to that, most women in the West are isolated from each other, each on her own treadmill.

Someone once told me that the Chinese symbol for war depicts two women in a kitchen (which, though funny, turns out not to be true). And it depends whether you believe it is *your* kitchen, your territory which is being invaded by an alien (and there are women who feel like that) or whether you think of it as a place for communal shared activity. The idea of a woman owning a kitchen is ludicrous in our society. It is more appropriate to a Greek village. But woman as queen of the kitchen is a convenient fiction by which men can ensure that they are fed regularly and looked after with minimal effort on their part.

Politics apart, I enjoy cooking with one or several daughters talking all the time, and '*oohing*' and '*aahing*' over the results. And I like best cooking festive food – not the usual festive dishes, though, but ones which remind me of special places and those kinds of gustatory experiences which come completely unexpected for any vegetarian on holiday who is anticipating yet another dreary mushroom risotto, omelette, vinegary mixed salad or boiled vegetables minus sauce and herbs.

There was the time, for example, when we discovered morilles, the convoluted black fungi which, I think, taste better than truffles. We were driving south from Strasbourg, where we were living then, and found a hotel in the little town of Arbois, nestling in the Jura, all twinkling lights, old oak beams and menus with mushrooms galore! Morilles remained a rare luxury until I was lecturing in Finland, when I found that the Finns enjoy them like any other mushroom and import dried morilles in vast quantities from Eastern Europe. Since then, the president of the Finnish midwives thrusts a box at me whenever we meet. They are gorgeous in an oniony, spicy cream sauce, either with toast or stuffed inside vol-au-vents. A touch of lemon juice and Madeira added at the last minute draws out their splendid flavour.

One year we were sailing with the children in the South of France and, arriving at the old harbour of Antibes, decided to eat out. We climbed the steps leading to the centre and came on a scene of bustling conviviality. Everyone was eating in the open at long tables which filled the square. We found a space and I told the waiter that the girls and I ate no meat or fish. Instead of the horror with which this information is often greeted, our waiter said that we must have soup. Well, soup and bread would fill our stomachs but it wasn't very exciting. And then he came up bearing huge white tureens and I tasted for the first time pistou soup. It was marvellous! It was unforgettable: mingled onions, courgettes, tomatoes, green beans and the magic of pistou sauce – ground pine kernels, garlic, Parmesan cheese and loads of fresh basil.

Lecturing at a conference of Italian obstetricians in Bologna, a doctor who had invited me out to dinner said rather ominously, on hearing that I was vegetarian, *'I shall take you to the place of goats. It is an inn up in the mountains.'* He explained. *'They are friends of mine and I will order in advance a menu for you based on goat milk and cheese.'* That was how I got to taste for the first time the pungent flavour of grilled goat's cheese.

Claude Giraud in Narbonne was one of the few chefs in Languedoc to have earned a Michelin star. Every year, with good warning, he produced a special menu for me. One dish was stuffed courgette flowers – baby courgettes with the blossom still attached, transformed into cheesy parcels. Delicious! But you have to grow your own courgettes or have a friendly nursery gardener nearby.

A memorable meal owes as much, of course, to the setting as to what is on your plate. I remember driving through the Camargue with a carload of angry, quarrelling girls, arriving at Arles and handing them money to explore and find places where they wanted to eat, while exhausted parents repaired to the peace and civilisation of the Hotel Jules César. There was nothing vegetarian on the menu so I decided to wait until the cheese course. And then I saw their raw vegetables, each arranged like a still life – courgettes, carrot fingers, red and green peppers, radishes, tomatoes and the greens of different lettuces – all the vegetables of high summer served with a mayonnaise so thick the spoon stood up in it. With crisp French bread, butter and black olives, it was a splendid meal.

Crudites are perfect for a garden lunch, varied with whatever is in season, and also asparagus (steamed) in May, artichokes, spears of chicory, miniature tomatoes, and very tiny raw broad beans.

Some Of My Own Recipes (Definitely Not Slimming!)

Though not addicted to food porn, I admit that I enjoy exploring and experimenting with recipes – adapting them to be vegetarian and using a variety of herbs and seasonings. I am grateful to all the chefs, past and present, from whom I have drawn my own recipes.

Potato Scones

You will need a cast iron girdle (or griddle) for this. Never wash it. Clean it with salt and kitchen paper. My father taught me how to make these – traditional Scottish scones.

> *450 g (1 lb) boiled or baked potatoes*
> *1 tsp sea salt*
> *flour*
> *butter*

Mash cold, skinned potatoes with salt. The mixture should be dry and smooth. Work in just enough flour to have a dough you can roll out. Knowing how much flour to add is a matter of practice and varies with the potatoes used. On a well floured surface roll the mixture until it is about the thickness of a 2p piece. Place a dinner plate over the dough and cut round it so that you have a large circle. Cut out the scone shapes as if making the spokes of a wheel. Have the girdle well heated so that when you throw on a few pinches of flour they go brown in about half a minute. Grease it with a very thin layer of butter. Prick the scones with a fork and place on the girdle, turning then with a metal spatula when brown blisters appear on the underside. When done they are the consistency of soft suede. Cool and eat with butter.

To manage the dough easily, keep your hands cool and lightly oiled. My father ate them with cheese but I prefer them plain.

Morilles à la Crème

> *6 morilles*
> *1 small onion, chopped*
> *1 clove garlic, chopped*
> *butter*
> *1 tsp flour*
> *salt and black pepper*
> *284 ml (1/2 pint) double cream*

If using dried morilles, soak in water overnight. Then wash thoroughly. Sauté onion and garlic in butter and when the onion is transparent, add the morilles. If served alone they are marvellous whole, but for vol-au-vents it is best to slice them. They take about 10 minutes to cook, but should not become sloppy. Sprinkle lightly with flour and stir till it forms a smooth paste with their juice. Season and gradually stir in double cream. It can also be served on a bed of rice.

Pistou Soup
This is a meal in itself. First make your pistou sauce. I make up a large quantity and keep it in the freezer.

Sauce
340 g (12 oz) pine kernels
3-4 cups roughly chopped fresh basil
6-8 roughly chopped garlic cloves
450 g (1 lb) finely grated Parmesan or other salty sheep's cheese
568 ml (1 pint) virgin olive oil
salt and black pepper

In a Magimix or blender (pestle and mortar if you have neither) grind the pine kernels. Throw in basil and garlic. Blend again. Add Parmesan or Feta cheese. While the machine is going, gradually pour in olive oil. Season and put in pots. You can add more or less garlic according to taste and if pine kernels are too expensive, you can either mix them with walnuts or, at a pinch, use walnuts instead. But don't use any other oil as green olive is best.

Soup
225 g (8 oz) haricot beans
olive oil
1 cup cubed potatoes
1 cup diced carrots
large cubed aubergine
4 or 5 cubed courgettes
13/4 litres (3 pints) water
225 g (8 oz) green stringless beans
142 g (5 oz) tin tomato puree
225 g (8 oz) diced mushrooms
few florets of cauliflower
4 or 5 peeled, chopped tomatoes

Soak haricot beans overnight and in the morning boil until they are barely cooked. In a large saucepan sauté the potatoes and carrots in olive oil. After about 20 minutes, add aubergine and courgettes. After another 15 minutes add water and let it come to the boil again. Add the strained haricot beans, green beans cut into inch lengths and tomato puree. Season well and cook for 10 minutes. Add mushrooms, cauliflower and tomatoes. Simmer until all vegetables are just cooked. Taste and season again. Serve with a dollop of pistou sauce in each bowl. The vegetables can be varied, but tomatoes, two kinds of beans and one root vegetable are essential.

Grilled Goat Cheese

> *Firm goat cheese*
> *Chopped walnuts*
> *Pepper*

Cut the goat cheese into thick 1 1/2-inch slices. Place each slice on a circle of foil, allowing space for it to melt. Press the chopped walnuts onto one side of it and place this down on to the foil. Pepper the upper side generously. Place under a very hot grill until golden. Serve on a watercress salad with a good French dressing and some crisp triangles of toast.

When my grandson Sam was five he made up a recipe for 'Nutty Nibbles'. Here it is in his own words:

Sam's Nutty Nibbles

> *Bread – brown and crusty – 2 cups*
> *Nuts – 1 cup*
> *Cheese – 1 cup*
> *Butter – 1 teaspoon*
> *Salt and Pepper – to taste*
> *Herbs – to taste: celery seeds, lemon, basil and dill*
> *1 macaroon*

Preheat oven to 200°c.

Break up the bread and put it in a Magimix. Turn it on. When the bread has turned into small crumbs turn it off. Put all the other ingredients in the bowl and turn it on again. When the mixture looks like fine crumbs again turn it off.

Take a spoonful of the mixture and squeeze it between your hands in the shape of a fat biscuit. Place these biscuits onto a baking tray and put them into the hot oven.

After 10 minutes, when the biscuits are brown at the edges, take them out of the oven. Allow the Nutty Nibbles to cool for five minutes before eating them.

Christmas

Preparing for Christmas well in advance is part of moving with the seasons – scenting the first whiff of frost in the air, seeing the brilliant pyracantha berries ripen on the wall opposite the kitchen window and cascade across in a sea of fire, and collecting nuts that have dropped on the lawn as branches of the big old walnut tree sway in the wind, before the excited squirrels get the lot. It started in early September, filling big bowls with white hyacinth bulbs and tucking them into the cool garden shed. As the days grew shorter, logs were sawn for fires and dried lavender tied in bunches to throw on the flames. Then there were presents to be found at craft fairs – and if I was lucky enough to be lecturing in south Germany or Austria, the magic of a night visit to the *Christkindlmarkt,* to find honey candles, straw and carved wooden baubles for the tree, to add to those dating from Uwe's childhood which are beginning to look a bit tatty now, and spices for mulled wine and cider.

Uwe was born in Germany so carrying on a German tradition we light the candles on the tree and open our presents on Christmas Eve.

I suppose that I am drawn back to some female ancestral role by these rituals, the rhythmic travail and comfort of tasks long familiar and deeply satisfying: kneading dough to cook special savoury rolls and cheese brioches; making polish from beeswax, lavender and turpentine so that the old oak floors will gleam; weaving raffia into long swags and wreaths to hang on doors to be studded with dried flower heads from the garden and pine cones and tied with ribbons; soaking fruit in jars of brandy; pounding pine kernels, garlic and fresh basil for pesto to spice our minestrone and pasta. It is a romanticisation of women's work, of course, thousands of years of female hard slog, the nurturing and sustaining of families, and making homes warm and welcoming. Yet it is a pleasurable counterpoint to writing, research and campaigning for women.

A Kitzinger Christmas is a vegetarian one, so there will be filo pastry stuffed with cheese, home-made hummus, goat cheeses marinated in olive oil and spiked with rosemary and other herbs from the garden, summer puddings rich with raspberries, tay berries and blackcurrants from Millets Farm down the road, stored in readiness in the freezer. We tuck into Nell's home-baked bread with artisan cheeses and shall savour morel mushrooms with cream and Madeira; cranberry sauce which goes well with a moist, garlicky nut loaf and with buckwheat pancakes and sour cream; tarte Tatin with apples from the paddock; loads of salads with oils and vinegars flavoured with herbs and lemon; potted Stilton with the added nip of Yugoslav plum brandy; and a mix of sesame seeds, hazelnuts and pine kernels, roasted in sesame oil and mixed with herbs and spices to sprinkle on vegetables and salads.

A big wrought-iron coffer that used to be in Uwe's grandfather's bank in Nuremburg is lined with evergreen branches and filled to overflowing with oranges, satsumas and clementines with their leaves still on. That way there will be a dramatic still life in the spicy dark against the linen-fold panelling and flickering candles, as tantalising parcels resplendent with glittering ribbons are piled under the pungent tree. Wooden bowls of chestnuts wait to be roasted, and daughters hunt through bookshelves for poetry to read aloud by the fireside.

Five of them come home, with partners and friends. When Sam was two and a half, Tess made him a puppet theatre (a very simple one, out of a big box) and I discovered a wicked-looking crocodile to add to the stock of characters. We found Sam fluffy wings, too, and one of Uwe's white shirts (to be worn back-to-front) for him to be a convincing angel when he handed us our presents after we had drawn the curtains on Christmas Eve.

One year I had a feminist tree – full of symbols of women's power to give life. At first I was going to make birthing women out of papier maché but it was incredibly difficult. I told Jenny about the problem, and she and her partner made birthing goddesses and birth symbols out of delicate ceramic, which they then painted. My tree was one of the more expensive ones that are not supposed to drop their needles. It was decorated in bronze and white, which suited the white and dark oak sitting room. The birthing symbols included the hooked diamond, which represents the woman giving birth, and the maze, a symbol of women's generative energy. There was also a wonderful Cretan snake goddess with a snake in each raised hand. I added golden and white balls and some traditional white angels.

I never thought of Christmas as just a family time when you bolt your doors, draw thick curtains and try to shut out other people. My mother always made it an opportunity to welcome anybody needing comfort and care; students from overseas, refugees from Nazi Germany, and others who were lonely, old, ill or unhappy. The smug, bourgeois, in-turned family Christmas, emotions simmering like a pressure cooker, can be a dreadful thing. I know from experience that women are most likely to phone me for urgent help with emotional difficulties at times of family gatherings. An open-hearted Christmas, with friends and others who find themselves away from home and who come to share ours, is much more fun. Christmas is a time for reaching out to other people.

The conventional Christmas is part of a tradition stemming from Prince Albert: middle-class Victorian society, with Father carving the turkey and lighting the brandy for the pudding while Mother fusses over the sprouts, tries to keep the children happy, and is up to her armpits in washing up.

Christmas is usually enacted as an expression of an intensely patriarchal society. Father Christmas holds centre stage as the giver of gifts, the spirit of benevolence, bringing the magic and excitement of a faraway glittering world into prosaic homes. He does this with much '*hoho-ing*' and great panache. Mother Christmas is invisible. Yet it is she who does all the backstage work, while this jack-booted, heavy-bearded Nordic father figure gets all the credit. A long time ago our Father Christmas caught fire as he reached across a candle to pluck a present from the tree. Uwe rushed across, flung him on the ground, and dragged him out into the garden and hosed him down. We rolled him on the wet lawn and finally extinguished his flaming beard by wrapping him in a rug from the hall. And there, instead of this sham figure of paternalistic authority, was revealed the children's kind and gentle grandfather, with eyebrows singed and a little shaky on his feet.

So maybe we should include the women who create Christmas, together with the central images of the tree and the birth of a Child, each of them symbols of life. I enjoy Christmas because it is the backdrop to the exhilaration of personalities meeting, meshing, sparking reactions from each other; to the laughter and heady arguments and sharing chores in the kitchen as women work together in an easy, steady rhythm. Christmas can strengthen bonds that link us, sharpening our perception, and helping us grow in understanding. It is not just a sentimental ritual, not only an affirmation of the importance of the family, but a celebration of the energy and creativity of the women who choreograph it.

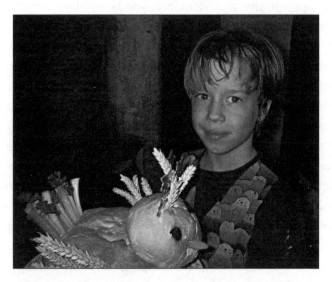

My grandson Josh holding our vegetarian christmas turkey of home made bread, wheat stalks, celery and carrot

CHAPTER SEVENTEEN

MY OBITUARY

Invited by a newspaper to contribute an advance obituary, this is how I tackled the task:

She died as she would have wished, flat on her back on a table with her legs in the air, in front of a large audience, demonstrating with vigour the dangers of making women lie down, hold their breath till their eyes bulge and strain as if forcing through a coconut to push a baby out. She claimed that treating the second stage of labour as a race to the finishing post did violence to a woman's spontaneous physiological rhythms, reduced oxygen flow, led to fetal heart deceleration and could result in cardiac arrhythmia and even a stroke. She made her point.

Sheila Kitzinger lived, and died, with zest. The media described her as a 'birth guru', 'earth mother', 'high priestess of the natural childbirth movement', 'the intellectual woman's Barbara Cartland' (she wrote about three dozen books), and a 'benign, fat broad making bread in a stripped pine kitchen'. Though there was some truth in such descriptions, the essence of her work was her feminism. She strove to validate women's experiences, to give words and meaning to female life events and transitions, and to challenge male autocracy and a medical system dictated and moulded by men.

She learned from her mother Clare Webster, midwife and worker in one of the first birth-control clinics, to question accepted 'truths' and to struggle for social justice – the basis of her books about emotional and social aspects of female sexuality, pregnancy and childbirth and the sociology of motherhood.

When she read social anthropology at Oxford in the 50s she discovered that academic anthropology ignored female realities and was dominated by a male view of the world. She pointed out that in her professor's studies of the Nuer there were many more references to cows than to women. Her M.Litt research project was on race relations in British universities. During this time she married Uwe Kitzinger, then a diplomat with the Council of Europe, and later president of Templeton College, Oxford. They had five daughters, and when her youngest was two the family went to Jamaica so that she could do field work on birth and motherhood among Jamaican peasant women, with further research on the Rastafarian politico-religious cult. Later, with a Joost de Blank Fellowship, she did research on Caribbean women's experiences of birth in Britain.

The radicalism of her book *The Experience of Childbirth* (1962) lay in her focus on women's experiences rather than on doctors' or psychologists' interpretations of these experiences. She wrote it after her fourth baby, Polly, was born and waking at 5.30 a.m. She continued this early morning writing and made it a precious space in her busy day. This was vital because there was a short time when she had three children under two, for Tess and Nell were twins, and Jenny, the youngest, was born when the oldest was still only seven.

She worked with gusto and, although she had a spell as a lecturer at the Open University, and created and helped set up the National Childbirth Trust's training scheme for antenatal teachers, she preferred to be free of the restraints of institutions. She lectured in many countries, and whenever she went sought the opportunity to be with women in childbirth rather than on official tours round hospitals.

Some of her earliest research projects concerned women's experiences of medical and surgical interventions in birth. Episiotomy, 'our Western way of female genital mutilation', is a usually unnecessary surgical wound. When a search of the medical literature revealed nothing on women's experiences of induced labour or episiotomy, she did the research herself – without funding. She threw herself into similar studies of women's experiences of antenatal care and was the first writer to indicate that many women suffer long-term backache after an epidural. Because it was impossible for most women to find out what was going on in maternity hospitals, she wrote *The Good Birth Guide*, based on women's own accounts of care in hospitals, on obstetricians' and administrators' answers to questions about rates of induction of labour and Caesarean section, and care on postpartum wards. The guide's publication opened the doors of maternity hospitals, made those who ran them 'consumer-conscious' for the first time, and initiated competition between hospitals to treat women with dignity and respect.

Many women sought her out after births in which they had been disempowered and which they described in imagery similar to that used about rape. So she started a Birth Crisis counselling network of women willing to listen to their experiences and help them find strength to cope.

The tradition of activism and love of challenges that she inherited from her mother she also shared with her daughters. She very much enjoyed being present when Tess gave birth in water in the family home, and her social and political awareness was sharpened by those of her daughters who are radical lesbian feminists. One of her books, *Talking with Children about Things that Matter,* she co-authored with her psychologist daughter, Celia.

For her the most important thing was that she passed on and shared with other women the courage, commitment and understanding needed in the struggle to enable women's voices to be heard.

POSTSCRIPT

Sheila did not get the melodramatic death she imagined in this scenario. She died at her home in Oxfordshire at the age of 86 on 11 April 2015 – shortly after completing this autobiography.

She approached death with the same attitude as birth – questioning the need for various medical interventions and making her own choices. She set down her wishes in an Advance Decision to Refuse Treatment and gave one of her daughters power to represent her should she lose the capacity to take decisions for herself at the time.

Her family carried her body in a brightly decorated cardboard coffin of her choice to a natural burial site. They read some of Sheila's own poetry at the grave and sprinkled in earth, sprigs of rosemary and camellia blossom from her beloved garden.

My special thanks

Lesley Page, CBE, President of the Royal College of Midwifery and an inspiring friend.

My assistant, Sue Allen, for her skills and commitment.

All the ideas contributed by Rosie Denmark and my new editor Jan Heron.

Hazel Wilce, who keeps the house shining so that I can concentrate on my work.

My husband, Uwe, for his superb long-term memory and his records of important events in our lives, of our international journeys and of hard facts. Whenever I seek a date Uwe can come up with it.

Dr Luke Zander, long-term friend and colleague, Founder of the Royal Society of Medicine Forum on Maternity and the Newborn.

Dr Ethel Burns for all her exciting work on labouring and giving birth in water.

Helena Kennedy QC for her tireless work for equality.

Celia and Jenny, sharing my struggle for social justice and helping create a feminist revolution.

My daughter, Tess McKenney, who has supported and nurtured me in every way possible. Without her this book would never have seen the light of day. She is responsible for the illustrations, for stimulating my energy, and keeping me focused.

REFERENCES

1 Torr H. A Matter of Life or Death, *Humanity*, vol.2, no.1, January 1948
2 The *Guardian*, 12 August 2003
3 Private correspondence, 1950
4 Garcia J. *The Politics of Maternity Care: Services for Childbearing Women in Twentieth Century Britain*, Clarendon Press, London, 1990
5 Kitzinger S. *Freedom and Choice in Childbirth,* Penguin, London 1988
6 Velvosky L., Platonov K., Ploticher V. and Shugom E. *Painless Childbirth through Psychoprophylaxis,* Foreign Languages Publishing House, Moscow 1960
7 Dick-Read G., *Childbirth without Fear* Heinemann Medical Books, London 1942
8 Karmel M. *Thank you Dr Lamaze* Harper & Row, New York 1959
9 Lamaze F. *Painless Childbirth* Burke, London 1958, p139–140
10 Guttmacher A. *Having a Baby*, Signet, USA, 1950
11 Leavitt J.W. *Brought to Bed: Childbearing in America 1750–1950* Oxford University Press, Oxford, 1986
12 *Hysterectomy Surveillance – United States, 1994–1999, available at* cdc.gov/mmwr/preview/mmwrhtml/ss5105a1.htm
13 Scully D. *Men Who Control Women's Health*, Houghton Mifflin, Boston 1980
14 Masters W.H. and Johnson V.E. *Human Sexual Response.* Bantam Books, New York 1966 and Masters W.H. and Johnson V.E. *Human Sexual Inadequacy* Bantam Books, New York 1970
15 Caldeyro-Barcia R. *et al* Bearing-down efforts and their effects *Journal of Perinatal Medicine*, 1981; 9 supple 1: 63–7
16 Edwards M. and Waldorf M. *Reclaiming Birth. History and Heroines of American Childbirth Reform.* The Crossing Press, New York 1984, p139
17 Newton N. *Maternal Emotions* Paul B. Hoeber Inc, New York 1955.
18 Mutwa V. *Indaba My Children: African Folktales*, 1st American Ed, Groves Press 1999
19 Kitzinger S. *Rediscovering Birth*, 2nd ed, Pinter & Martin, London 2011
20 Pankhurst S. *The Suffragette: The History of the Women's Militant Suffrage Movement: 1905–1910* Sturgis & Walton 1911, available at archive.org/details/suffragettehisto00pankuoft

21 Kitzinger S. *Giving Birth: Emotions in Childbirth*, Gollancz, London, 1971, p5

22 Kitzinger S. *Women as Mothers*, Fontana Books, Glasgow, 1978, p142–143, 162

23 *Spare Rib*, Issue 36, 1975

24 *Expectant Fathers*, National Childbirth Trust, London 1974

25 O'Driscoll K. and Meagher D. Active Management of Labor, Sanders W (ed), *Clinical and Obstetric Gynecology Supplement* 1, 1980.

26 Chalmers I., Enkin M. and Keirse M. (eds) *Effective Care in Pregnancy and Childbirth*, Oxford University Press, Oxford, 1989

27 Chard T. and Richards M., eds. *Clinics in Developmental Medicine No. 64: Benefits and Hazards of the New Obstetrics* Spastics International Medical Publications, London 1977, p72

28 Chalmers I., Lawson J.G. and Turnbull A.C. Evaluation of different approaches to obstetric care *British Journal of Obstetrics and Gynaecology*, 1976, p921-929, p930-933

29 *Winterton Report* House of Commons Health Committee, London 1992

30 *Changing Childbirth* Department of Health, London 1993

31 Micklethwait L., Beard R., and Shaw K. Expectations of a Pregnant Woman in Relation to Her Treatment *British Medical Journal*, 1978;2:188

32 Kitzinger S. *The Good Birth Guide*, Fontana, London 1979 and Kitzinger S. *The New Good Birth Guide*, Penguin, London 1983

33 O'Driscoll K., *et al.* Active Management of Labour – care of the fetus *British Medical Journal*, December 1977

34 Chalmers I. Confronting therapeutic ignorance *British Medical Journal* 2008;337:a841;246-247

35 Klaus M., Kennell J. *Maternal–Infant Bonding*, Rosby, 1976

36 Department of Health and Social Security *Report on Health and Social Subjects 9 'Present day practice in infant feeding'* HMSO, London 1974

37 Garcia J. *Community Health Council News* 70, 72, 1981

38 Bowlby J. Psycho-Analysis and Childcare in Sutherland J. (ed) *Psycho-analysis and Contemporary Thought*, Hogarth Press, 1958

39 Kitzinger S., and Nilsson L., *Being Born*, Dorling Kindersley, 1986

40 *Guardian Women*, 1986

41 Medical Defence Union *Consent to Treatment* London 1974

42 Bourne G. *Pregnancy* Pan Books, London 1984

43 Thompson W.I., *The Time Falling Bodies Take to Light* Palgrave Macmillan, 1996

44 *Toronto Globe* 25 June 1982

45 Velvovsky I., *et al. Painless Childbirth from Psychoprophylaxis*, Foreign Languages Publishing House, Moscow 1960

46 Wood P., Foureur M. A clean front passage: dirt, douches and disinfectants at St Helens Hospital, Wellington, New Zealand, 1907-1922 in Kirkham M. ed. *Exploring the Dirty Side of Women's Health*, Routledge, London 2007

47 Tao Te Ching translated by Heider J. *The Tao of Leadership*. Wildwood House, London 1986

48 Information booklet for EU applicants: Registering as a nurse or midwife in the UK. NMC, November 2010

49 Case of Dubská and Krejzová v. The Czech Republic hudoc.echr.coe.int/sites/eng Applications 28859/11 & 28473/12

50 House of Commons Health Committee, 1992: para 49

51 Ternovsky v Hungary. Application No: 67545/09

52 Dubská and Krejzová v. The Czech Republic. Application Nos. 28859/11, 28473/12

53 www.freegereb.org

54 Communique of the Ministry of Justice, Budapest, Hungary, 12 November 2010

55 Kerry D., International Spokesperson, Freebirth Support Group, www.freegereb.org

56 Broz, S. Our Campaign for Civil Courage, lecture Sarajevo, 19 November 2010; www.gariwo.org

57 Brown S. and Lumley J. *Missing Voices: The Experience of Motherhood*, Oxford University Press, Melbourne 1994, p83

58 *op cit*, p37

59 Garcia J. Women's Views of Antenatal Care, in Enkin M., Chalmers I. (eds), *Effectiveness and Satisfaction in Antenatal Care* Spastics International Medical Publications 1982, p. 81–91

60 Simkin P. *Pregnancy, Childbirth and the Newborn*. Meadowbrook, Minnesota USA 1979

61 Oakley A. *Women Confined: Towards a Sociology of Childbirth*, Martin Robertson, Oxford 1980

62 *British Medical Journal* 2011;343:d7400

63 Paul C. The New Zealand cervical cancer study: Could it happen again? *British Medical Journal* 297: 533–539, 1988

64 Page L (ed). *The New Midwifery: Science and Sensitivity in Practice*, Churchill Livingstone, Edinburgh 2000

65 Audit Commission. *First Class Delivery: improving maternity services in England and Wales*, HMSO, London, 1997; Green J., Coupland V., Kitzinger J. *Great Expectations: a prospective study of women's expectations and experiences of childbirth* Child Care and Development Group, Cambridge, 1998; Mccourt C., Page L., Hewison J., Vail A. Evaluation of one-to-one midwifery: women's responses to care *Birth*, 1998;125:2; Simkin

P. Just another day in a woman's life? Part II: Nature and consistency of women's long-term memories of their first birth experiences, *Birth* 1992;19:2

66 Page L. and McCandlish R. *The New Midwifery: Science and Sensitivity in Practice*, Elsevier, 2006

67 Kitzinger S. *Having a baby in a major teaching hospital: Some women's experiences*, unpublished, 1998

68 Kitzinger S. Birth and violence against women: generating hypotheses from women's accounts of unhappiness after childbirth. In Roberts H (ed) *Women's Health Matters*, Routledge, London 1992

69 Gaskin I.M. *Spiritual Midwifery*, The Book Publishing Co, USA, 1977

70 Gaskin I.M. *Birth Matters: A Midwife's Manifesta*, Pinter & Martin, London 2011

71 Sherr L. *The Psychology of Pregnancy and Childbirth*, Blackwell Science, Oxford 1995

72 *ibid* p91

73 *ibid* p92-95

74 *ibid* p115

75 Rothman S. cited in Wertz R.W. *Lying-In: A History of Childbirth in America* The Free Press, New York 1977

76 Gabbe S.G. and DeLee J.B. cited in Wertz R.W. 1977 *Lying-In: A History of Childbirth in America*. The Free Press, New York 1977

77 Beynon C. The Normal Second Stage of Labour – a plea for reform in its conduct, *Journal of Obstetrics and Gynaecology of the British Empire*, 64: 815-820, 1957

78 Kitzinger S. (ed) *Episiotomy: physical and emotional aspects*, NCT, London, 1981

79 Tselem B. The Israeli Information Center for Human Rights in the Occupied Territories www.btselem.org/english

80 United Nations *Towards a More Secure Future: UN Agencies Operating in the Occupied Palestinian Territory Call for Action in Improving the Situation of Palestinian Women*. UN Press Release, International Women's Day, 2005

81 Amnesty International. *Israel and the Occupied Territories – Conflict, Occupation and Patriarchy – Women carry the burden.* www.amnesty.org/library/index/engmde150162005. 2005

82 McNabb M. Pregnancy and Childbirth in Palestinian communities under military occupation *International Midwifery*, 2003;16(1)

83 Amnesty International *Israel and the Occupied Territories – Conflict, Occupation and Patriarchy – Women carry the burden.* www.amnesty.org/library/index/engmde150162005, 2005

84 Amnesty International. Israel and the Occupied Territories – Conflict,

Occupation and Patriarchy – Women carry the burden. www.amnesty.org/library/index/engmde150162005. 2005

85 United Nations. *Report of the UN Special Rapporteur on violence against women, its causes and consequences: Mission to Occupied Palestinian Territories* February 200

86 Prison Reform Trust 2004 Fact File. In *Lacking Conviction*, London, Prison Reform Trust.

87 Kitzinger C., Kitzinger S. Birth Trauma: talking with women and the value of conversation analysis, *British Journal of Midwifery*, May 2007;15:5

88 Kitzinger S. *Birth Your Way*, Freshheart Publishing, London, 2011

89 Quoted from Wordsworth's *Ode: Intimations of Immortality from Recollections of Early Childhood*

90 Kitzinger C. Afterword: *Reflections on Three Decades of Lesbian and Gay Psychology, Feminism and Psychology*, 2004, 14(4) 523-530

91 *ibid*

92 World Health Organization, Women's Health: Fact Sheet No. 334, updated 2013

93 *The Sunday Times*, 16 March 2014

94 Family Experiences of Vegetative and Minimally Conscious States, www.healthtalk.org

INDEX